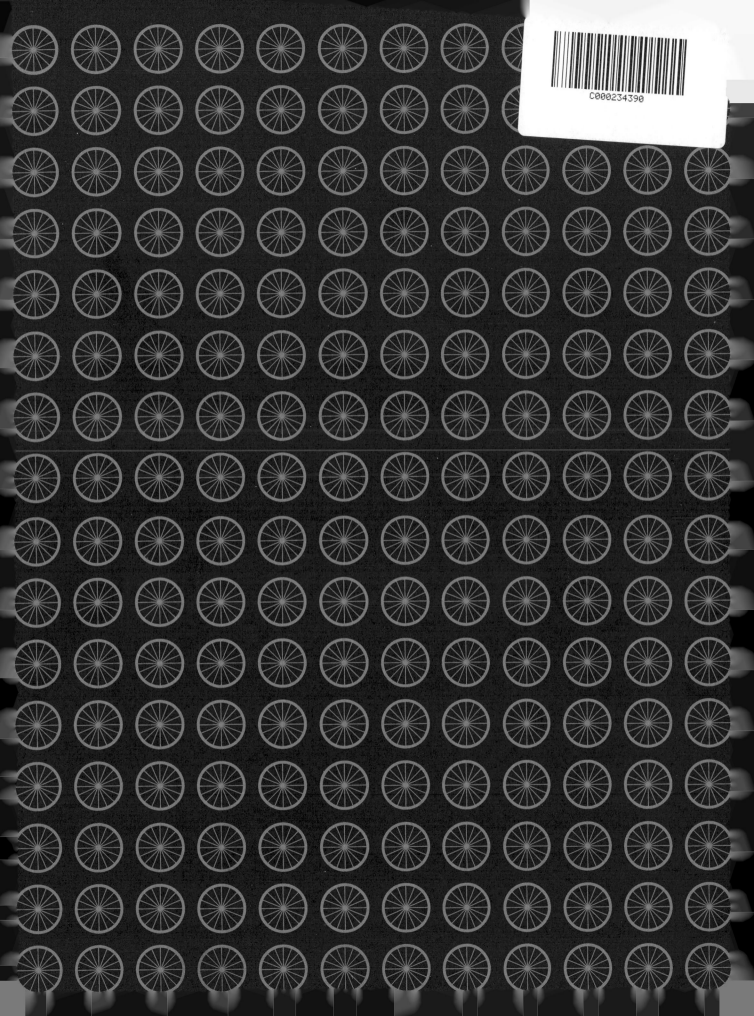

C000234390

THIS BOOK BELONGS TO:

The Grand Tour Cookbook
Translated from the original Danish version.
© Hannah Grant and Musette Publishing Aps. 2015

www.hannahgrantcooking.com
Follow us on: @dailystews

Photos: Hannah Grant
Portrait photos of the riders: Tim de Waele, TDWsport.be, Bettini Photo
Art Direction & Design: Johannes Torpe Studios Denmark ApS
www.johannestorpestudios.com

Editor: Musette Publishing ApS
Proofreading: Hamilton Chase Shields, Chris Calvert

Printed by Narayana Press
Paper quality: Galerie Art Volume 150 g
1st edition, 2nd impression
Printed in Denmark 2016
ISBN 978-87-998169-0-3

THE *Grand* TOUR COOKBOOK

HANNAH GRANT

M U SETTE
PUBLISHING

CONTENTS

FOREWORD BY BJARNE RIIS — 8

INTRODUCTION BY HANNAH GRANT — 10

PERFORMANCE COOKING BY ANNE DORTHE TANDERUP — 12

FOOD, DIET AND NOURISHMENT BY DR. STACY SIMS — 16

PRACTICE AND PRINCIPLES BEFORE YOU START — 22

CONVERSION TABLE — 28

INFORMATION FOR THE RECIPES — 29

THE 21 DAY CYCLE — 31
PROLOGUE — 33
STAGE 1 — 43
Chris Anker Sørensen — 54
STAGE 2 — 57
STAGE 3 — 67
Matti Breschel — 78
STAGE 4 — 81
STAGE 5 — 91
Roman Kreuziger — 102
STAGE 6 — 105
STAGE 7 — 115
Nicolas Roche — 124
STAGE 8 — 127

STAGE 9	**137**
Alberto Contador	144
Michael Mørkøv	145
REST DAY 1	**147**
A day in the kitchen truck	162
STAGE 10	**167**
STAGE 11	**179**
Nicki Sørensen	188
STAGE 12	**191**
STAGE 13	**201**
Michael Rogers	210
STAGE 14	**213**
STAGE 15	**223**
Ivan Basso	228
REST DAY 2	**231**
STAGE 16	**247**
Peter Sagan	256
STAGE 17	**259**
STAGE 18	**269**
Michael Valgren	278
STAGE 19	**281**
STAGE 20	**291**
Christopher Juul Jensen	294
RACE SNACKS & RECOVERY FOODS	**297**
BREAKFAST	**305**
Kristoffer Glavind Kjær	318
SAUCES, DRESSINGS, PICKLING LIQUIDS & BREAD	**321**
RECIPE INDEX	**342**

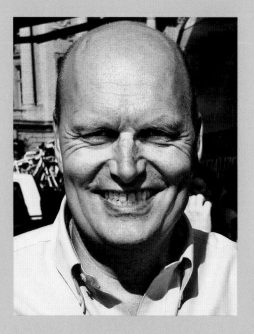

FOREWORD *by*
BJARNE RIIS

Time after time, I found myself in this situation: The day's race or stage has finished, I'm exhausted and tired from my labour and a new hotel with a menu of unknown quality awaits. Sometimes, I was pleasantly surprised. But, on far too many occasions, the food simply did not satisfy my basic nutritional needs as a professional athlete.

Even as a team manager, I found myself in the same situation. Over the years, I saw how my cyclists had to accept the luck of the draw in terms of the quality of their diet – a crucial factor in achieving peak performance. Needless to say, that situation finally became untenable.

In 2006, the team decided to employ a professional chef to accompany us on the road and ensure the quality of all our meals. Ever since, we have consistently increased our focus on diet and the impact it has on performance. As far as I know, we were the first team to introduce the concept of a mobile kitchen, consisting of a truck equipped with a state-of-the-art professional kitchen.

In 2010, we kick-started the dietary project which is known today as Performance Cooking. In 2012, we invested a large sum of money in an upgraded catering truck and our wonderful chef, Hannah Grant, acquired an assistant. Last, but

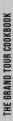

not least, this year we have started what is undoubtedly the most modern and individualised diet and test programme in cycling. Everything aims to guarantee our cyclists are in the best possible physical and mental condition for peak performance.

The last decade has been a journey; from the desire to guarantee the quality of the cyclists' diets, to a broader focus on how quality food affects performance and what elite athletes should eat on an individual level. This work has been incredibly exciting and rewarding, and I am very proud that we are now ready to take the next step and share some of our many experiences and recipes with you.

Enjoy the book and have fun!

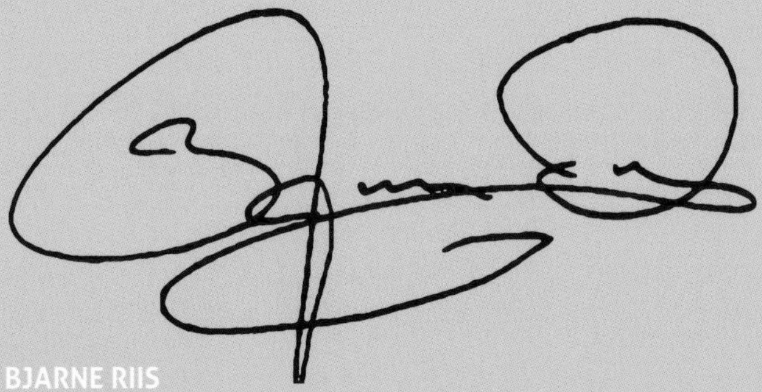

BJARNE RIIS
Founder
Riis Cycling A/S

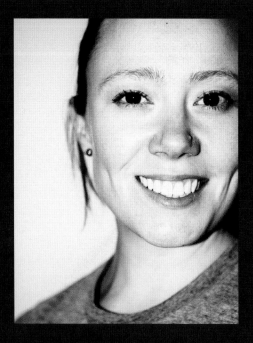

INTRODUCTION
BY HANNAH GRANT

This book is about healthy, exciting and nutritionally beneficial food for both professional athletes'and physically active individuals. Food fuels the body, so your performance is enhanced when you fill your body with the proper fuel. In broad terms, "proper fuel" means that, if you want to achieve your optimal energy yield, you must select the highest quality ingredients.

Proper fuel is not just about food. It is about the correct food for every single meal. Proper food is made from scratch and devoid of refined products such as white sugar, white pasta and ready-made sauces, dressings, breads, or desserts. Once you start cooking from scratch, using fresh whole vegetables and fresh, top quality fish and meat (all preferably organic), things will start to fall into place.

The Grand Tour Cookbook follows a 21-day "Grand Tour" (Tour de France, Vuelta a España, or Giro d'Italia). Every single one of the cyclists' meals, big or small, is made from scratch, primarily using local organic ingredients. This book is specifically based on a menu for a Tour de France. Between the various stages, you can read the cyclists' own thoughts about the food and the difference it makes for them, both when performing and back home.

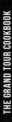

The Grand Tour Cookbook consists of 21 evening meals, each of three, four, or five recipes. Of course, you do not have to make as many courses for yourself every evening as I make for the riders. When we do so, it is because there must be something to suit a range of tastes. It takes a bit of effort to make food for an entire cycling team that collectively represents most of the world!

Since many people have a slight intolerance to dairy or gluten, most of the recipes have been devised to suit a dairy- or gluten-free diet. By minimising dairy and gluten in our riders' diet, they can increase their body's capacity to fight off sickness and resist other non-food allergies (e.g. hay fever).

As in all recipe books, some recipes are more demanding than others, so I advise you read through the whole recipe before you start. If you find it impossible to source specific fresh fruits, vegetables or herbs that are used in the recipes, you can replace them with others according to taste and availability. Additionally, you can always replace milk with rice milk or vice versa, if you prefer one to the other.

I hope you will share our riders' enthusiasm for these dishes and enjoy creating your own "proper fuel" with the basic principles outlined in the recipes enclosed.

HANNAH GRANT
Chef
Tinkoff-Saxo

PERFORMANCE COOKING *by*
ANNE DORTHE TANDERUP

WHAT IS THE "RIGHT" DIET?

Over the years there have been many opinions on what is the right diet for professional cyclists and other elite athletes. Innumerable types of diets have been tried – everything from red-meat-based diets to carbohydrate-heavy diets and vegetarian diets. Perhaps you have already tried to replicate the diets of top cyclists, or have leafed through some scientific studies and tried to translate the results into your own practice. However, discovering what works for you usually requires simply giving it a go. Some cyclists are lucky enough to discover the right diet for them, but others fumble around, changing direction again and again, because they do not achieve any long-lasting effects.

Professional road cycling is a physically demanding sport. In order to achieve success, there are several criteria that must be fulfilled. First, you need the genes and the talent. Next, you need extraordinary commitment, hard work and mental strength. It's not just a sport, it's a way of life that involves knowing what choices to make and, more importantly, what choices not to make. Except for the rare off-season time you have to relax, you must be a professional all day, everyday and all year, constantly focused on your goals. Every aspect of a cyclist's life is planned so they can achieve peak performance: sleep, practice, rest, travelling, races and diet.

UNDERSTAND YOUR BODY, INDIVIDUALISE YOUR DIET

To plan your diet and get the very best out of it, you need to analyse and understand your own body and then, on that basis, optimise and individualise your diet. We are all built differently. Therefore, something that works well for one person may not necessarily work for another. The body is made up of millions of cells. The majority of them are replaced on an on-going basis: some after a couple of days (stomach cells) others after a couple of weeks (skin cells), others after a few months (blood cells) and then others after six months (muscle cells). The new cells are affected by what we eat. If we are aware of this, we can help determine the quality of our new cells. But, an improvement of the quality of our cells is not something that happens the moment we put food in our mouths. It is a process in which the body gradually adapts to utilising more nutrients, thereby building a better, stronger body.

THE SIGNIFICANCE OF DIET FOR BODY AWARENESS

According to nutritional research, diet plays a major role in body awareness, function and reconstruction. During high performance activity, such as cycling at the elite level, the body uses extra resources. Not only does it consume an extreme amount of energy (professional cyclists can burn up to 8,000 calories during a tough mountain stage in the Tour de France), but it also needs far more minerals, vitamins, healthy fats and antioxidants.

As a result, the body requires large amounts of excellent nourishment, so it can heal, repair and reconstruct itself with the right building blocks. You will not get very far in your car if you use the wrong fuel. Your body is the same. I cannot put it more simply than that. If your body is to function and perform at its best, the quality of what you put in your mouth is a crucial factor.

I am a former world and Olympic champion, a mother to four boys and a trained dietician specialising in optimal performance. That means I am all too familiar with the frustration of being unable to consume my optimal individual diet because of the fluctuating quality of food at the restaurants and hotels I had to stay in during competitions. It dawned on me that professional cyclists were more than lucky if the food they ate on the road had any more value than sating their immediate hunger and filling their stomachs.

Each country has its own problems. In my time in France, the pasta and the few available vegetables were boiled to death. In Belgium, most of the food was deep-fried. In Spain, the chips from the day before were blended into the tomato soup the following day. To find something satisfying, in terms of both nutrition and flavour, was just about impossible.

FROM HOTEL FOOD TO PERFORMANCE COOKING
In my work with Riis Cycling, I soon became aware that, in the world of professional cycling, there was more focus on the quantity than the quality of food. I was soon convinced that something could be done for the performance and general well-being of the cyclists by optimising their diet and in particular, the quality of the food.

The first step on the road to providing the cyclists with a more nutritious diet was to hire a chef to travel with the team and cook for them in the hotels' kitchens. Gradually the cyclists began to see and feel the difference between the food our chef made and the food in the restaurants.

However, it turned out to be difficult to gain full control over the cyclists' diets because our chef could not always be guaranteed access to the hotels' kitchens. We had a new plan: work with our sponsors to convert a truck into a kitchen-on-wheels. That meant we would have 24-hour access to a mobile kitchen, optimising most of the food we served to the cyclists and controlling everything they consumed in the course of a day. So from 2010 when we realised this plan, we started demanding more of the food we cooked ourselves.

In the course of the following year, Performance Cooking took shape, starting with the basic idea that all individuals are composed differently and thus have fundamentally different needs.

WE WORK ON THE BASIS OF THE FOLLOWING GUIDELINES:

- Options for individual diets and adaptation to the cyclists' actual needs
- All made from scratch
- No additives, preservatives or artificial sweeteners
- Varied, colourful, visually impressive and surprising food
- Gluten- and dairy-free foods must always be available
- Lots of good sources of protein: fresh vegetables, fresh fruit, whole grains and healthy fats
- The option to avoid carbohydrate-rich foods
- Priority to superfoods and ingredients rich in antioxidants
- Minimal use of refined foods
- Preference for organic ingredients
- Healthy fats as a source of energy to complement carbohydrates

THE CHALLENGE: CHANGING THE DIET OF AN ENTIRE CYCLING TEAM

For many of the cyclists on the team, Performance Cooking meant having to eat foods and combinations they had never experienced before. Professional cycling teams are composed of cyclists from many different cultures and it takes time to change the eating habits of a lifetime. To put it mildly, we were facing a major revolution and challenge.

The appointment of Hannah Grant for the 2011 season marked the kick-off of the Performance Cooking programme. Thanks to Hannah's fantastic food and strong personality, she won the trust of the cyclists. She, together with her assistants, started to break old habits and build a bridge between Performance Cooking and the individual tastes and needs of the cyclists. She spends a great deal of time adapting and improving recipes, often based upon direct discussions with the cyclists.

In 2012, we took Performance Cooking one step further and invested in a truck equipped with a state-of-the-art professional kitchen. We now have an even greater capacity to individualise diets and make food that is hard to find on the road, such as freshly-pressed juices and gluten-free bread.

THE RIGHT DIET IS VITAL

Almost every single day, professional cyclists subject their bodies to extremely tough physical activity. Shattering their bodies time and time again, they need extra protection against inflammation and cell death. Therefore, the antioxidants in vegetables and fruits must be central in diet planning. Other anti-inflammatories, such as Omega-3 fatty acids, freshly-pressed ginger, turmeric and lots of fresh herbs, also play a more important role in Performance Cooking than in a regular diet. Such a diet takes care of an athlete's body's need for reconstruction and protection. Beyond recovery, in order to train and perform at the highest level over a long period of time, cyclists need substantial quantities of nutrients. That is why paying attention to the nutrients in food, their quality and the effects of preparation is essential.

A CYCLIST'S WEIGHT

A cyclist's body weight is extremely important. Cycling can basically be reduced to watts per kilo, i.e. how many watts a cyclist can pedal with the lowest possible body weight. Top-seeded cyclists in the major Grand Tours have about 4-6% body fat. Meanwhile, the Cobblestone Classics in the spring, such as the Tour of Flanders and Paris-Roubaix, are dominated by cyclists with about 6-8% body fat. That makes it essential for a cyclist to keep their weight down without starving the body and missing out on essential nutrients.

A common misconception is that it is easy for cyclists to lose weight because they train hard and burn off so many calories. For some cyclists, yes, it is easy. But for others it is a daily struggle, just like for the rest of us. There are always some people who look slim and healthy, regardless of what they eat and how little they exercise. Then there are those for whom weight is always a bit of a struggle.

Almost half of the cyclists on the team find it difficult to lose the weight they need to. We have cyclists who, despite extreme physical activity and low calorie intake, still find it hard to lose the last percentages of fat they need to. We have found that for these cyclists, radically cutting down on carbohydrate intake and increasing protein and healthy fat intake works best. Performance Cooking takes care of this by providing the cyclists with the option of avoiding carbohydrate-rich foods and offering alternatives in the form of meat, vegetables and healthy fats at every meal.

When you burn off 4,000-6,000 calories in the course of a day, it is easy to indulge oneself by eating whatever you feel like. But professional cyclists must be professionals 24 hours a day. A body's performance capacity in the long run depends on whether its building blocks are made from McDonald's and Mars bars or vegetables, meat and superfoods.

The sport of cycling is all about precision and optimisation. It is important to have precisely calibrated equipment, an optimised training schedule, the most efficient recovery and the greatest mental reserves. Without the right fuel and proper engine maintenance though, it is impossible to be a winner. Now more than ever, diet is a deciding factor in victory.

There are still many opinions about what a cyclist should and should not eat. All agree, though, that the right nutrition can make a substantial difference in terms of strength, stamina, speed and mental preparedness. In this book, Hannah provides a glimpse of what the team has achieved since beginning the Performance Cooking programme.

FOOD, DIET AND NOURISHMENT
BY DR. STACY SIMS

Aside from serving as fuel for our bodies, food is connected to our bodies in many ways. The psychological impact of taste, smell and texture supersedes the conscious voice that says, "This food is good for me so I should eat it." In the globalised western culture and vocabulary, "diet" has become associated more with weight management and marketing than the actual nourishment.

When I first met Hannah, she understood that food is not just energy and macronutrients, and each rider's body may react differently to the same diet. She also understood that food is functional and can be used as medicine. For example, turmeric and ginger are powerful anti-inflammatory agents; FODMAPs (Fermentable Oligo-, Di-, Mono-saccharides and Polyols), not gluten, might be the underlying cause of gastro-intestinal issues; and protein is essential to exercise recovery and performance improvements.

With this knowledge of how food affects the body, we started to think about two new concepts: lifestyle nutrition and training and racing nutrition. Lifestyle nutrition encourages the selection of nutritious foods that enhance liver and muscle glycogen storage and body fat loss, and broadens the selection of foods for greater micronutrient intake. Lifestyle nutrition is the base of the pyramid on which you build specific training and racing nutrition.

The seasons of a pro-cyclist's year (recovery, endurance, intensity, competition) are like nature's seasons: a time to recover, a time to build, a time to grow and accelerate and a time to be fierce. Understanding the dynamic demands on athletes over the course of a year, we can manipulate athletes' diets to allow them to perform at their peak. Racing nutrition builds on lifestyle nutrition to make sure athletes are at the peak of the pyramid when they need to perform.

BODY COMPOSITION, PERFORMANCE WEIGHT AND CARBOHYDRATES

In sports performance nutrition there has been a recent movement toward higher-fat, higher-protein and lower-carbohydrate intake diets in which the kind of food matters as much as, or more than, the macronutrient aspect content of the food. The increased interest in the use of nutrition and nutrient timing to improve general health and wellness fits with our focus on performance nutrition.

There's substantial debate about the efficacy of a lower-carbohydrate, low-grain diet and its relationship to athletic performance. You may have heard that low-carbohydrate, high-fat diets substantially improve performance. The short answer is "sort of". Yes, low-carbohydrate diets do increase fatty acid oxidation during exercise and encourage intramuscular fat storage. The body is smart. If there isn't enough primary fuel to support the stress it's under, it will use a secondary source and store more of that for the next time it encounters stress. However, this does not translate into improved performance, as it compromises the ability to maintain high-intensity or prolonged endurance. Yes, the body does need carbohydrates to exist, but it needs the right carbohydrates to perform in the professional cycling and endurance competition world.

It is important to understand the basic physiology around carbohydrates. Firstly, the roles of carbohydrates in the body include providing energy for working muscles, providing fuel for the central nervous system, enabling and perpetuating fat metabolism and preventing the use of protein as a primary energy source. Remember, carbohydrates, specifically glucose, are the preferred source of energy for muscle contraction and biologic work.

Secondly, the body's storage capacity for glycogen (the storage form of glucose in the muscles and liver) is limited to about 300 grams of muscle glycogen and 40 to 45 grams of liver glycogen in a non-obese 60-kilogram woman. The glycogen stored in the muscle is used directly by the muscle during exercise. It cannot borrow glycogen from other, resting muscles. Hence, it becomes critical for the endurance athlete to replenish glycogen stores.

Thirdly, the minimum intake of carbohydrates necessary for survival is 130 grams per day to support the central nervous system, red blood cell production, the immune system and tissues dependent on glucose. 130 grams per day does not support additional physical activity.

In regards to the effects of aerobic exercise on muscle glycogen utilization, the intensity and duration of the exercise directly affects the amount of glycogen used. It's common knowledge that low-intensity exercise (e.g., 20 to 30 percent O2max) uses minimal glycogen. But when the intensity approaches 75 percent of VO2max, muscle glycogen is almost completely depleted after 2 hours of excerise. It is interesting to note that the rate of glycogenolysis is higher in type IIa and IIb muscle fibres at intensities greater than 75 percent VO2max. Usually, type I fibres deplete first. Therefore, in a race situation when it's go from the gun, the actual rate of total muscle glycogen depletion will be faster, increasing the probability of early fatigue.

It appears that glycogen availability is the primary limiting factor with respect to sustaining intensity during prolonged exercise, with the initial amount of glycogen stored in the muscle directly proportional to the athlete's ability to sustain work rates greater than 70 percent VO2max over time. Since dietary carbohydrates are a significant contributor to muscle glycogen stores and thus performance, how does an athlete maximise their stores on a low-carbohydrate, low-grain diet? The best answer is to use your body's natural windows of glycogen replenishment and specific types of carbohydrate to maximise glycogen stores.

Muscle glycogen synthesis is more rapid if carbohydrates are consumed directly after exercise, as opposed to several hours later. Several pro-athletes I've worked with had the idea that if they delayed eating post-exercise, they would maintain fat burning and lose weight more effectively. In fact, the opposite occurs. Delaying eating put them in a catabolic state that perpetuated weight gain and led to inadequate recovery. The difference between eating within 30 to 60 minutes post-exercise and 2 to 2.5 hours post-exercise is a 50 percent reduction in glycogen synthesis. As those minutes tick away, insulin sensitivity declines, slowing muscle glucose uptake and overall glycogen storage. Eating immediately after exercise delays the decline in insulin sensitivity. You can extend the ability to rapidly store glycogen by up to 8 hours with a hit of carbohydrates every couple of hours.

Perhaps you have heard that you need to mix protein and carbohydrate post-exercise. There are three key reasons for this. Firstly, protein intake within 30 minutes of exercise shifts the body from the catabolic state (breakdown) of exercise into the anabolic state (muscle repair and synthesis). Carbohydrates assist this process by increasing muscle insulin sensitivity.

Secondly, the ingestion of carbohydrates and protein post-exercise can reduce inflammation and positively affect the immune system. Thirdly, and most interestingly, carbohydrates and proteins work synergistically to increase glycogen storage rates. In a comparison of glycogen storage rates in the first 40 minutes following exhaustive cycling (3 hours at greater than 75 percent VO2max), glycogen storage was four times faster after carbohydrate-protein supplementation (2:1 carbohydrate to protein; 80 grams carbohydrate, 40 grams protein, 6 grams fat) than after an iso-carbohydrate supplement (80 grams carbohydrate, 6 grams fat) and twice as fast than with an iso-caloric treatment (120 grams carbohydrate, 6 grams fat).

The important thing to take away is this: if you are eating a lower-carbohydrate diet, maximise your glycogen resynthesis by eating protein with carbohydrate within the first 30 to 40 minutes post-exercise.

SOURCES OF CARBOHYDRATES
Many people believe that the best sources of post-exercise carbohydrates are grain based (e.g. oatmeal, pasta, bread, cereals), but this isn't exactly true. The best sources of carbohydrates are those that have a greater composition of glucose, sources that are high on the glycemic index. Starchy veggies such as sweet potatoes, yams, butternut squash and root vegetables like parsnips are just a few good options. They are moderate to high on the glycemic index and moderate to high in carbohydrate content. Raw cassava has 78 grams carbohydrate per cup; mashed plantains have 62 grams per cup; and mashed sweet potatoes have 58 grams per cup. Compare this to cooked oatmeal at 27 grams per cup; quinoa at 39 grams per cup; and the ever-popular cooked pasta at 43 grams per cup.

WHAT ABOUT FRUIT?

The critical difference between starchy vegetables and fruit is the type of carbohydrates in each. Vegetables are composed of longer chains of glucose, whereas fruit is primarily fructose. Glucose is more efficient at muscle glycogen resynthesis, as fructose is preferentially used by the liver.

WHAT'S THE BOTTOM LINE?

The metabolic window of opportunity is the time after exercise in which the muscle is most capable of responding to the anabolic effects of insulin with the ingestion of carbohydrate and protein. Without any nutrient intake, this window begins to close 45 minutes post-exercise. By taking advantage of this post-exercise window and extending insulin sensitivity with the ingestion of specific carbohydrates with protein, individuals who adhere to a lower-carbohydrate diet can maximise glycogen storage.

HANNAH, PROFESSIONAL CYCLISTS AND PERFORMANCE COOKING

Performance Cooking is more than just supplying carbohydrates, fat and protein to the professional riders of Tinkoff-Saxo. It is about providing nourishing, functional food for high performance athletes. Hannah is an amazing chef with a strong grasp of the physiology of the body under extreme exercise stress. She has fused this with innovative cuisine, empowering athletes' bodies and minds to reach their performance potential. In this book, you too can experience the fusion of real food and real nourishment to achieve your performance potential.

DR. STACY SIMS, MSC, PHD
Exercise Physiologist and Nutritional Scientist

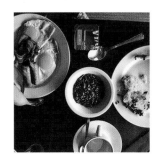 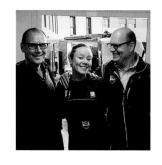 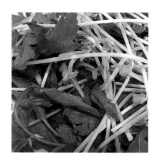 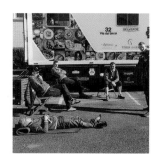

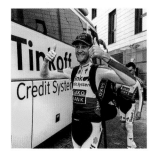 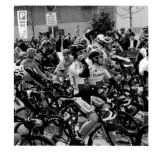 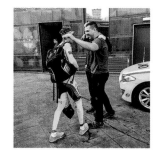 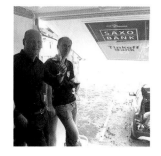

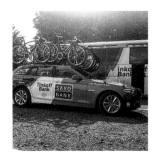 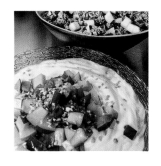 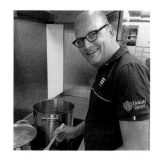 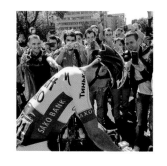

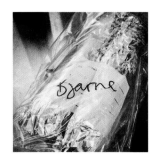 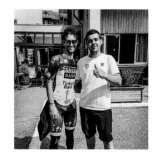 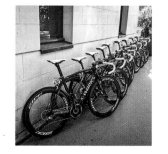 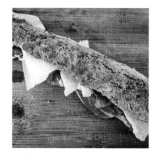

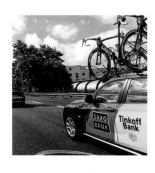 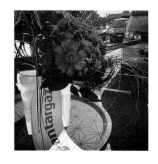 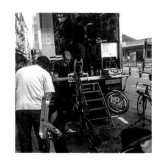 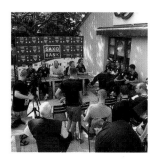

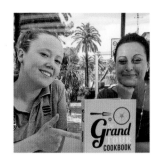 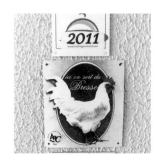 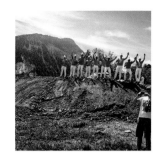 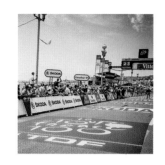

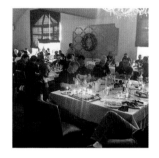 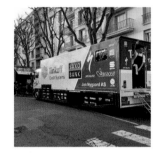 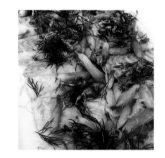 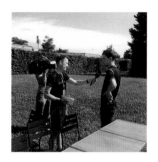

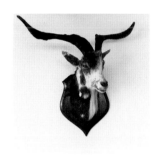 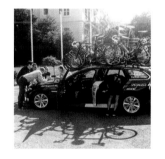 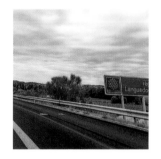 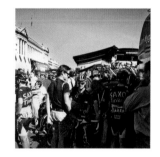

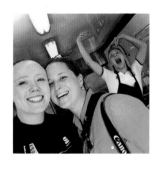 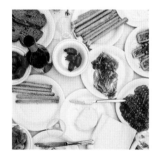 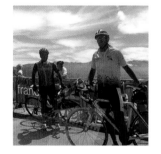 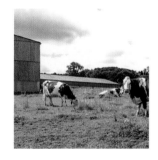

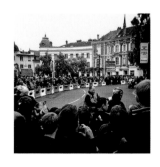 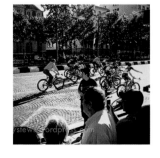 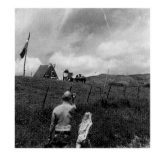 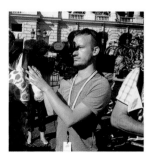

PRACTICE AND PRINCIPLES
BEFORE YOU START

THE DIETARY PRINCIPLES AT THE HEART OF PERFORMANCE COOKING
More fruit and vegetables
More healthy fat
More protein
Less starch and sugar

MORE FRUIT AND VEGETABLES

We work on the principle that with the right diet, you can optimise recovery, reduce inflammation and increase energy. That is why we pay a great deal of attention to fruits and vegetables. They contain all the minerals and vitamins needed to keep a professional cyclist going. The majority of our recipes are based on large portions of fruit and vegetables, together with a suggestion for a type of carbohydrate you should eat, if necessary. Getting athletes to eat pasta, rice and potatoes is not exactly difficult, but it can be a challenge to persuade them to eat enough fruit and vegetables.

MORE HEALTHY FAT

We favour the good fats: cold-pressed flaxseed, olive and sunflower seed oils for dressings and smoothies. Cold-pressed flaxseed oil is rich in omega-3 and omega-6 fatty acids, which are essential for the functioning of the brain, nervous system and digestive system. Healthy fat in a diet is also essential for the absorption of vitamins. Of course, you must find the balance that works best for you. All people, including athletes, are different. Athletes at all levels need different combinations of healthy fat depending on the type and intensity of their performance.

MORE PROTEIN

Protein covers animal protein, which we get from eggs, chicken, veal, pork, lamb and fish and vegetable protein, e.g. beans, quinoa, lentils and chia seed. When you practise sport at such an intense level, it is extremely important for your diet to supply you with adequate protein. Protein provides the building blocks for rebuilding muscle fibres after a hard training session. In a diet with few carbohydrates – a low carb diet – your body operates on energy from fat. So, along with good fat and green vegetables, protein is a critical element in covering your energy needs. Protein sates the appetite for longer periods of time, which is especially important for endurance athletes.

LESS STARCH AND SUGAR

Starch covers the type of carbohydrates that, in the cooking world, we call satiation garnish. Potatoes, pasta, rice, cereals and noodles are compact sources of carbohydrates. They contain a greater amount of energy per 100 g than aqueous vegetables. When we choose starches, we tend to select the gluten-free varieties, i.e. potatoes, rice, rice noodles, tapioca and corn (polenta), in order to avoid possible discomfort caused by minor gluten intolerances. Some cyclists choose to eat less compact carbohydrate in order to keep their weight down during the season and during periods when their activity is lower than usual, rest days and the off season.

A lower starch and sugar intake stabilises blood sugar, minimising fluctuations of energy during the day. By sugar, I mean refined sugar such as sweets, cakes, castor sugar, breakfast cereals, ketchup, gels (consumed during training), Nutella, jams and carbonated drinks etc. Because a cyclist consumes huge amounts of energy in the course of a day, we believe it is sensible to reduce the intake of unnecessary sugar. We strictly limit the consumption of sugar outside of races, due to the fact that cyclists only need an extra energy boost while riding.

ORGANIC PRODUCE
We choose organic produce, whenever possible. We believe it is better both for us and for nature. We seek out products with no artificial sweeteners, no growth stimulants and, above all, more flavour and nutrients.

SLOW VERSUS FAST CARBOHYDRATE
Every morning, three hours before the start of a race, the cyclists eat a hearty meal consisting of porridge (preferably made from gluten-free oatmeal), whole grain bread, rice or pasta. These carbohydrates are located at the 'slowly absorbed' end of the spectrum. Energy is released little by little, maintaining a stable level of energy from the start of the race. During the race, the cyclists switch to fast carbohydrates (e.g. bars of chocolate, gels and sugary drinks) to get a boost of energy for the long, tough stages when instant energy is required. These quickly absorbed carbohydrates can make the difference as to whether or not a cyclist completes a stage, so be sure to pack some good race snacks for a long day of training.

WHOLE GRAINS
Whole grains are great for sating the appetite and have a higher fibre content than refined grain products. A high fibre-content is good for the digestive system, so if cyclists consume sufficient amounts, they can avoid constipation and other digestive problems.

USING THE RECIPES
We make a distinction between race days and rest days. In this book there are recipes for 19 race days and 2 rest days. There are also recipes for breakfast, race snacks, bread, dressings and more. All the dishes can be combined to suit your performance needs and you can choose whether or not to eat starchy accompaniments. The symbols next to the recipes show whether the recipe is gluten-free, nut-free and/or dairy-free (see guidelines for the recipes on Page 27).

1. ON RACE DAYS

Breakfast
A race day starts with a breakfast consisting of protein and carbohydrates. Every cyclist has his favourite source of carbohydrates in the morning, e.g. rice, soaked muesli or porridge. Other cyclists do not eat any starchy carbohydrates in the morning. To avoid going cold or hitting a wall and to feel comfortable on a ride, you need to know your body well and know what works for you. Many riders suffer from bloated stomachs if they consume gluten-rich starch, so they choose gluten-free alternatives in order to perform better. All riders consume protein in the morning, usually from eggs.

Race snacks – during the race

After breakfast, the next meal is consumed on the bike. Cyclists are supplied with feedbags (musettes) on their bikes. They contain small, simple sandwiches, cakes and bananas: no strong flavours – a little savoury and a little sweet – and are packed to be eaten in quick mouthfuls to maintain energy levels. Many cyclists stick to real food instead of energy gels, which have very high sugar content. The balance is delicate. Once again, it is up to the individual cyclist to find out what works best.

Recovery foods – after the race

Immediately after the race, cyclists consume a protein drink to help kick-start recovery. On the bus on the way back to the hotel, the cyclists are served food boxes, which contain carbohydrates and protein in different combinations: e.g. Danish omelette with potato and a mixture of leftovers from the night before. Food boxes are a great way to make use of leftovers.

Dinner

The last meal of the day is dinner. We always serve two kinds of protein (one of which is always chicken), a large selection of fresh vegetables in salads and at least two kinds of carbohydrates – one of which is gluten-free. Of course, you do not need to make five courses for yourself every evening, but in our case it is important to provide a wide range of choices to keep all the taste buds happy. It is not the same at home, where you know what you like and need.

2. ON REST DAYS

On a rest day, we eliminate starchy carbohydrates from breakfast and lunch. The cyclists only cycle a short route so they do not require as much energy as on a race day. Dinner, however, is the same as on race days because their batteries need to be charged for an entire day in the saddle the next day.

HOW DO YOU FIND OUT WHAT WORKS?

There is only one way: give it a try. Remember, it takes time before you can determine if and how a diet works for you. Also, remember that all people are different and that what works for one person does not necessarily work for another. One thing is certain: being able to recover more quickly day in and day out can make a big difference in the long run. The small margins help you stay on top over the course of a Grand Tour.

We believe that you can prevent injuries and other physical problems by eating correctly. Medication eliminates pain and symptoms but blocks the body's natural healing processes and reduces the benefits of training. On the other hand, proper food helps prevent many problems and is the best source of energy available.

OUR PERFORMANCE COOKING CONCEPT IS NOT A STEP BY STEP GUIDE TO HELP YOU IMPROVE IN YOUR SPECIFIC SPORT. RATHER, IT SERVES AS INSPIRATION TO SHOW YOU HOW TO OPTIMISE YOUR NUTRITION AND HELP YOU DISCOVER WHAT SUITS YOU BEST AS AN ATHLETE.

SUPERFOODS

All green vegetables: e.g. broccoli, cabbage, parsley, spinach etc.
They contain Vitamin K and Vitamin B9, which are important for producing red blood cells.
Green vegetables, nuts, seeds and grains contain high levels of potassium and magnesium, which relax muscles and are excellent for the metabolism and stabilise blood sugar.

Ginger, galangal and turmeric
Anti-inflammatory
10-15 g a day for maintenance and prevention
100-200 g a day for 7 days as treatment for inflammatory conditions
(not appropriate for people with stomach ulcers)
Ginger leads to better blood circulation and warmth.
All are excellent for preventing nausea and digestive problems.
The active substances in ginger, galangal and turmeric are stable and can be heated and dried.

Beetroot
Optimises oxygen uptake, improves blood flow
½ litre beetroot juice or 5½ tbsp beetroot crystals taken daily optimises the body's ability to use oxygen.

Brazil nuts
Source of selenium
Good for the thyroid, metabolism, immune system, the body's antioxidant defences and detoxification in the liver and kidney
Reduces the risk of joint infection

Garlic
Antibacterial
Leads to better blood circulation
Source of selenium and Vitamin C

Goji berries and blueberries
Rich in antioxidants
Source of Vitamin C

Kombu seaweed
Neutralises the enzymes in beans, which cause flatulence

Flaxseed oil
Contains omega-3 and omega-6 fatty acids
Good for regeneration of joints and a faster metabolism
Omega-3 fatty acids are important for the joints, skin, brain and metabolism

PREPARATION AND EQUIPMENT

Having the right equipment in the kitchen makes cooking much easier. There is no need to spend unnecessary hours cutting carrots into long strips when you can do this in no time using a food processor or a mandolin. It should be easy to cook good food.

Efficiency is good, so try cooking large portions of food twice a week. When you are preparing food and have your equipment out, you might as well grate a lot of carrots, slice a lot of cabbage, chop a lot of herbs and so on. If you know that potatoes and quinoa are good for you, always make sure you have boiled quinoa and potatoes ready in the fridge. The same goes for vegetables. All this helps make the cooking process much easier and, more importantly, much shorter. Prepared vegetables can be kept in re-sealable containers in the refrigerator. Herbs can be kept covered with a regularly dampened cloth.

Make a weekly meal schedule

Plan your week so you can cook easily and quickly. The Grand Tour Cookbook is aimed at a three-week period with several different combinations a day, so every day you can select a protein dish and a salad, while combining them in various ways to suit your tastes.

THE KITCHEN CUPBOARD

It is also a good idea to have a well-stocked kitchen cupboard with a variety of spices, oils and vinegars as well as dry goods, so you are always able to make a decent meal. I suggest that you tidy up your kitchen cabinets and remove all the products that might tempt you when you are hungry. This means sweetened breakfast cereals, artificially sweetened goods, instant products and products with a high sugar content such as ketchup and Nutella. You should instead fill your cabinets with good, easy to use and useful products:

PRESERVED AND SEMI-PRESERVED
Peeled tomatoes
Tomato paste
Albacore tuna in water
Cornichons
Capers
Dijon mustard
Olives
Tahini
Honey

SPICES
Salt flakes
Sea salt
Dried oregano
Bay leaves
Curry powder
Ground coriander
Turmeric
Ginger
Paprika
Ground cumin
Ground cloves
Ground cinnamon
Cinnamon sticks
Cardamom
Ground allspice
Star anise
Nutmeg
Five spice
Dried yeast
Baking powder
Bicarbonate of soda

OILS AND VINEGARS
Cold-pressed virgin olive oil
Cold-pressed flaxseed oil
Coconut oil (flavourless)
Hazelnut oil
Apple vinegar
Balsamic vinegar
Sherry vinegar
A variety of flavoured
vinegars: e.g. raspberry,
elderflower, tarragon etc.

DRY GOODS
Quinoa
Brown rice
Basmati rice
Dried beans
Dried chickpeas
Couscous
Bulgur wheat
Wholemeal pasta
Gluten-free pasta
Buckwheat noodles
Rice noodles
Flaxseed
Sunflower seeds
Pumpkin seeds
Hazelnuts
Almonds
Dried fruit

EQUIPMENT LIST FOR A GOOD BASIC KITCHEN
Fine grater (e.g. Microplane)
Mandolin
Spiralizer (optional)
Food processor
Thin peeler (transverse blade)
Whisk
Rubber spatula
Pepper grinder
Salad spinner
Chef's knife
Peeling knife
Paring knife
Sharpening steel
Oven-proof thermometer

CONVERSION TABLE

MILLILITERS	US CUPS	GRAMS	OZ.	CELSIUS	FAHRENHEIT
1	0.0042	1	0.04	1	33.8
50	0.21	50	1.76	50	106
100	0.42	75	2.65	75	159
125	0.5	100	3.53	100	212
150	0.63	125	4.41	110	230
200	0.84	150	5.29	125	257
250	1.05	175	6.17	150	302
300	1.26	200	7.05	160	320
350	1.47	250	8.82	165	329
400	1.68	300	10.58	170	338
450	1.89	400	14.11	180	356
500	2.1	500	17.64	185	365
600	2.52	600	21.16	190	374
700	2.94	700	24.69	200	392
800	3.36	800	28.22	210	410
900	3.78	900	31.75	220	428
1000	4.2	1000	35.27	225	437

From milliliters to cups:
milliliters x (1/250)

From grams to oz.:
grams x 0.035

From Celsius to Fahrenheit:
Celsius x 9 / 5 + 32

INFORMATION *for* THE RECIPES

ALL THE RECIPES ARE FOR 4 PEOPLE, UNLESS OTHERWISE NOTED.

The recipes are accompanied by symbols which indicate that they are GLUTEN-FREE, DAIRY-FREE or NUT-FREE:

 GLUTEN-FREE

 DAIRY-FREE

 NUT-FREE

IMPORTANT INFORMATION ABOUT THE SYMBOLS:

Certain recipes contain nuts, gluten and dairy. In that case, they will not be accompanied by any of the above symbols. At the back of the book, there is a complete, alphabetical list of the recipes that are gluten-free, nut-free and/or dairy-free.

Recipes containing pine nuts, sunflower seeds and sesame are classified as nut-free since intolerance to them differs from one nut allergy sufferer to another.

Recipes that contain nut oil are not classified as nut-free.

Recipes that contain coconut (coconut milk or coconut fat) are not classified as nut-free.

Recipes that call for either milk or rice milk are classified as dairy-free recipes, since the milk can be substituted with rice milk.

Recipes that contain soy sauce are classified as gluten-free but this depends on the particular soy sauce used. Check the sauces before using them. Tamari is always gluten-free.

Recipes with chocolate listed as nut-free do not account for traces of nut that may be in the chocolate you use.

Please be aware that some recipes require preparation the day before.

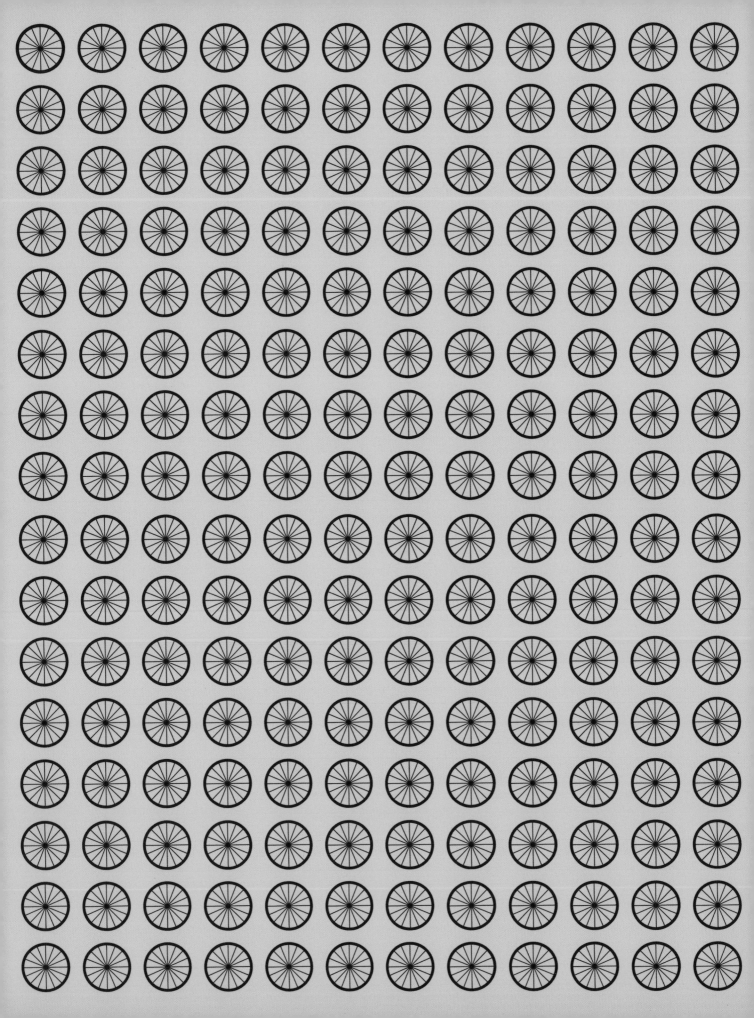

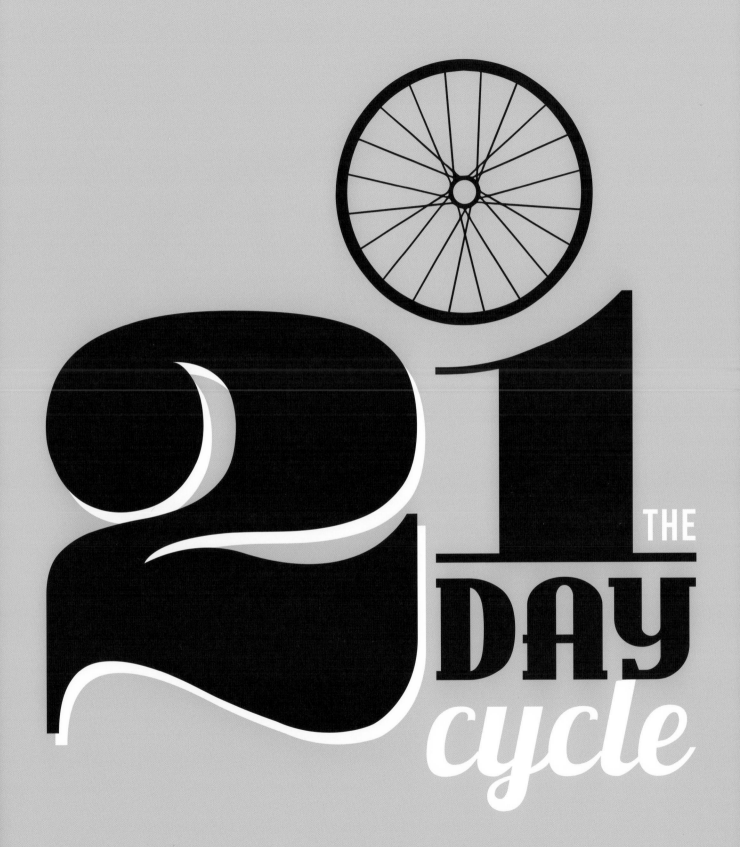

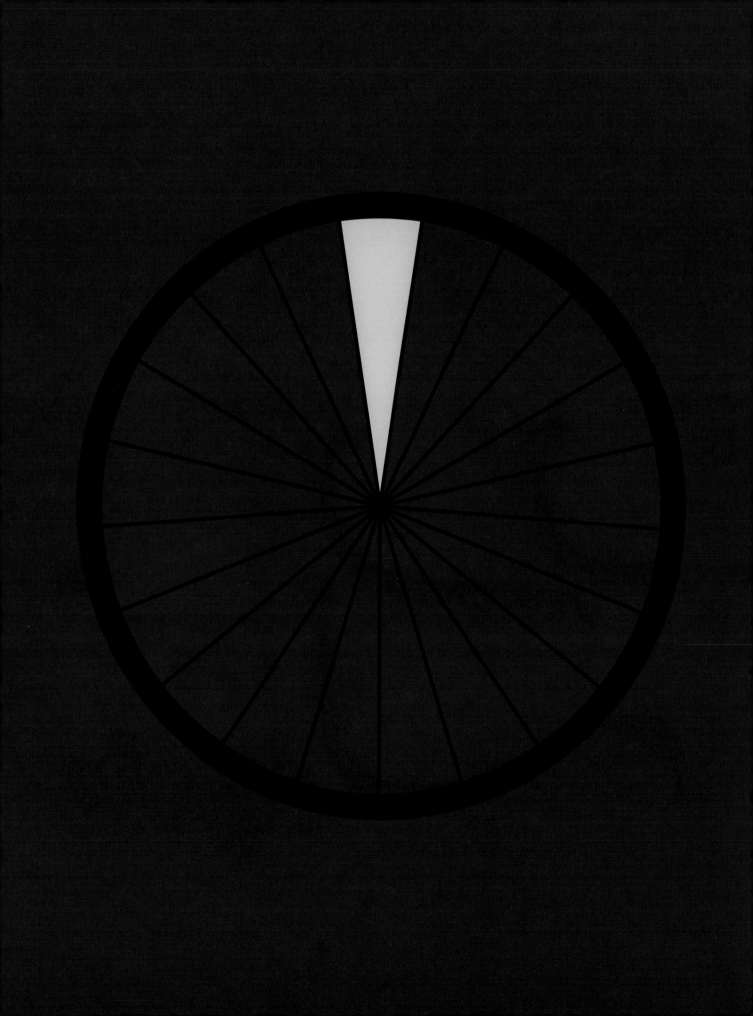

1

DAY

PROLOGUE

TOMATO, *avocado,* PINE NUTS AND FETA

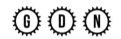

6 PLUM TOMATOES
¼ BUNCH PARSLEY
JUICE AND ZEST OF 1 ORGANIC LIME
100 G PINE NUTS
2 AVOCADOS
200 G FETA
4 TBSP OLIVE OIL
½ TSP SALT
FRESHLY GROUND BLACK PEPPER

Preheat the oven to 170°C.

Wash the tomatoes, trim off the stalks and cut each into 8 wedges. Sprinkle with a little salt.
Rinse and chop the parsley and grate the lime zest using a fine grater. Toast the pine nuts in the oven until golden – about 5-6 minutes. Halve the avocados and scoop out the flesh with a spoon. Slice and marinate in the lime juice. Drain the tomatoes and toss with the parsley. Crumble the feta into bite-sized pieces.

Serve everything on a platter, drizzle with olive oil and sprinkle with the pine nuts. Season with freshly ground pepper.

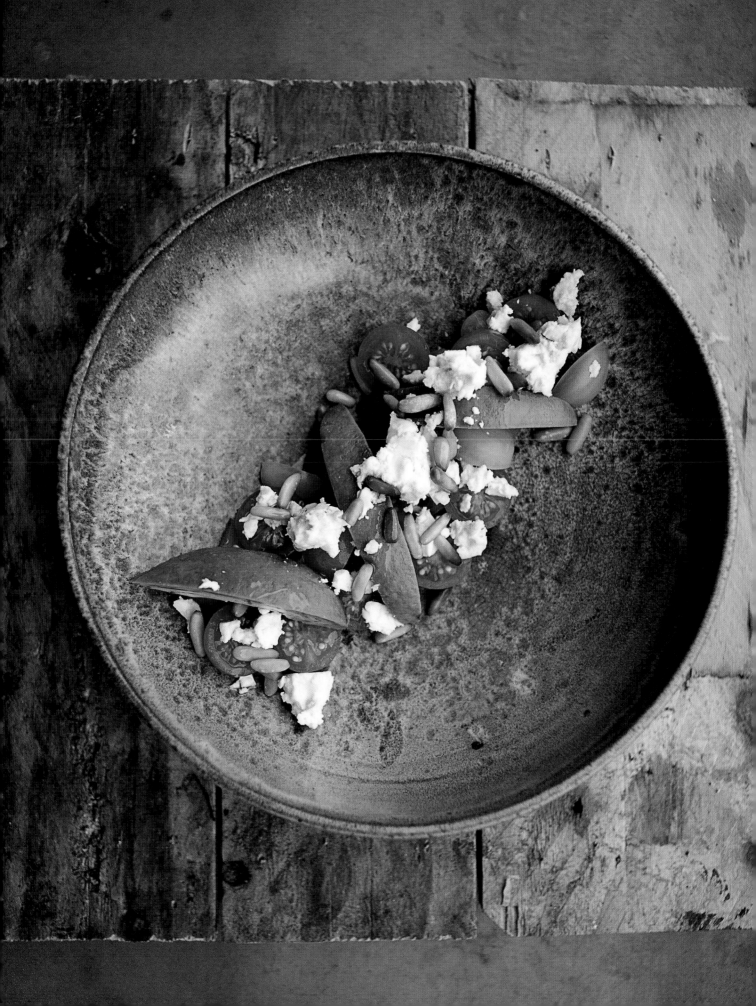

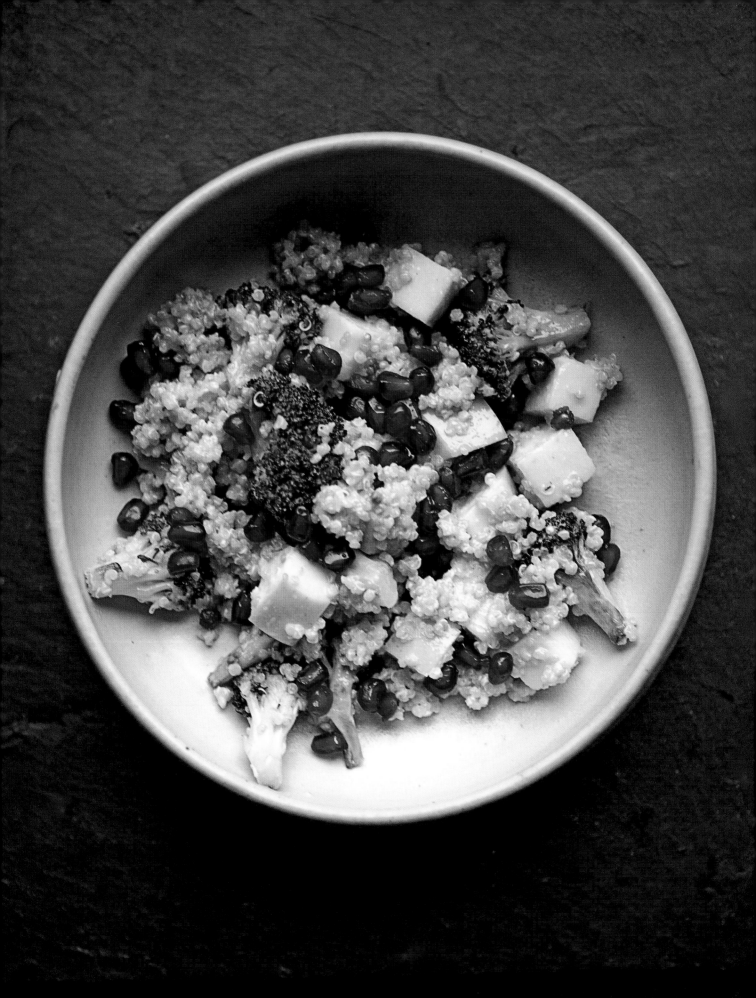

QUINOA, *broccoli,*
APPLE AND POMEGRANATE

1 HEAD OF BROCCOLI
2 TBSP OLIVE OIL
½ TSP SALT
2 APPLES
JUICE AND ZEST OF 1 ORGANIC LIME
1 POMEGRANATE
500 G WHITE QUINOA,
BOILED AND LEFT TO COOL
100 ML LIME VINAIGRETTE
(SEE PAGE 325)

Separate the broccoli into small florets. Peel the stalk and chop into bite-sized pieces. In a frying pan, roast the broccoli in olive oil until nicely browned, but still has bite and a vibrant green colour. Season with salt.

Quarter the apples, remove the cores, cut into small cubes and toss with the lime juice and zest. Halve the pomegranate. Line the bottom of a large bowl with a paper towel. Hold half the pomegranate over the bowl (cut surface facing down) and tap the pomegranate with a wooden spoon so the seeds drop out. Continue with the other half and remove any remnants of the white membrane from the bowl.

Toss the quinoa with the broccoli, apples and lime vinaigrette. Arrange the salad in a bowl and sprinkle with the pomegranate seeds.

SALAD with
DUCK, PICKLED SHALLOTS, RED CURRANTS AND WALNUTS

2 FRESH DUCK BREASTS (CAN BE SUBSTITUTED WITH SMOKED DUCK BREAST)
1 HEAD ROMAINE LETTUCE
50 G RED CURRANTS
50 G WALNUTS
100 ML RASPBERRY VINAIGRETTE (SEE PAGE 323)
SALT AND FRESHLY GROUND BLACK PEPPER

PICKLED SHALLOTS
2 SHALLOTS
100 ML PICKLING LIQUID #2 (SEE PAGE 334)

Start by pickling the shallots. Peel, halve and slice into thin rings. Boil the pickling liquid and pour over the shallots. Rest for 20 minutes.

Preheat the oven to 180°C.

Trim the duck breasts and score the skin with a knife. Rub with salt. Slowly brown the duck breasts skin side down in a frying pan over medium heat until the skin is browned and a substantial portion of the fat has rendered. Transfer the breasts to an ovenproof dish. Roast until firm and the juices run red – about 8 minutes. Let the breasts rest for 8 minutes or let them cool completely. If you are using smoked duck breasts, they need no preparation.

Tear the lettuce into bite-sized pieces and rinse thoroughly. Rinse the red currants. Slice the duck breast, lightly dry with a paper towel and arrange on the lettuce leaves. Season with salt and pepper. Garnish with the red currants, pickled shallots and walnuts. Top with the raspberry vinaigrette or serve it on the side.

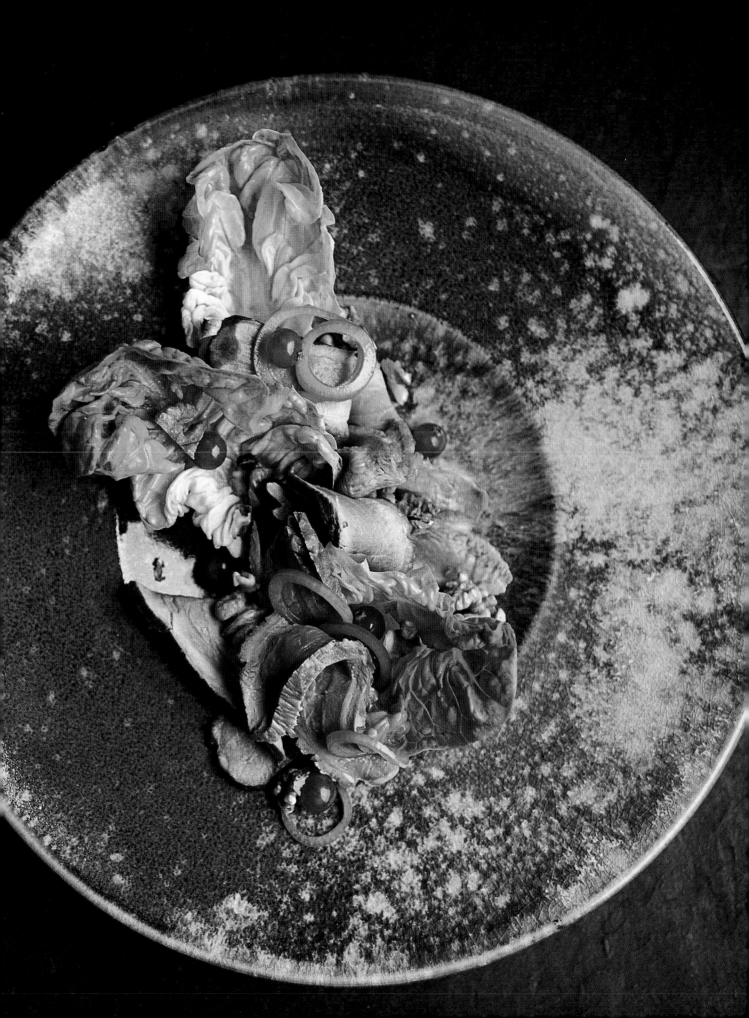

CHICKEN *with*
PICKLED AND ROASTED MUSHROOMS AND SAUTÉED LEEK

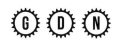

4 WHOLE CHICKEN LEGS
4 LEEKS
200 G SHIITAKE MUSHROOMS
2 SPRIGS THYME
1 TSP SALT
OLIVE OIL
FRESHLY GROUND BLACK PEPPER

PICKLED MUSHROOMS
200 G SHIMEJI MUSHROOMS
2 SPRIGS ROSEMARY
3 CLOVES GARLIC
2 STAR ANISE
50 ML OLIVE OIL
50 ML CIDER VINEGAR

Start by pickling the shimeji mushrooms. Rinse and chop off the bases. Rinse the rosemary sprigs and peel the garlic cloves. Transfer the mushrooms to a saucepan with the rosemary, garlic, star anise, olive oil and cider vinegar. Bring the mixture to a boil over medium heat and skim off any impurities. Remove the pan from the heat and let the mushrooms infuse while preparing the chicken.

Preheat the oven to 175°C.

Chop the leeks into ½ cm slices, rinse and spin in a salad spinner. Split the chicken legs into drumsticks and thighs. Season with salt and brown, skin side down, in olive oil over medium heat until the skin is a nice golden colour. Lay the chicken pieces on a baking tray covered with baking paper and roast in the oven for 20-25 minutes, until the juice runs clear.

Drain the mushrooms and clean the pan with paper towel. Pan-roast the shiitake until caramelised in a little olive oil with salt and thyme sprigs. Sauté the leeks in olive oil until tender. Season with salt and pepper. Mix the leeks and mushrooms and plate with the chicken.

Serve with whole grain pasta or brown rice.

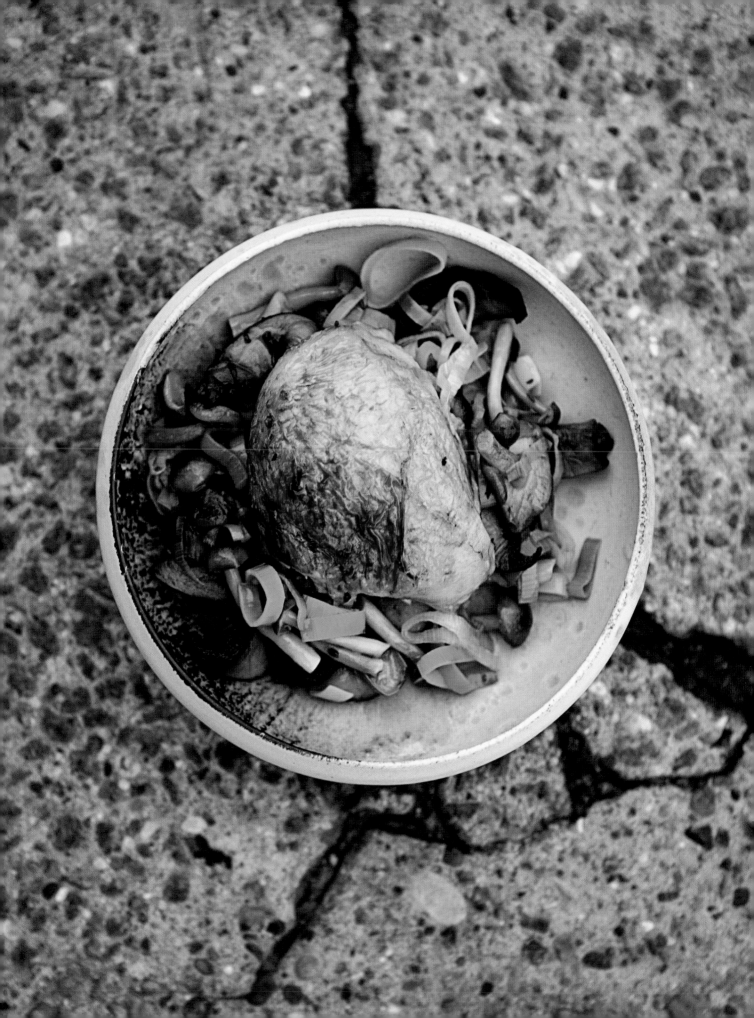

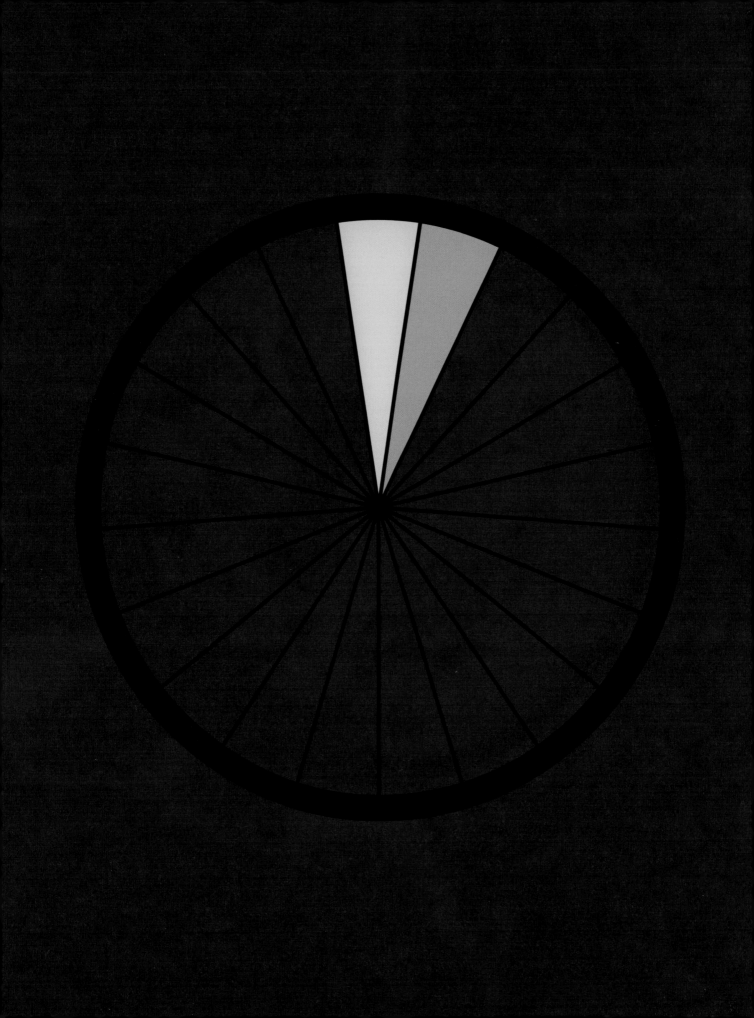

DAY

STAGE 1

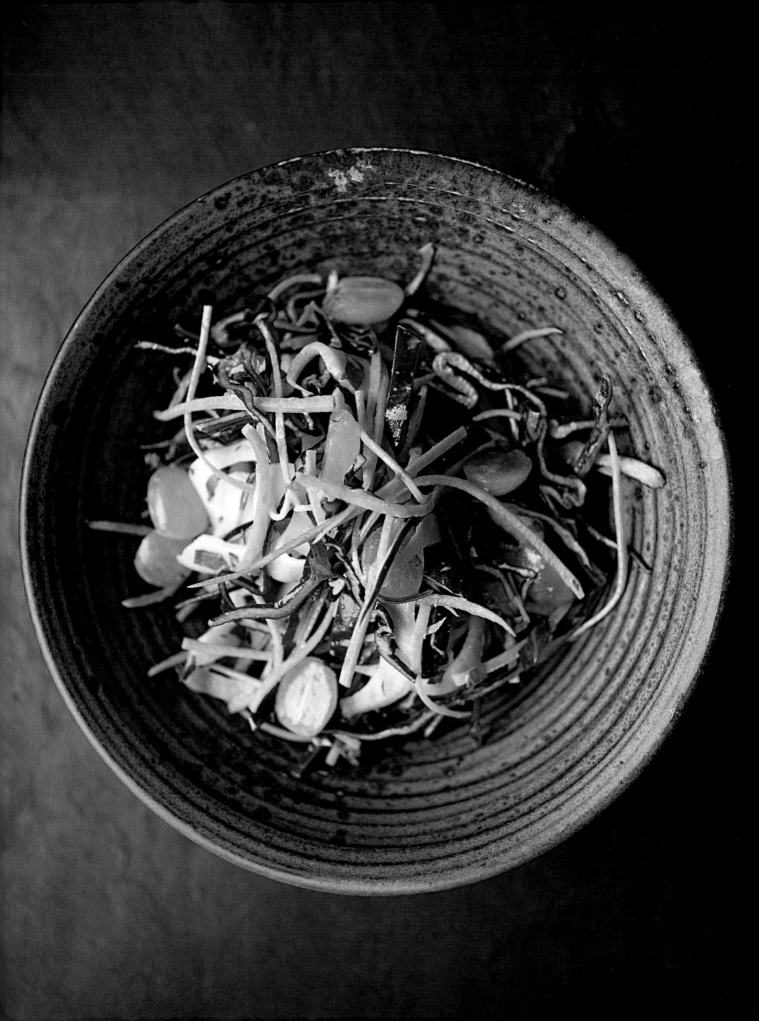

RED CABBAGE,
FENNEL AND GRAPES

½ HEAD OF RED CABBAGE
4 LARGE CARROTS
200 G GREEN, SEEDLESS GRAPES
2 FENNEL BULBS
JUICE OF 1 LEMON
50 ML HAZELNUT VINAIGRETTE
(SEE PAGE 322)

Peel the outer leaves off the red cabbage. Chop the cabbage in half lengthwise and reserve one half for later. Cut the other half in two, cut off the stalk and finely shred (1-2 mm) using a mandolin or a food processor.

Peel the carrots, cut off the tops and bottoms and finely grate using a grater or a food processor. Rinse the grapes and halve lengthwise. If not using seedless grapes, remove the seeds.

Rinse the fennel bulbs, cut off tops in a wedge shape and trim bottoms. Cut crosswise on a mandolin into 2 mm slices. Place the slices in a bowl of cold water and lemon juice to prevent oxidation.

Gently mix the cabbage, carrots, fennel and grapes in a bowl with the hazelnut vinaigrette.

The coleslaw can be made ahead of time and kept in the refrigerator for a couple of days. Make a big batch and marinate it just before serving.

ROASTED *broccoli,*
BLACKBERRIES AND WALNUTS

1 HEAD OF BROCCOLI
OLIVE OIL OR FLAVOURLESS COCONUT OIL
SALT
50 G WALNUTS
100 G FRESH BLACKBERRIES
50 ML HONEY VINAIGRETTE (SEE PAGE 324)

Separate the broccoli into small, bite-sized florets. Peel the stalk and cut into 2x2 cm cubes. Rinse both the florets and the stalk thoroughly and drain in a sieve. Pan-roast the florets a few at a time in oil and salt until they are a patchy nut-brown but still have a bite and a vibrant green colour.

Coarsely chop the walnuts. Rinse the blackberries and halve half of them. Mix the broccoli and walnuts. Toss with the vinaigrette and serve on a platter. Add the blackberries.

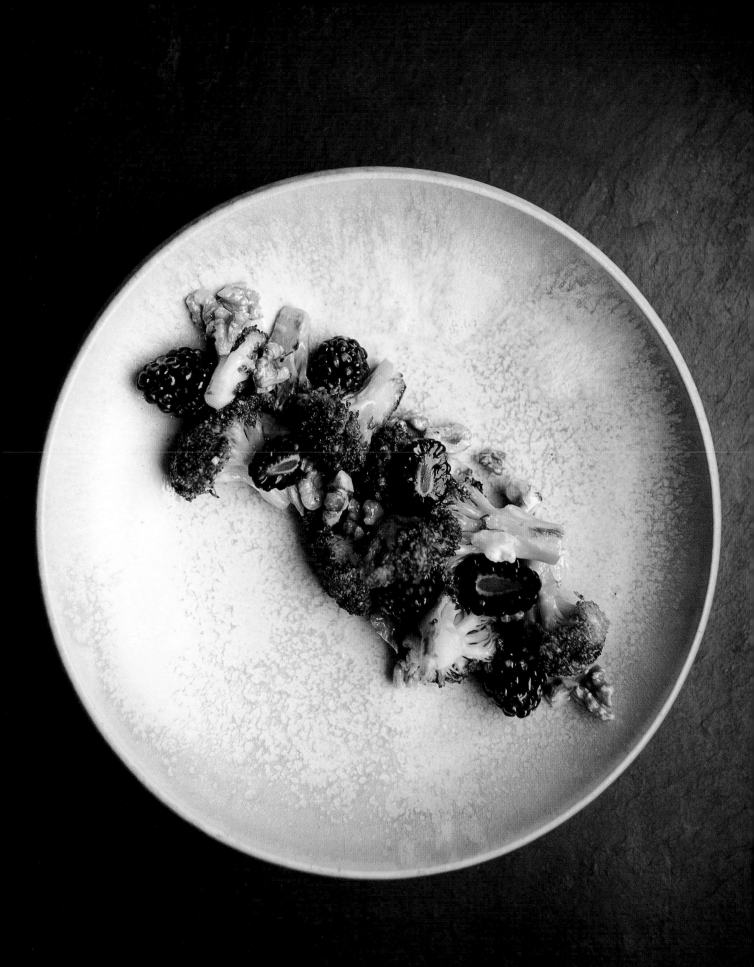

POACHED CHICKEN,
LEEKS AND FRIED APPLE

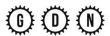

1 CHICKEN (1.2-1.4 KG)
50 G SEA SALT
1 TBSP SMOKED SALT (MALDON)
2 STAR ANISE
6 SPRIGS ROSEMARY, RINSED
½ HEAD OF CELERIAC
1 ONION
3 TBSP OLIVE OIL
500 ML WATER
500 ML WHITE WINE
50 ML CIDER VINEGAR
1 LITRE CHICKEN STOCK (SEE PAGE 332)
WHOLE BLACK PEPPERCORNS
WHOLE CORIANDER SEEDS
4 BAY LEAVES
5 CLOVES GARLIC

PARSLEY OIL
1 BUNCH PARSLEY
100 ML OLIVE OIL
JUICE AND ZEST OF 1 ORGANIC LEMON
SALT

Clean the chicken. Cut off the wings and the tail. In a spice mill or mortar, crush the sea salt, smoked salt, star anise and the leaves from 3 sprigs of rosemary into a uniform salt mixture. Place the chicken in an ovenproof dish and rub with the salt mixture. Cover the dish in cling film and refrigerate for at least 2 hours, preferably overnight.

Peel the celeriac and chop into chunks. Peel the onion and split lengthwise. In a frying pan, roast the celeriac and onion in olive oil over a high heat. In a large, heavy-based saucepan, boil the water, wine, stock and cider vinegar with the whole black peppercorns, coriander seeds, the last three sprigs of rosemary, garlic, onion and celeriac.

Remove the chicken from the dish and wipe dry with a paper towel. Carefully transfer it into the large saucepan, bring it to a boil over a medium heat and then turn down to a simmer. Simmer for 30-35 minutes. The internal temperature should be 65 degrees. Measure by inserting a thermometer in the leg, right into the bone. Remove the chicken and place in a dish or on a cutting board and cover with cling film so it does not dry out. Strain the stock, discard the herbs and reduce by a quarter. Season with salt and cider vinegar.

PARSLEY OIL
Rinse the parsley thoroughly and tear the leaves off the stalk. Wash and zest the lemon. Squeeze the juice into a container. Blend the parsley, lemon zest, lemon juice and olive oil thoroughly. Season with salt and strain.

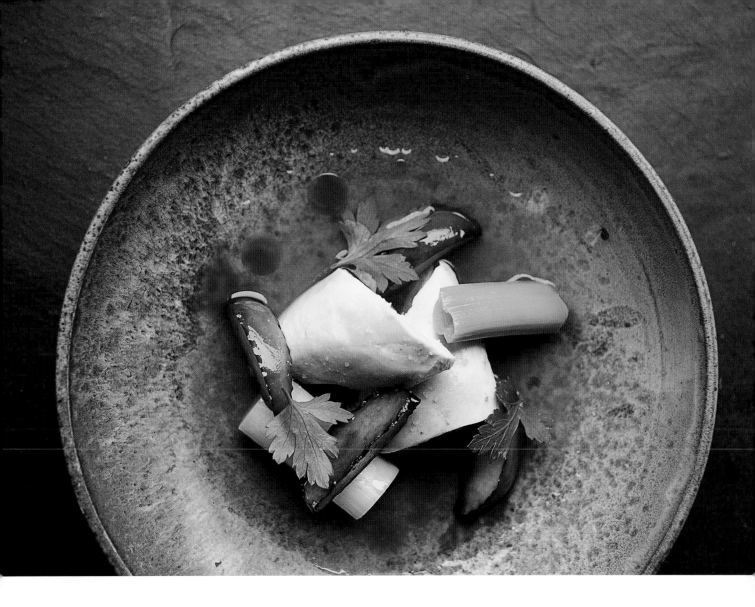

4 LEEKS
4 APPLES
2 SPRIGS ROSEMARY
OLIVE OIL
SALT

LEEKS AND APPLE

Chop the leeks into 5 cm long pieces and rinse thoroughly. Wash the apples, quarter and remove the cores. Cut each quarter into three equally thick slices. Rinse the rosemary, tear off the leaves and finely chop them.

Poach the leeks in the reduced chicken stock for 6-7 minutes until tender. Sauté the apples in olive oil over medium heat until golden and tender on both sides. Sprinkle with salt and rosemary and sauté for another 2 minutes.

Drain the chicken and cut into 8 pieces. Serve in soup bowls with the stock, leeks, apples and parsley oil.

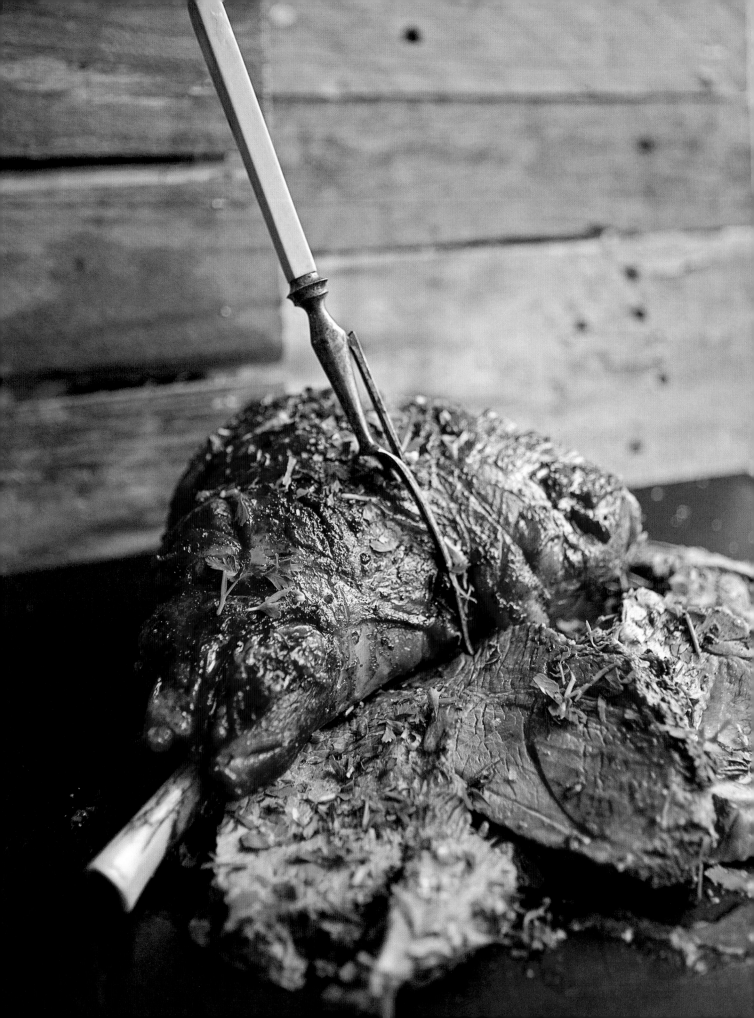

LEG OF LAMB *with* PARSLEY, LEMON AND CRUSHED POTATOES

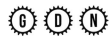

1 BONELESS LEG OF LAMB (APPROX. 2 KG)
½ BUNCH PARSLEY
JUICE AND ZEST OF 2 ORGANIC LEMONS
4 CLOVES GARLIC
5 TBSP OLIVE OIL + A LITTLE EXTRA FOR RUBBING ON THE MEAT
SALT AND FRESHLY GROUND BLACK PEPPER
MEAT STRING

CRUSHED POTATOES WITH HERBS
600 G POTATOES
100 ML OLIVE OIL
½ TSP SALT
½ BUNCH CHIVES, CUT
ZEST OF 2 ORGANIC LEMONS
2 CLOVES GARLIC, CHOPPED

Preheat the oven to 200°C.

Rinse the parsley, remove and coarsely chop the leaves. Rinse the lemons, zest and squeeze the juice into a bowl. Peel and chop the garlic. Stir the lemon juice together with the olive oil, garlic, lemon zest and parsley. Season with salt and pepper.

Lightly score the lamb and rub thoroughly with the marinade. Fold the meat together and tie with meat string. Don't tie too tightly – the flesh will pull itself together while cooking. Rub the roast with olive oil and sprinkle with salt and freshly ground pepper.

Roast the leg of lamb for 15 min at 200°C, then turn down the temperature to 150°C and cook until the internal temperature is between 54 and 56 degrees. Check the temperature regularly to avoid over cooking. While roasting, periodically baste the roast with its juices. After removing the roast from the oven, rest for 20 minutes before slicing and serving with chopped parsley. Reduce the juices from the pan and the resting meat, season with the lemon juice mixture and salt.

Clean the potatoes and boil them in unsalted water until tender. Drain the potatoes, then crush them with a metal whisk and mix in olive oil, chives, lemon zest and garlic, season with salt.

Serve the lamb with the crushed potatoes or with coarse bulgur wheat.

POLKADOT
MOUNTAIN JERSEY DESSERT

4 EGG WHITES
250 G CANE SUGAR
1 TSP RASPBERRY VINEGAR
¼ TSP SALT
110 G GROUND ALMONDS
200 ML WHIPPING CREAM
SEEDS OF 1 VANILLA POD
200 G FRESH STRAWBERRIES
50 G FRESH BLUEBERRIES
50 G FRESH RASPBERRIES
50 G FRESH BLACKBERRIES

Preheat the oven to 150°C.

Whisk the egg whites to soft peaks with sugar, vinegar and salt. Fold in the almond flour and divide the mixture into four equally large portions on a baking tray covered with baking paper. Bake for 30 minutes.

Whip the cream lightly with vanilla seeds. Rinse the berries and remove the tops from the strawberries. Cut into halves and quarters.

Plate the merengue with whipped cream and berries and serve straight away.

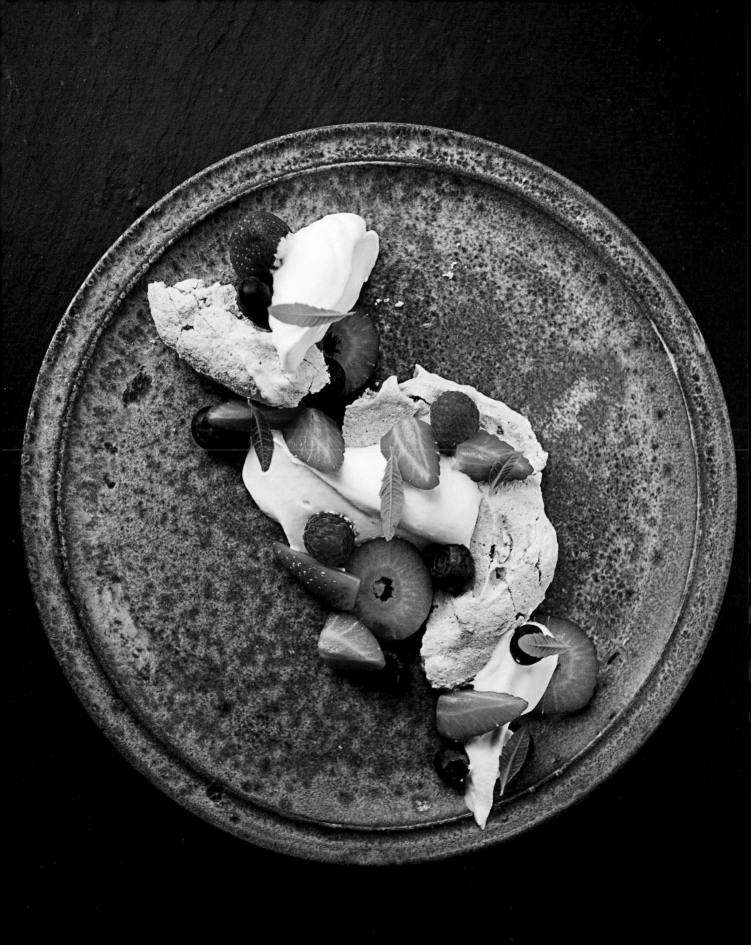

CHRIS ANKER SØRENSEN

"FOOD IS THE ALPHA AND OMEGA"

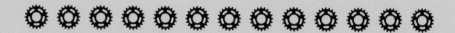

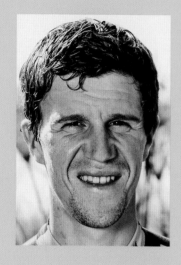

BORN: 5th September 1984
NATIONALITY: Danish
EXPERIENCE: Professional
since 2007
FAVOURITE RACE: Liège-
Bastogne-Liège

Hannah (H): What difference does food make for you physically and/or mentally during a long season or race?

Chris Anker Sørensen (CAS): Food is the alpha and omega. It's what gives us energy. Getting the right food helps the body's capacity to recover and it provides energy for the next day because food recharges your batteries. In a long race like the Tour de France, I can't really be bothered to eat during the final week. I'm simply so wrecked by that point. That's why it's important for the food to look delicious so you really feel like eating it. It doesn't take much for the stomach to give up and then, before you know it, you're out of the race. Of course, the taste is crucial! Breakfast is particularly important. You fill your stomach and get ready for a long day in the saddle. But in the morning, there's always a bit of time pressure because we have to be on our way. On the other hand, dinner is the only time of the day when we have time to sit and enjoy a bit of a chat. So that meal also has a unifying value. In this context, it would be appropriate to challenge people with smartphones not to check them every second, but to wait until after the meal. The rest of the day, we eat either on our bikes or on the bus on the way back to the hotel.

H: In what way do you think food can change an athlete's performance?

CAS: Food gives us what the body needs for survival, for regeneration, for warmth etc. So, if you don't eat properly, you cannot perform. If you put regular petrol in a diesel car, you don't get very far. Cyclists are extremely concerned about weight. That's why a varied and properly composed diet is very important.

H: What has a proper diet meant for you personally as a cyclist?

CAS: I can feel the difference from day to day in terms of whether I've eaten properly or not. I'm really interested in food. Occasionally I sin a bit and I can feel it in my level of cycling. I hit the wall more easily, my mental reserve is not as large and I often find it difficult to complete the training session. Even in terms of cyclists, I'm pretty thin, which is an advantage in the mountains.

This is thanks to a strict diet that gives me exactly what I need so I can perform or train the following day with no problems.

H: In what way has your opinion on food for athletes changed over the past year?
CAS: The importance of a proper diet has really hit home for many of us. There are still lots of different views on what it is. But what's right for one person isn't necessarily right for another person. The body is a complex entity and you have to learn to listen to yourself. Personally, porridge works best for me in the morning while others prefer rice or bread with ham and cheese.

H: Have you found that food can improve or worsen your condition?
CAS: Absolutely. As I said, the right building blocks are necessary for the body to regenerate.

H: How do you see the future of cycling in terms of food?
CAS: I think there'll be more and more attention paid to the subject and, in the future – I am thinking maybe about 100 or 200 years down the line – we'll get all our energy, vitamins and minerals from shakes and pills.

H: What is your favourite food?
CAS: I love food and there are very few things I don't like. Anything, apart from curried meatballs, tripe, black pudding and brawn. I live in Italy and, if I had to choose, my favourite meal would be caprese with buffalo mozzarella for *antipasti*, risotto with porcini mushrooms for *primo* and pork from a pata negra pig with *sformatini di verdure* for *secondo*. For dessert, a tiramisu, washed down with San Pellegrino sparkling water and a 2005 Percarlo from San Giusto a Rentennano. And, if it had to be Danish food, it would have to be my mum's meatballs with stewed cabbage and potatoes.

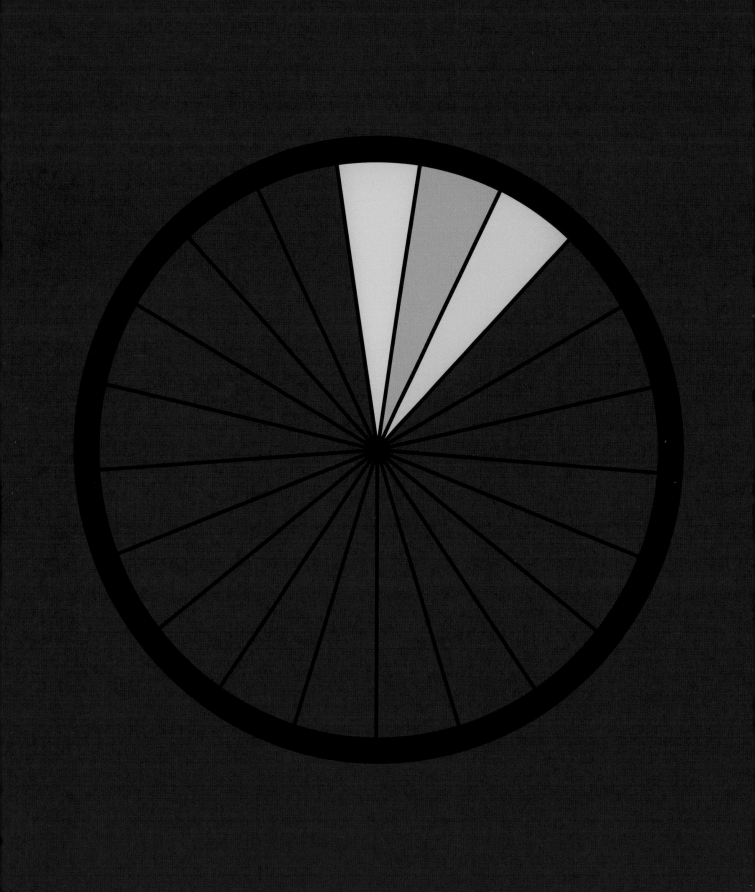

DAY

5

STAGE 2

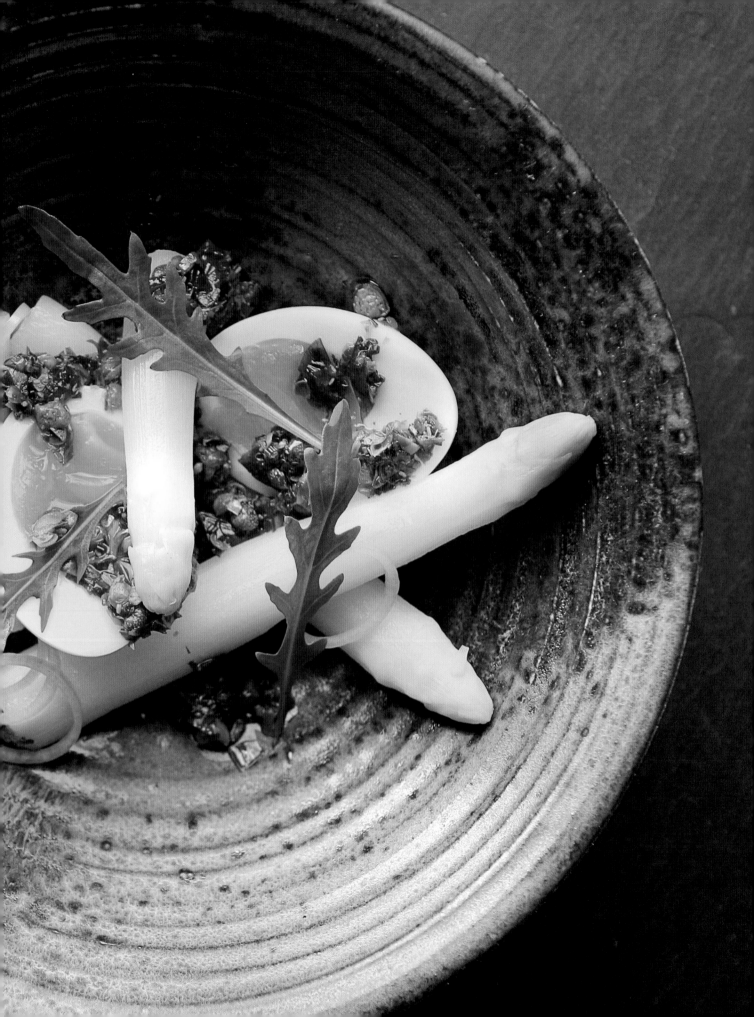

PICKLED *white* ASPARAGUS, SOFT-BOILED EGGS AND CAPER VINAIGRETTE

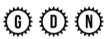

20 WHITE ASPARAGUS SPEARS
200 ML PICKLING LIQUID #2, CHILLED
(SEE PAGE 334)
8 EGGS
¼ BUNCH OF TARRAGON
4 TBSP CHOPPED CAPERS
1 SMALL SHALLOT
100 ML CIDER VINEGAR VINAIGRETTE
(SEE PAGE 323)
ZEST OF 1 ORGANIC LEMON
100 G ROCKET, WASHED

Snap off the bottom of the white asparagus spears and peel evenly and straight. Bring 1 litre of salted water to a boil and blanch the asparagus until it is cooked but still has bite – about 15 seconds depending on the thickness. Immediately cool the asparagus spears in cold water, drain, place in a separate container and cover with the cold pickling liquid. Refrigerate for at least 1 hour.

Bring a pot of water to a rolling boil. Boil the eggs for 8 minutes and quickly cool under cold tap water. Peel and halve the eggs. Tear off the tarragon leaves, rinse, dry and chop with the capers. Peel the shallot and cut into thin rings. Stir together the cut shallot, caper/tarragon mixture, lemon zest and cider vinegar vinaigrette.

Drain the asparagus, serve with the soft-boiled eggs and garnish with vinaigrette and rocket.

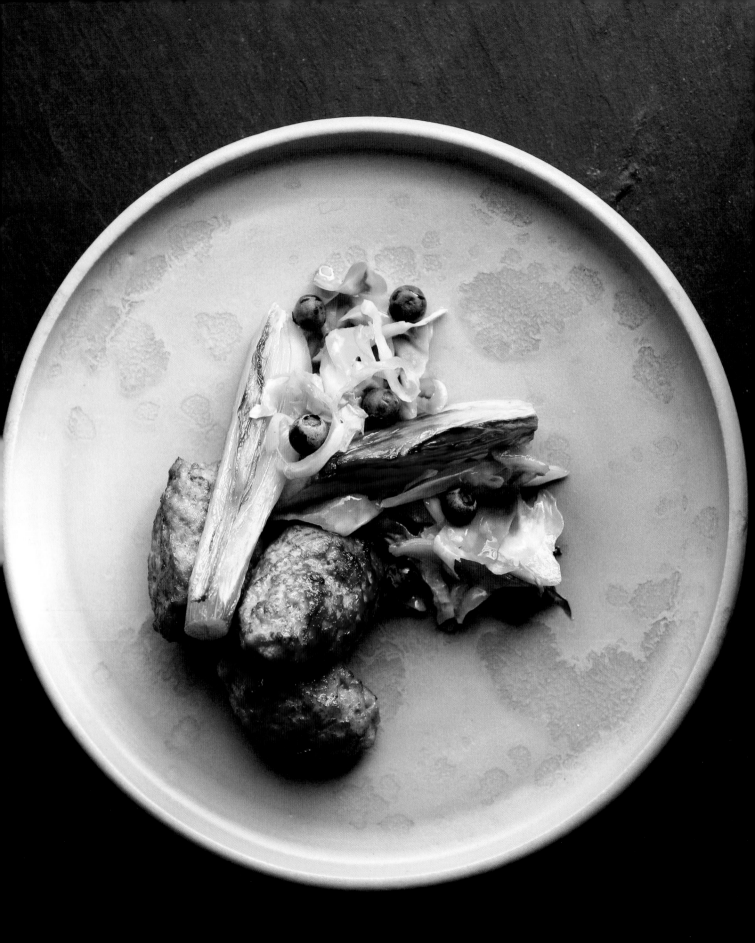

MEATBALLS *and*
SAUTÉED CABBAGE WITH FENNEL AND BLUEBERRIES

250 G MINCED VEAL
250 G MINCED PORK
½ TSP SALT
2 EGGS
200 ML GLUTEN-FREE OATMEAL
200 ML RICE MILK OR WHOLE MILK
2 ONIONS
2 CLOVES GARLIC
1 TBSP GROUND CORIANDER
1 PINCH GROUND CUMIN
FRESHLY GROUND BLACK PEPPER

SAUTÉED CABBAGE WITH FENNEL AND BLUEBERRIES
½ WHITE CABBAGE OR POINTED CABBAGE
2 FENNEL BULBS
2 TBSP COCONUT OIL
SALT AND FRESHLY GROUND BLACK PEPPER
OLIVE OIL
ZEST OF 2 ORGANIC LEMONS
100 G FRESH BLUEBERRIES

Mix the minced veal and pork thoroughly with salt, preferably in a food mixer. Add the eggs and oats and mix the mince until homogeneous. Heat the milk until bathtub warm, pour into the mince a little at a time and mix until the mixture has a soft, homogeneous consistency. Peel the onions and garlic, finely chop both and add them to the mince mixture along with the ground coriander, cumin and pepper. To achieve the best taste and texture, rest the mince mixture for 30 minutes in the refrigerator.

Preheat the oven to 200°C.

Fry a mini meatball in a frying pan to test the seasoning. Cover a baking tray with baking paper brushed with olive oil. Shape the meatballs with a tablespoon and place them on the tray. Bake until the meatballs are cooked through and firm – about 8-10 minutes. Serve with the sautéed cabbage with the fennel and blueberry and, if you wish, boiled or roasted potatoes.

SAUTÉED CABBAGE WITH FENNEL AND BLUEBERRIES
Halve the cabbage and slice into 1 cm strips. Halve the fennel bulbs lengthwise and cut each half into three wedges of equal size. Heat the coconut oil in a pan and sauté the cabbage until tender. Season with salt and pepper.

In a separate pan, roast the salted fennel wedges in olive oil over medium-high heat until caramelised on both sides.

COCONUT CHICKEN
with GINGER AND LIME

150 G FRESH GINGER
2 STALKS OF LEMONGRASS
4 ORGANIC LIMES
2 COURGETTES
3 RED ONIONS
4 SMALL BOK CHOY
50 ML OLIVE OIL
6 KAFFIR LIME LEAVES,
PREFERABLY FRESH
1 TBSP CORIANDER SEEDS
1 STAR ANISE
4 CHICKEN BREASTS (APPROX. 200 G)
2 CANS COCONUT MILK (2 X 400 ML)
1 BUNCH CORIANDER, RINSED AND
LEAVES REMOVED

Scrub the ginger and chop it into large pieces. Rinse the lemon grass stalks and cut them into ½ cm slices. Rinse and peel the limes with a thin peeler. Set the peel aside and juice the limes. Rinse the courgettes, split lengthwise and chop into 2x2 cm cubes. Peel the onions, halve lengthwise and cut into 1 cm thick slices from top to bottom. Slice each bok choy into 6 wedges and rinse them thoroughly.

Sauté the onions until tender in a little olive oil. Set aside in a bowl. Chop the chicken breasts into 3x3 cm cubes.

In a blender, blend the oil, ginger, lemon grass, kaffir lime leaves, coriander, star anise and lime zest into a homogeneous mixture and pour into a thick-bottomed saucepan. While stirring, sauté over medium heat for 3 minutes.

Add the chopped chicken breasts to the ginger mixture. Pour in the coconut milk and allow the chicken to simmer over a low heat for 5 minutes. Add the onion, courgette and bok choy and let the dish simmer until the chicken is cooked through.

Serve with brown rice and top with fresh coriander.

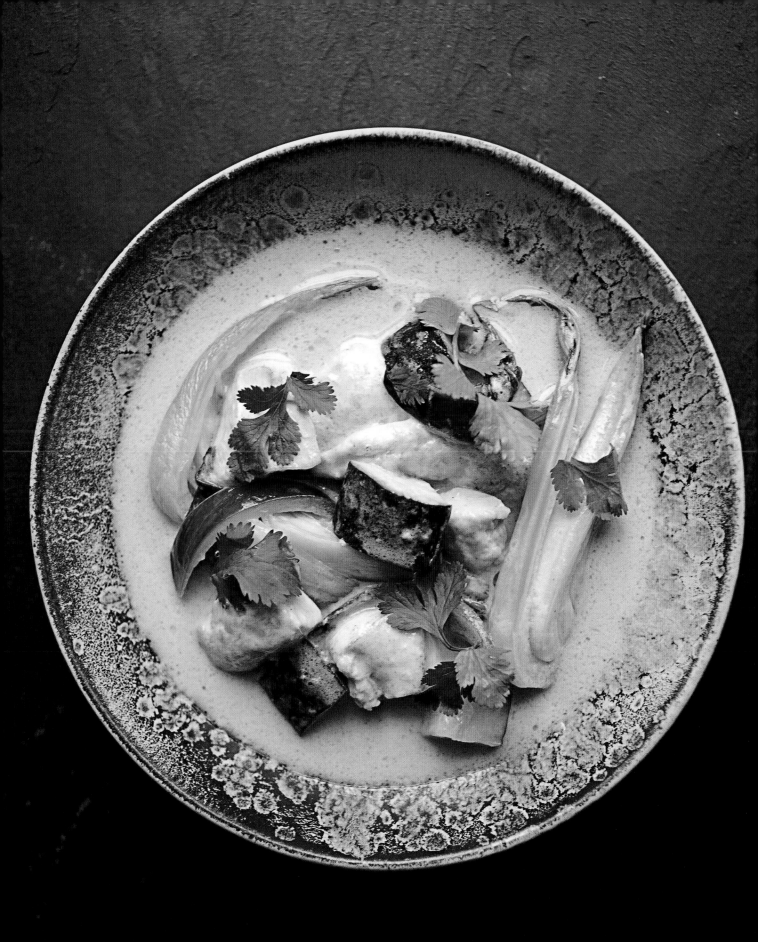

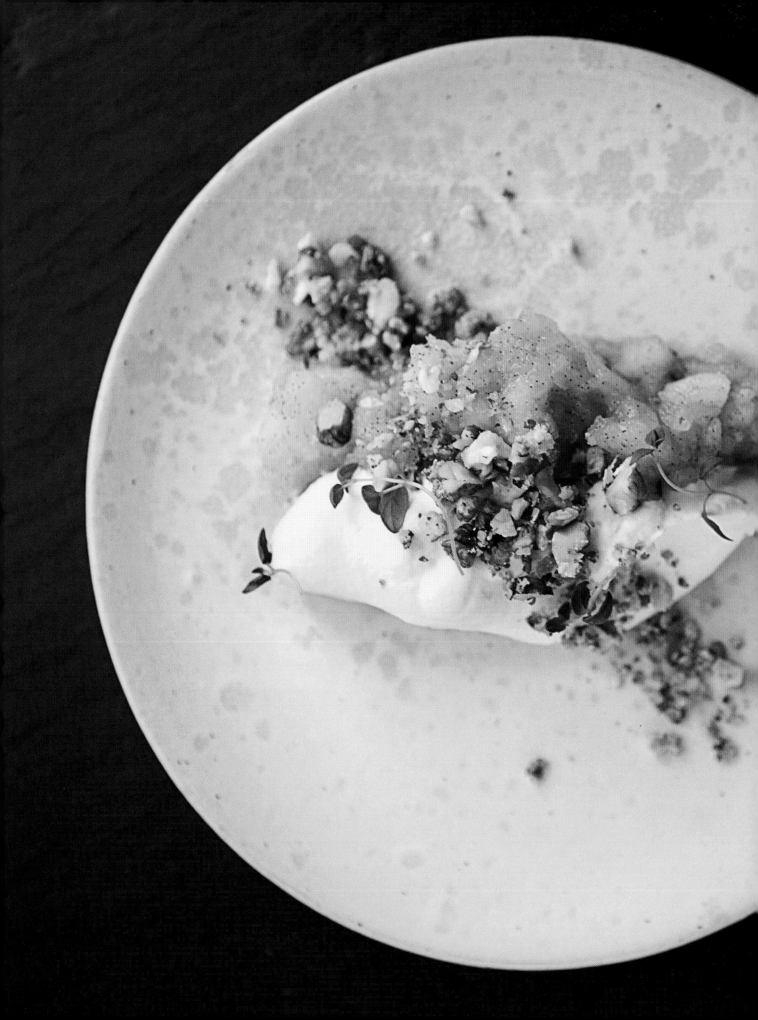

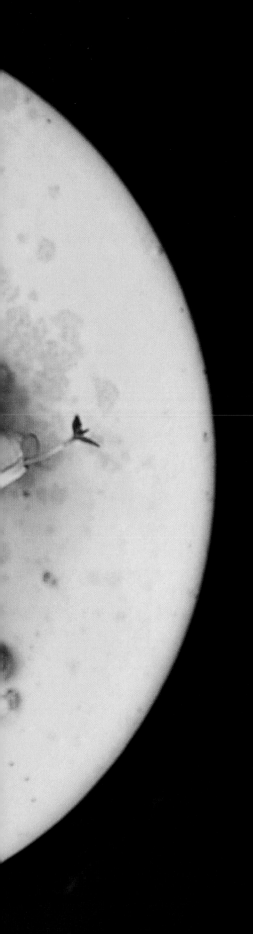

OLD-FASHIONED
APPLE CAKE

**10 TART APPLES (E.G. BELLE DE BOSKOOP,
COX'S ORANGE OR INGRID MARIE)
50 ML WHITE WINE
SEEDS OF 1 VANILLA POD
2 TBSP CREAMED HONEY
200 G HAZELNUTS
¼ BUNCH FRESH SOFT THYME
200 ML WHIPPING CREAM**

Preheat the oven to 170°C.

Peel and quarter the apples. Remove the cores and chop the wedges into cubes. Soften the honey in a thick-bottomed saucepan. Add the apples, wine and vanilla seeds. Cover the pan and simmer over medium heat for 5 minutes. Turn down the heat and simmer for another 15-20 minutes. Stir regularly.

At the same time, toast the hazelnuts in the oven until golden – about 8-9 minutes. Let them cool and then chop coarsely.

Tear the soft top shoots off the thyme stalks and rinse them. Whip the cream lightly.

Serve the apple compote – warm or chilled – on the plate with the whipped cream, chopped hazelnuts and thyme.

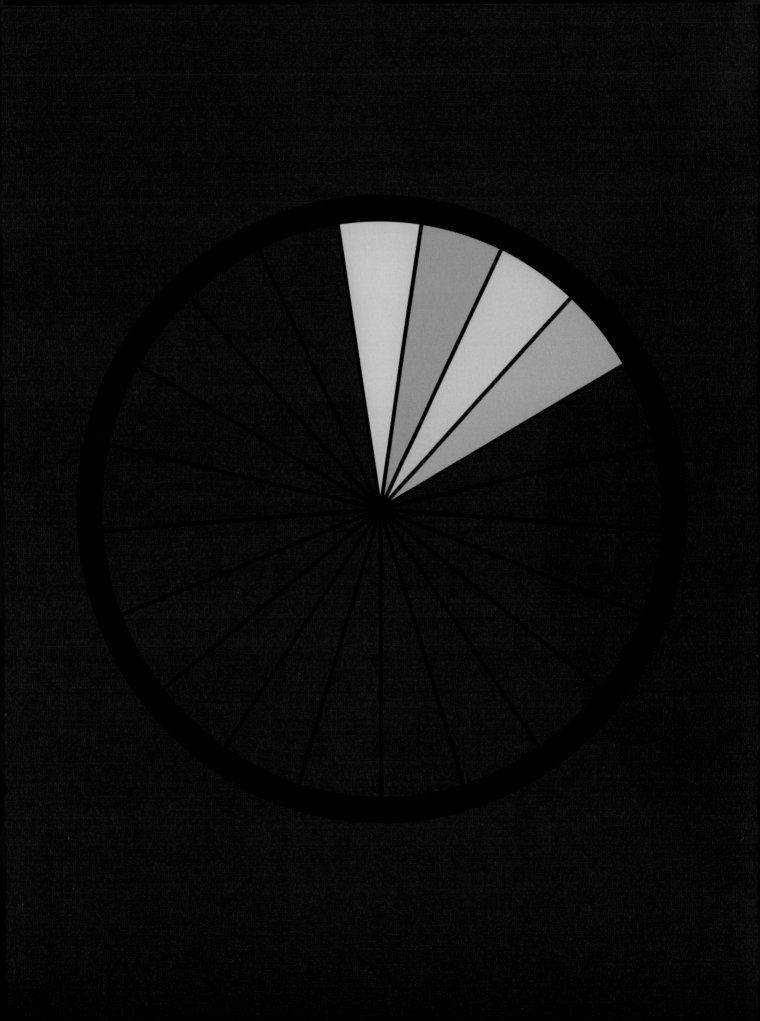

DAY 4

STAGE 3

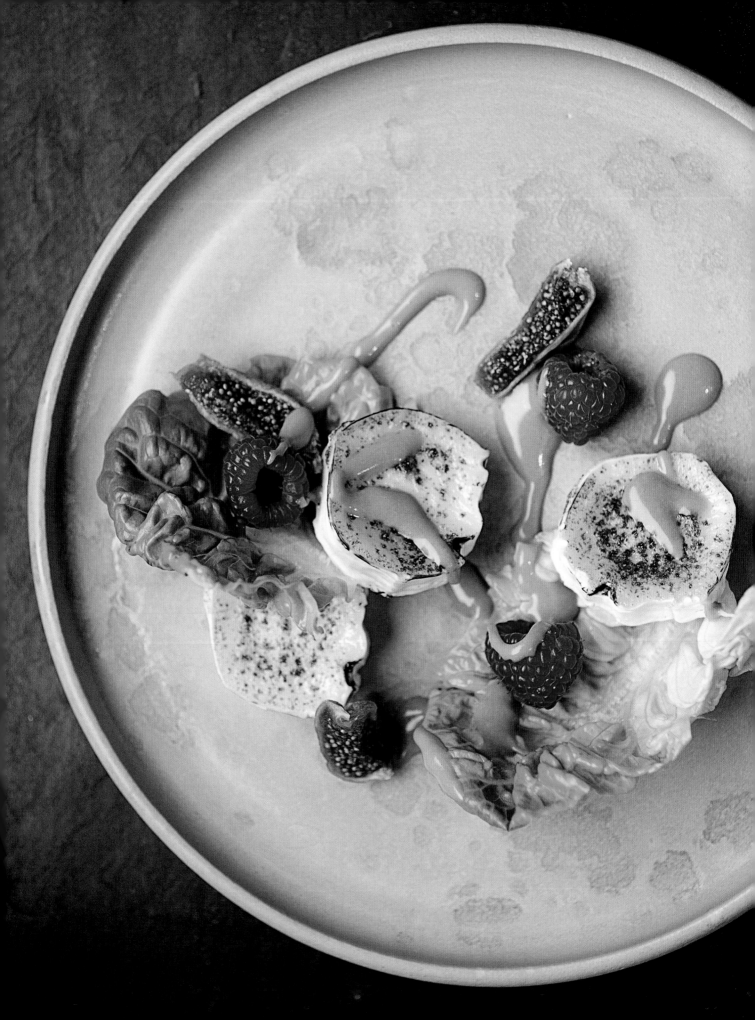

GOAT CHEESE,
FIGS AND RASPBERRIES

8 FIGS, DRIED OR FRESH
200 G GOAT CHEESE LOG
2-3 HEADS ROMAINE LETTUCE
50 G FRESH RASPBERRIES
100 ML BALSAMIC VINAIGRETTE (SEE PAGE 324)

If using dried figs, soak in boiling water for 10 minutes.

Quarter the figs. Warm the blade of a knife under hot tap water or in a cup of hot water and cut the goat cheese into 1 cm slices. Cover a baking tray with baking paper, place the slices on it and grill for 2-3 minutes until the tops are caramelised. You can also use a gas torch.

Tear the lettuce into bite-sized pieces, rinse and spin in a salad spinner.

Plate the lettuce leaves, figs, goat cheese and raspberries on a platter and drizzle with the dressing.

BULGUR WHEAT SALAD
with NECTARINE AND YELLOW PEPPER

500 G COARSE BULGUR WHEAT,
PREFERABLY WHOLE GRAIN
750 ML WATER
1 TSP SALT
1 STAR ANISE
3 RIPE NECTARINES
2 YELLOW PEPPERS
½ BUNCH PARSLEY
100 ML ELDERFLOWER VINAIGRETTE
(SEE PAGE 323)

Bring the water to a boil with the salt and star anise, add the bulgur wheat and boil over a low heat until the bulgur wheat has absorbed the water – about 15 minutes. Pour the bulgur wheat into a large bowl to cool.

Rinse the nectarines and peppers and chop into 2x2 cm cubes. Rinse the parsley, pick and chop the leaves. Toss the cooled bulgur wheat with the nectarine, pepper, parsley and vinaigrette.

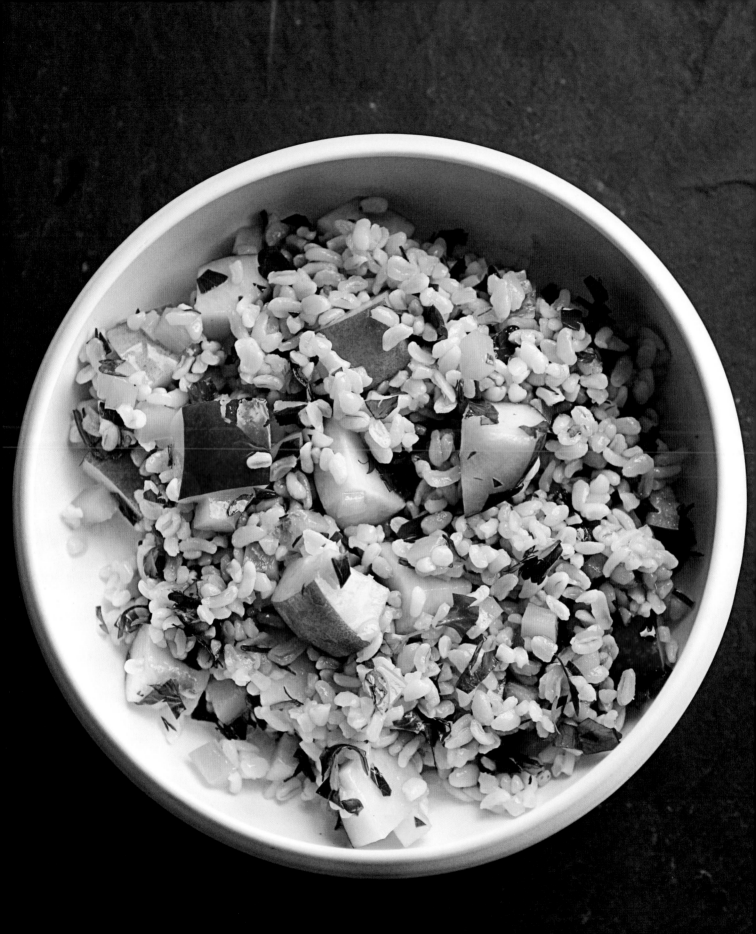

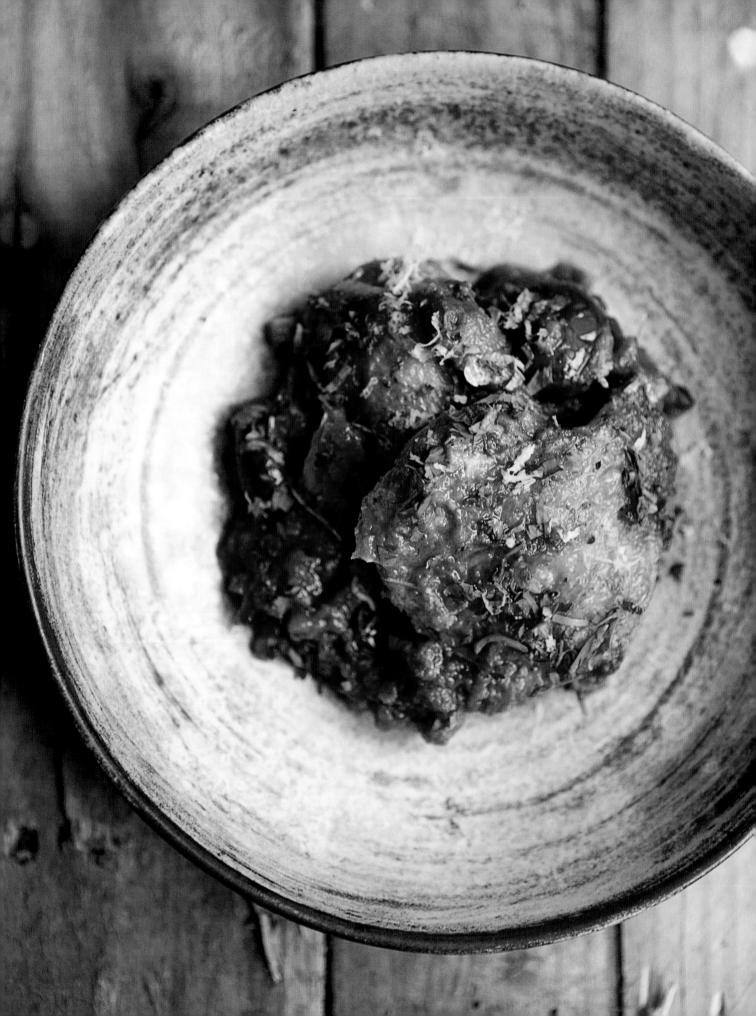

MOROCCAN-STYLE
CHICKEN WITH BLACK OLIVES

1 CHICKEN (1.2-1.4 KG)
OLIVE OIL FOR FRYING
SALT AND FRESHLY GROUND
BLACK PEPPER
1 TSP CUMIN
1 TSP CINNAMON
1 TSP GROUND CORIANDER
3 ONIONS
1 TBSP COCONUT OIL
100 G BLACK PITTED KALAMATA OLIVES
1 LITRE TOMATO SAUCE OF YOUR
OWN CHOICE (SEE PAGES 330-331)
¼ BUNCH PARSLEY
ZEST OF 2 ORGANIC LEMONS

Preheat the oven to 175°C.

Divide the chicken into 8 pieces (2 thighs, 2 drumsticks and 2 halved breasts) and brown over medium heat in olive oil. Season with salt and pepper. Place the chicken in an ovenproof dish and season with cumin, cinnamon and coriander.

Peel and dice the onion. Heat the coconut oil in a frying pan, sprinkle with salt, add the onion and caramelise. Arrange the caramelised onions and black olives on the chicken. Cover with the tomato sauce and roast for 30-35 minutes. While the chicken cooks, rinse and chop the parsley and zest the lemons.

Once finished, garnish the chicken with chopped parsley and lemon zest and serve with brown rice or couscous.

You can replace the tomato sauce with 2 cans of peeled tomatoes and 1 can (70 g) of concentrated tomato purée.

BAKED COD *with* RADISH CRUDITÉ, DILL AND SAMPHIRE

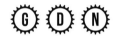

8 PIECES OF 100 G COD
SALT
200 G RADISHES
50 G SAMPHIRE
½ BUNCH DILL
50 G CAPERS
100 ML HONEY VINAIGRETTE
(SEE PAGE 324)
ZEST OF 2 ORGANIC LEMONS
OLIVE OIL

Place the cod on a plate or dish covered with baking paper, sprinkle with salt, cover with cling film and refrigerate for half an hour.

Preheat the oven to 170°C.

Wash the radishes, trim off the roots and finely shave into a bowl of cold water with a mandolin. Discard the tops. Tear the samphire into bite-sized pieces and rinse well. Pick the dill into small 3 cm pieces, rinse and spin in a salad spinner. Coarsely chop the capers and mix with the vinaigrette and lemon zest.

Drizzle the fish with olive oil and bake on a baking tray covered with baking paper until a carving fork/cake tester slides through the flesh with no resistance – about 8 minutes.

Plate the fish and pour over the vinaigrette. Top with the radish crudité, dill and samphire. Serve with boiled new potatoes.

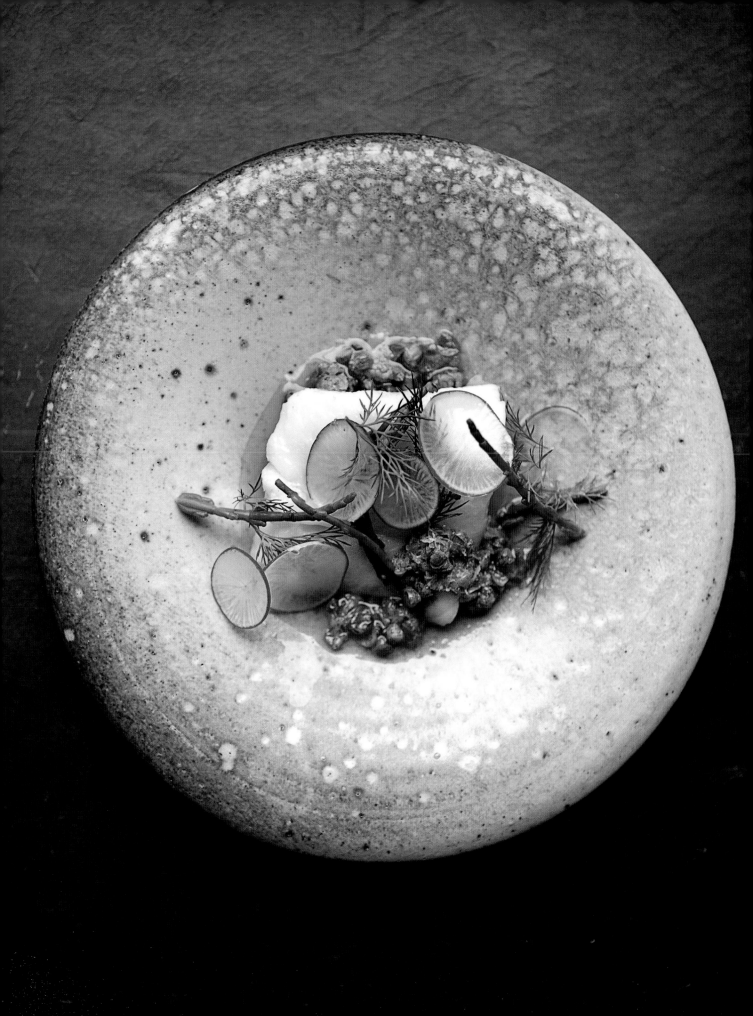

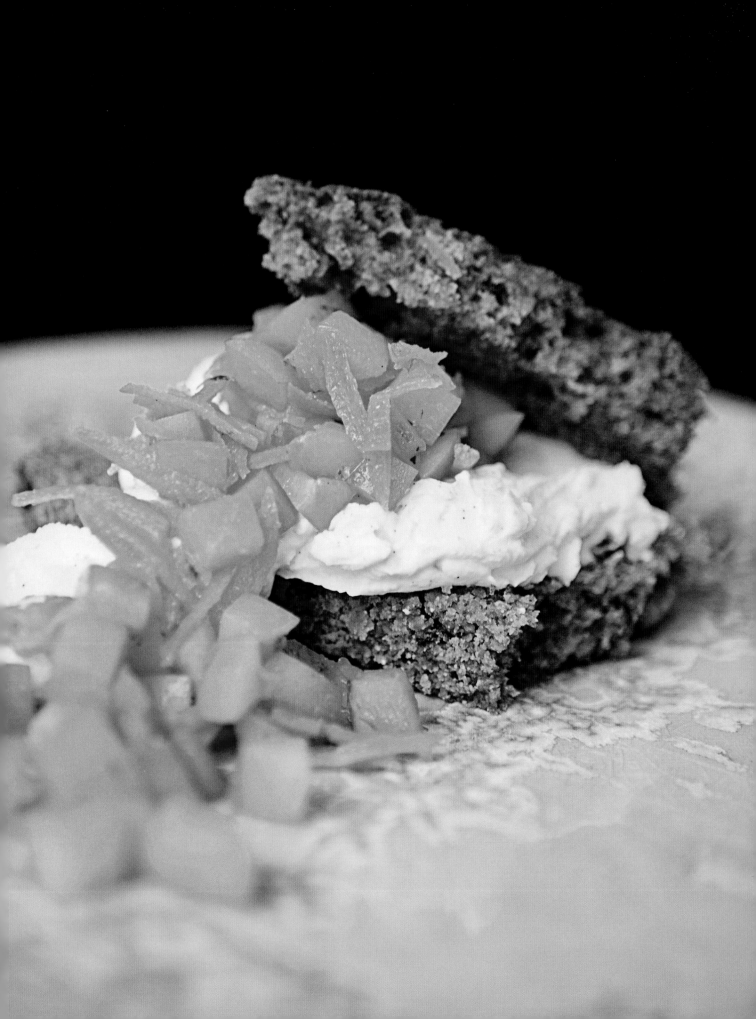

CARROT CAKE *with*
VANILLA YOGHURT AND APRICOTS

285 G WHOLE WHEAT FLOUR
2 TSP BAKING POWDER
1 TSP BICARBONATE OF SODA
1 TSP CINNAMON
½ TSP GROUND CLOVES
1 TSP SALT
170 G DARK BROWN SUGAR
55 G CHOPPED WALNUTS
3 EGGS
2 BANANAS
200 G GRATED CARROT
JUICE AND ZEST OF 1 ORGANIC ORANGE

VANILLA YOGHURT AND APRICOTS
200 ML GREEK YOGHURT (10% FAT)
1 TBSP CLEAR HONEY
SEEDS OF 1 VANILLA POD
JUICE AND ZEST OF 1 ORGANIC LEMON
4 APRICOTS
2 CARROTS
JUICE AND ZEST OF 1 ORGANIC LIME
1 TBSP CLEAR HONEY

Preheat the oven to 170°C.

VANILLA YOGHURT AND APRICOTS

Mix the yoghurt, honey, lemon zest and vanilla. Flavour the cream with lemon juice. Rinse the apricots, halve and remove the stones. Cut into cubes. Peel and grate the carrots. Mix the apricot, carrot and lime zest. Toss in the lime juice and honey.

CARROT CAKE

Sift the flour, baking powder, bicarbonate of soda, cloves and salt together in a bowl. Add the sugar and walnuts. Mix the eggs and mashed banana together with the dry ingredients and stir well.

Add the grated carrot, orange juice and orange zest. Stir the batter well and pour into two cake tins greased with oil and sprinkled with flour.

Bake the cakes for about 35 minutes. Check the cake by inserting a sharp knife into the middle of one cake and when no dough sticks, it's done.

Let the cakes cool completely, remove from the mould, cut lengthwise and fill with the vanilla yoghurt, apricots and shredded carrot.

MATTI BRESCHEL

"REAL FOOD MAKES MY JOB MUCH MORE ENJOYABLE"

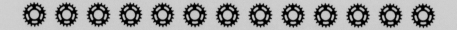

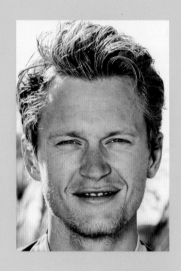

BORN: 31st August 1984
NATIONALITY: Danish
EXPERIENCE: Professional
since 2005
FORMER CYCLING TEAMS:
Team PH, CSC,
Rabobank, Saxobank
FAVOURITE RACES: World
Championship, the Tour of
Flanders and Paris-Roubaix

Hannah (H): What difference does food make for you physically and/or mentally during a long season or race?
Matti Breschel (MB): I can definitely feel it in my body if I've been eating poorly for a while or haven't been consuming the right amount of protein, fat, carbohydrates and, most importantly, vitamins. My head gets tired and sluggish and my body hurts. I become inept and ineffective. On the other hand, if I get the right food or even just eat a healthy and varied diet, I find it easier to do my best when training or in a race. Overall, good food makes my job much more enjoyable.

H: In what way do you think food can change an athlete's performance?
MB: Whether you're a top athlete or a recreational athlete, I am in no doubt that proper food is the key to progress and success as a cyclist. A Snickers bar or a big burger might be nice sometimes but if you time and time again pollute your body with empty calories and fill your stores with something from the local take away, you will never seriously raise the bar in terms of training and results in cycle racing. Instead, your potential just stagnates.

H: What has the proper diet meant for you personally as a cyclist?
MB: It has meant that I have the energy to get out on the bike every morning and I find it easier to keep my weight down. When I started cycling at the age of 10, I could eat what I wanted to and had absolutely no interest in diet and healthy food. I would eat two large meatballs during breaks at school and munch crisps and cakes after every cycling race. When I got older, alcohol and junk food entered the picture and that worked for me too for a while. But, of course, the result was that one winter I gained 7 kilos and got stumped every time we approached anything that even resembled a hill. My teammates didn't wait for me at the top so I had to pull myself together and pay more attention to healthy food. As a professional cyclist, you don't need to live like a monk year round. But everything is much easier if you eat healthy, nutritious food. Anyway, eating fish, chicken, salad and vegetables needn't be boring.

H: In what way has your opinion on food for athletes changed over the past year?

MB: Cyclists generally have a greater understanding of what proper food is and how a healthy diet can make a difference in terms of competitions. For my part, I try not to get carried away when some diet guru discovers a new kind of edible grass that is brilliant at burning fat or a potato root that you can put in your smoothie and instantly get 2% stronger. I've tried out a lot of different diets, everything from the Zone diet to a pure protein diet, to weighing each and every meal to the last gram. It became too much – too hard in the long run. Now, if I just maintain a healthy and varied diet, I think my body gets the right balance. I believe that many athletes have had a similar experience.

H: Have you found that food can improve or worsen your condition?

MB: In early 2011, I had two knee operations because of inflammation. When I finally came back, I was constantly ill with a high temperature and upset stomach. Things were just not going well in terms of cycling and I absolutely believe it had something to do with diet. I was paying far too much attention to being thin and lean and forgot everything about eating the right food and the right fats. It wasn't until I changed my diet that things started to go well again.

H: How do you see the future of cycling in terms of food?

MB: In the world of professional cycling, a lot has happened in the field of diet and nutrition and in the last five years, we've seen a plethora of nutritionists and dieticians on many of the major cycling teams. In contrast to the 80s and 90s, there's much more focus on diet and I absolutely believe that diet and nutrition are the way forward. In addition to training, diet is something you can continue to optimise.

H: What is your favourite food?

MB: Clam chowder and venison marinated in beer.

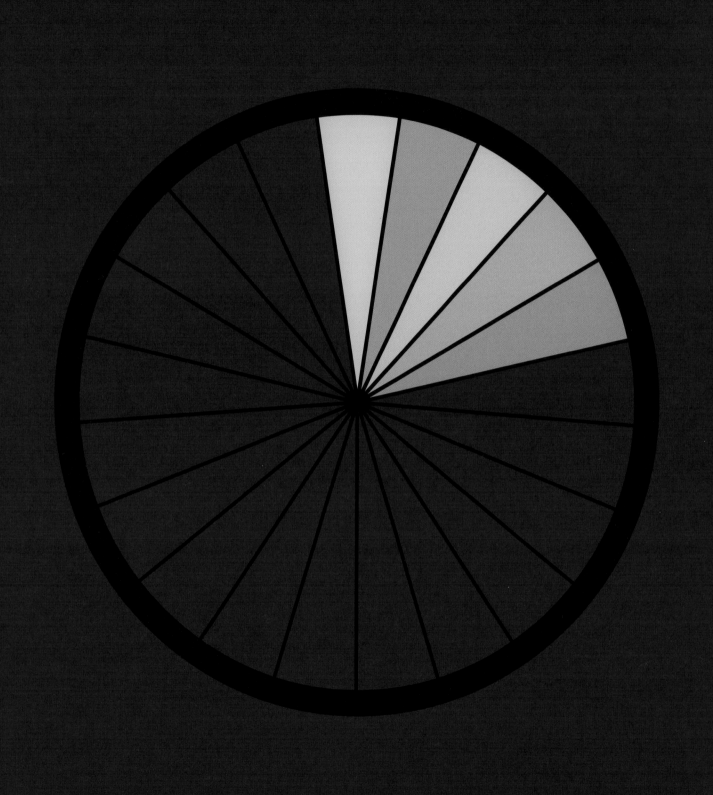

5

DAY

STAGE 4

CAULIFLOWER SOUP
with DILL AND ROASTED CAULIFLOWER

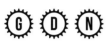

6-8 SERVINGS

1 CAULIFLOWER
2 ONIONS
2 CLOVES GARLIC
3 SPRIGS THYME
½ BUNCH DILL
3 TBSP OLIVE OIL
¼ TSP SALT
1 STAR ANISE
750 ML RICE MILK
750 ML CHICKEN STOCK (SEE PAGE 332)
FRESHLY GROUND BLACK PEPPER
JUICE AND ZEST OF 2 ORGANIC LIMES
200 ML COLD-PRESSED OLIVE OIL

Rinse and drain the cauliflower and separate it into florets, saving a third of the smallest florets for garnishing the soup. Coarsely chop the rest. Peel the onions and garlic and cut into thin slices. Rinse the thyme and dill. Pluck the dill sprigs, place them in a bowl and refrigerate for later.

Heat the 3 tbsp of olive oil in a thick-bottomed pan and sauté the onion, garlic and cauliflower until tender. Season with salt, star anise and thyme. Add the rice milk and stock, bring the soup to a boil and then turn down the heat. Allow the soup to simmer for 15-20 minutes until everything is tender.

Remove the thyme stalks and star anise and blend to a thin purée. Season to taste with salt, pepper, lime juice and lime zest. Add half of the dill, then blend again until the soup has a beautiful green colour. Strain the soup back into a clean saucepan, carefully heat through before serving.

Over a medium heat, pan-roast the remaining florets in olive oil and salt until they are tender and caramelised. Serve the soup garnished with the cauliflower florets, dill and a good olive oil. Accompany with fresh bread.

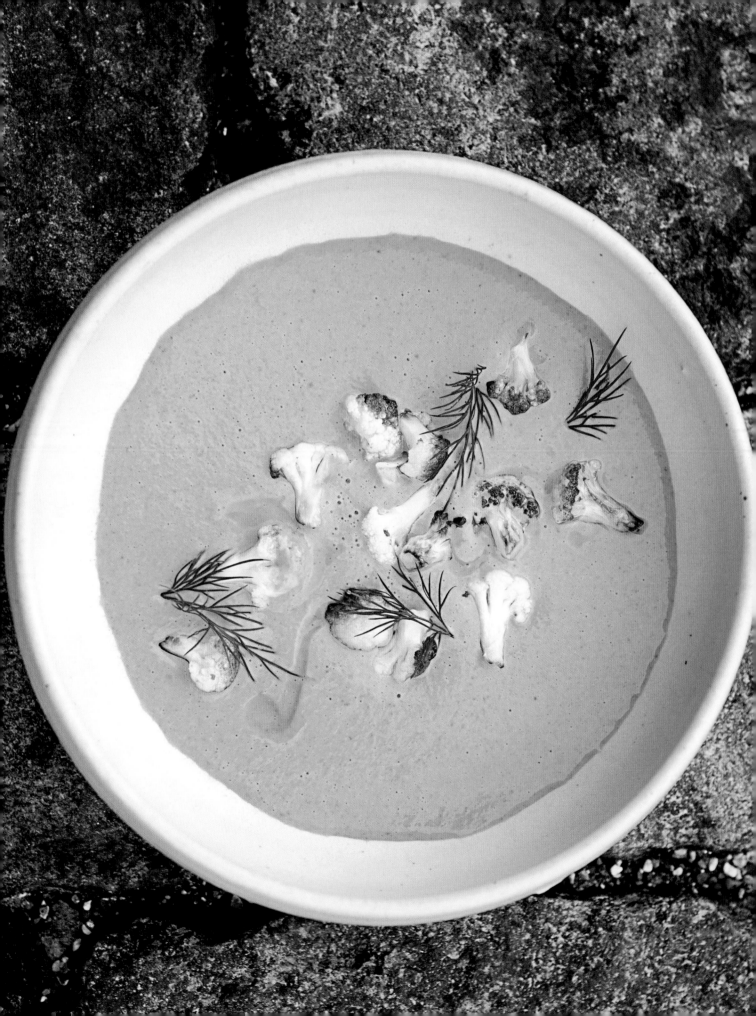

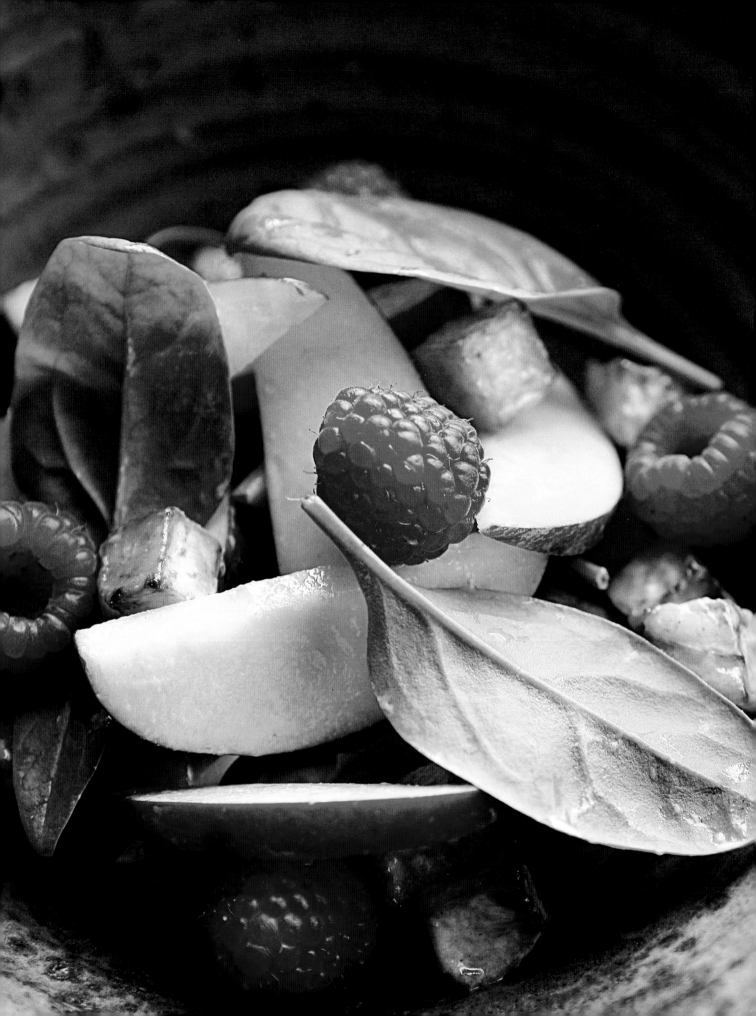

ROASTED *celeriac,*
APPLE, SPINACH AND RASPBERRIES

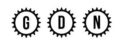

1 HEAD OF CELERIAC
3 APPLES (E.G. PINK LADY)
200 G FRESH RASPBERRIES
200 G BABY SPINACH
JUICE OF 1 LEMON
3 TBSP OLIVE OIL
SALT AND FRESHLY GROUND
BLACK PEPPER
100 ML RASPBERRY VINAIGRETTE
(SEE PAGE 323)

Peel the celeriac and cut into 2x2 cm cubes. Pan-roast over medium heat in olive oil and salt until caramelised, sweet and tender. Cool before using.

Cut the apples into quarters and remove the cores. Cut the wedges into slices and toss them in lemon juice to prevent discolouration. Gently rinse the raspberries and let them drain on two layers of paper towel. Rinse and spin dry the baby spinach.

Toss the celeriac, apples and spinach with the raspberry vinaigrette. Garnish with the fresh raspberries just before serving.

BOLOGNESE
SAUCE

500 G MINCED BEEF OR VEAL
4 TBSP OLIVE OIL
2 SHALLOTS
5 CLOVES GARLIC
½ BUNCH THYME
3 SPRIGS ROSEMARY
1 TBSP DRIED OREGANO
1 TBSP HONEY
100 ML BALSAMIC VINEGAR
70 G CONCENTRATED TOMATO PURÉE
3 CANS PEELED TOMATOES
3 BAY LEAVES
2 STAR ANISE
SALT AND FRESHLY GROUND
BLACK PEPPER

Peel and chop the shallots and garlic. Rinse and drain the thyme and rosemary. Brown the meat in olive oil over high heat, season with salt and set aside.

In a thick-bottomed saucepan, sauté the shallots, garlic, thyme, rosemary and oregano in olive oil. Stir until the shallots are tender but have not taken any colour. Add the honey. When the honey starts to bubble, add the vinegar and reduce by half.

Stir in the tomato purée and bring to an even heat. Add the browned meat, peeled tomatoes, bay leaves and star anise. Quickly bring to a boil, cover, reduce the heat and simmer for 30 minutes.

Remove the thyme, rosemary and star anise and season with salt, pepper and balsamic vinegar. Serve with freshly cooked pasta and parmesan.

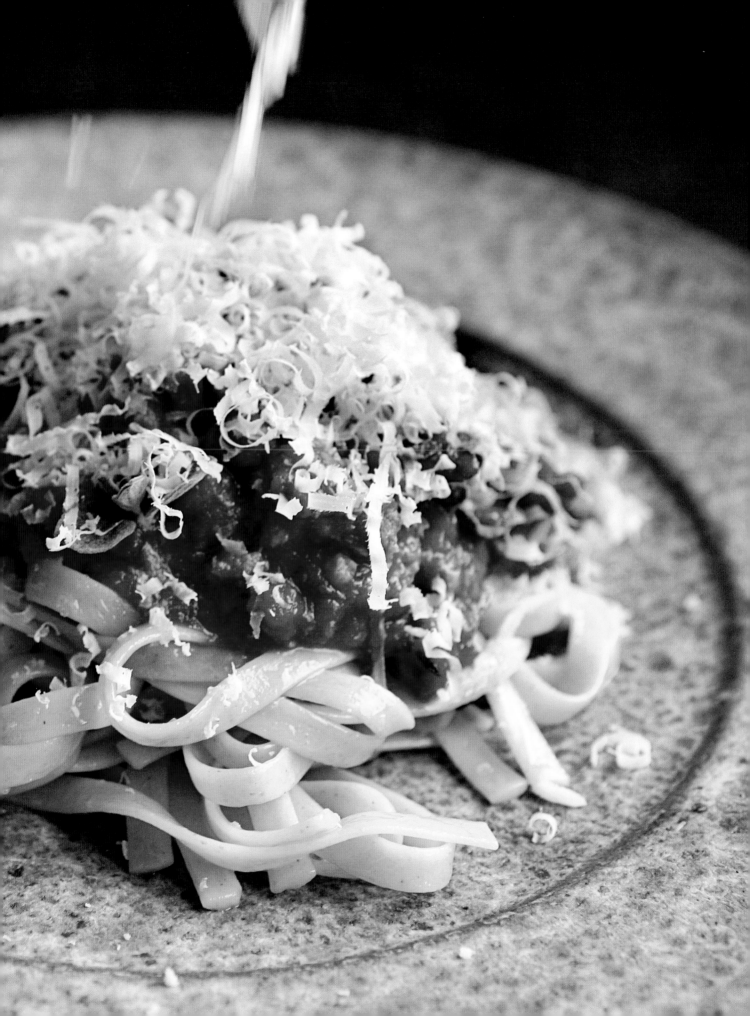

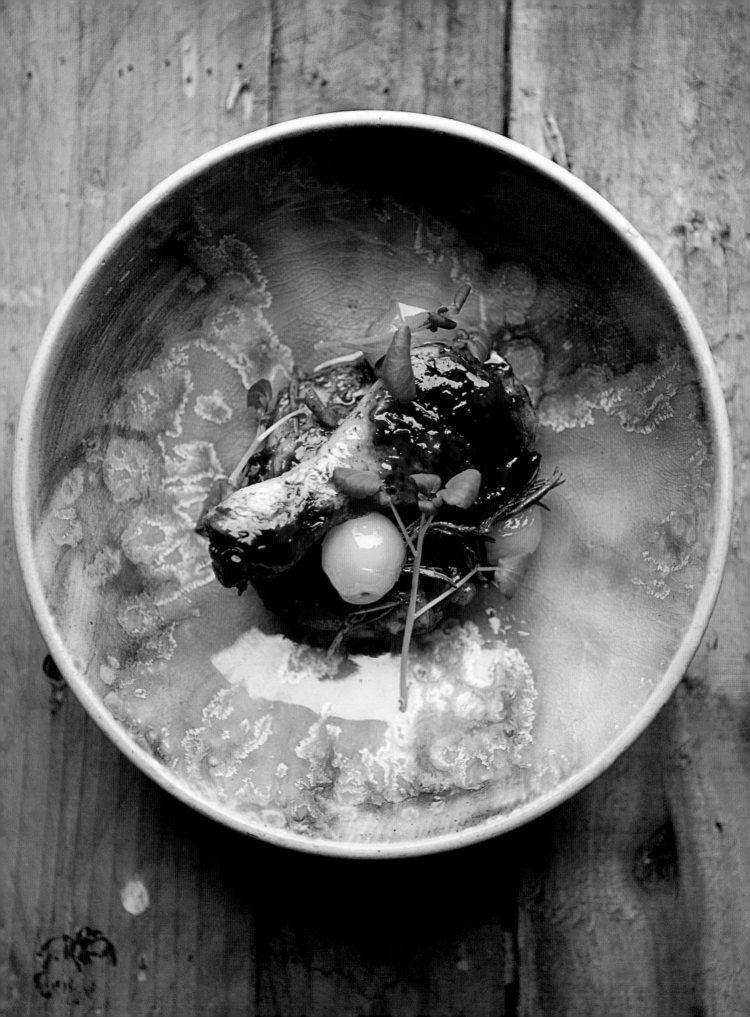

BALSAMIC *and*
HONEY MARINATED CHICKEN

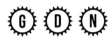

1 CHICKEN (1.4-1.6 KG)
5 SPRIGS ROSEMARY
5 CLOVES GARLIC
300 ML BALSAMIC VINEGAR
100 G HONEY
1 TSP SALT
FRESHLY GROUND BLACK PEPPER
200 ML OLIVE OIL

PICKLED YELLOW CHERRY TOMATOES
500 G YELLOW CHERRY TOMATOES
200 ML BALSAMIC VINEGAR
200 ML OLIVE OIL
1 TSP SALT
2 STAR ANISE
3 BAY LEAVES
4 SPRIGS THYME, RINSED
1 SPRIG ROSEMARY, RINSED

Clean the chicken and divide it into 8 parts (2 thighs, 2 drumsticks and 2 halved breasts).

Rinse the rosemary and pluck off the leaves. Peel the garlic. With a hand blender, blend the rosemary, garlic, balsamic vinegar, honey, salt, pepper and olive oil to the consistency of a pesto.

Place the chicken and the marinade in a resealable plastic bag. Squeeze out the air, seal and refrigerate. Let the chicken marinate for at least 1 hour, preferably overnight.

Preheat the oven to 175°C.

Place the chicken in an ovenproof dish and cover with the marinade. Turning the chicken regularly, roast until cooked through – about 35-40 minutes.

PICKLED YELLOW CHERRY TOMATOES
Rinse the tomatoes, poke a hole with a sharp knife and place in a saucepan. Add the vinegar, oil, herbs and salt and simmer for 2 minutes over medium heat. Remove the pan from the heat, cool and allow the tomatoes to infuse.

If possible, prepare the tomatoes several days in advance and refrigerate. The longer they infuse, the better they taste.

Serve with roasted potatoes or brown rice.

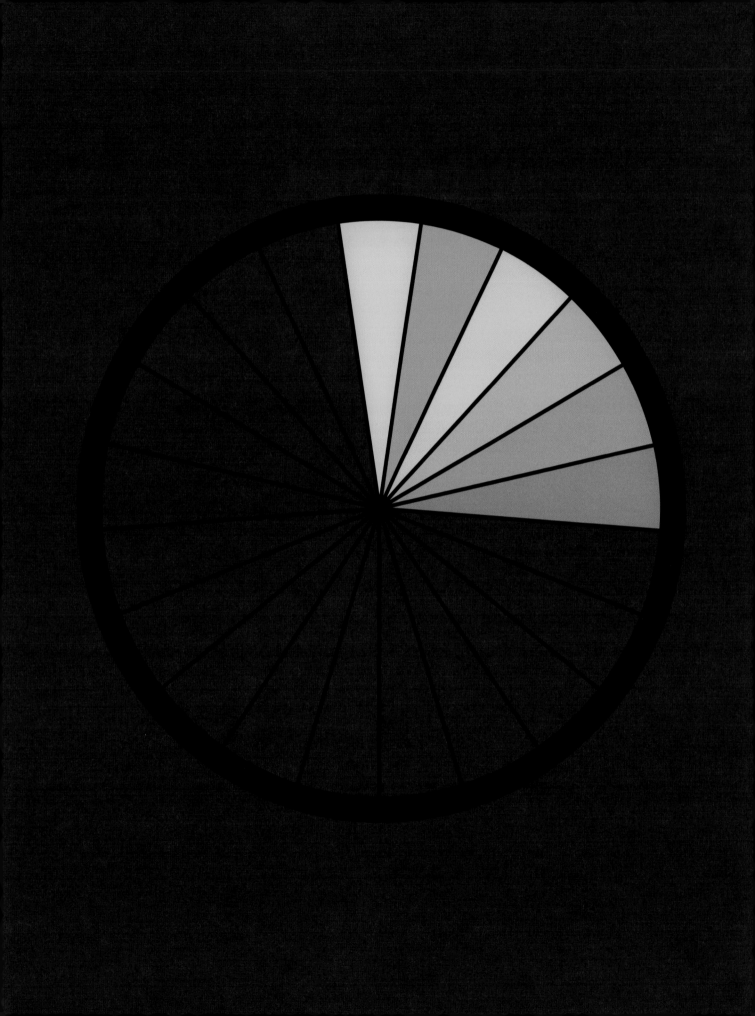

DAY

STAGE 5

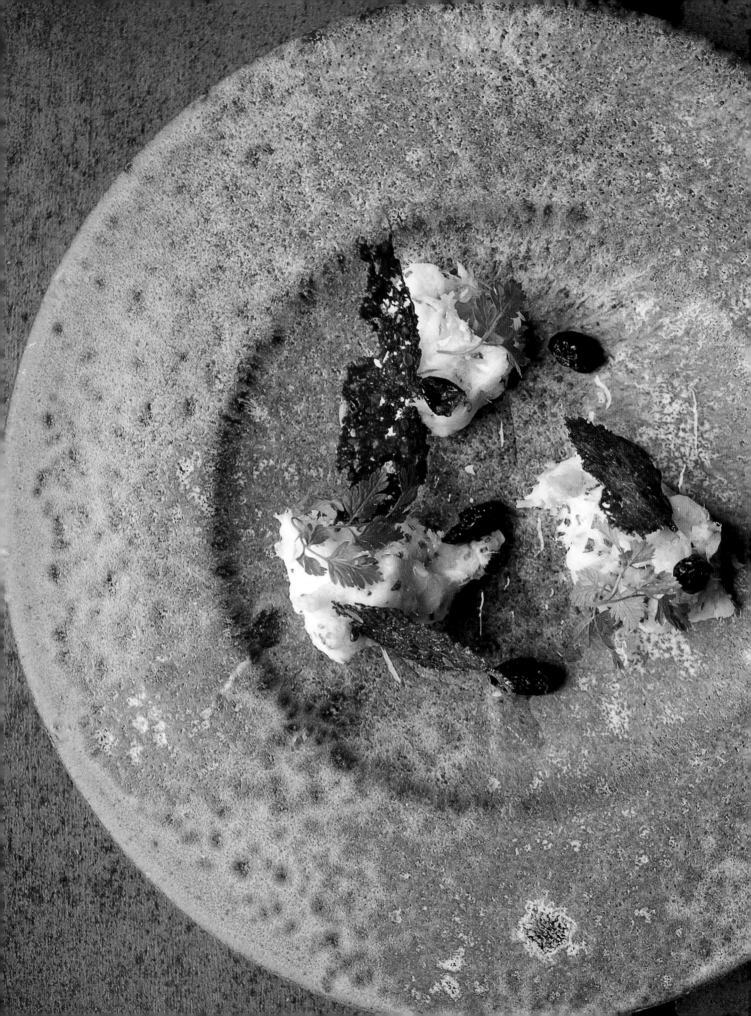

COD BRANDADE,
CHERVIL AND CRANBERRIES

**200 G COD FILLET,
NO BONES OR SKIN
200 G POTATOES
200 ML WHOLE MILK
1 TSP CORIANDER SEEDS
3 SPRIGS THYME
6 BLACK PEPPERCORNS
¼ BUNCH DILL
1 BUNCH CHERVIL
50 ML OLIVE OIL
JUICE AND ZEST OF 1 ORGANIC LEMON
DAY OLD SOURDOUGH OR RYE BREAD
3 TBSP OLIVE OIL
½ TSP SALT
50 G DRIED CRANBERRIES**

Place the cod in a resealable container, season with salt, cover and refrigerate for at least 1 hour, preferably overnight.

Preheat the oven to 170°C.

Peel the potatoes and boil in unsalted water until tender. Remove from the heat and leave until the fish is ready. Rinse and finely chop the dill and chervil. Refrigerate the chervil until needed.

Pour the milk into a thick-bottomed saucepan and add the coriander, thyme, pepper and cod. Gently warm the milk until it starts to simmer. Simmer for 2 minutes, remove the pan from the heat and allow the fish to rest until ready.

Drain the potatoes and crush over low heat for 1 minute to steam dry. Carefully remove the fish from the milk and mash into a homogenous mixture with the potatoes. Add the olive oil, chopped dill and grated lemon zest. Season the Brandade with salt, pepper and lemon juice. Refrigerate until serving.

Cut the day old bread into 1-2 mm slices and spread on a baking sheet covered with baking paper. Drizzle the slices with olive oil and sprinkle with salt. Bake for 6-8 minutes until golden and crispy.

Serve the Brandade with the bread. Garnish with chervil and cranberries.

WATERMELON, *feta* AND BLACK CUMIN

Ⓖ Ⓝ

½ SEEDLESS WATERMELON
250 G FETA
200 G ROCKET
100 ML OLIVE OIL
SALT AND FRESHLY GROUND
BLACK PEPPER
1 TBSP BLACK CUMIN SEEDS

Chop the watermelon into 3x3 cm chunks. Remove any seeds. Rinse and spin the rocket. Carefully toss the watermelon with the rocket. Crumble the feta into bite-sized pieces and garnish the salad with them. Drizzle with olive oil and season with salt, pepper and sprinkle with black cumin seeds.

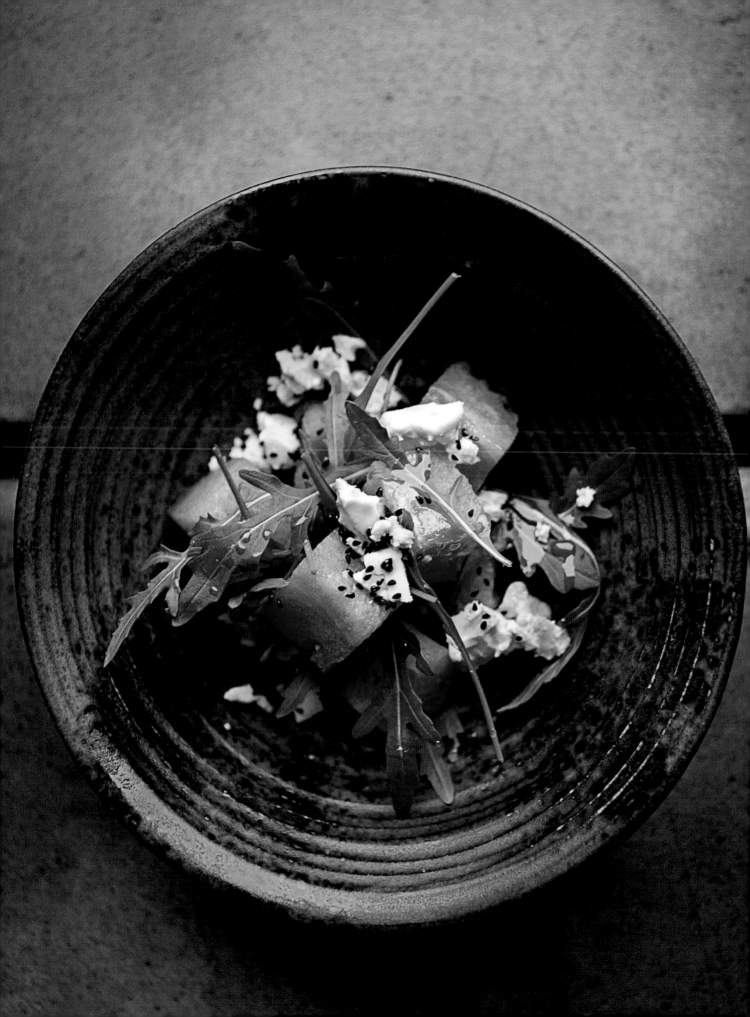

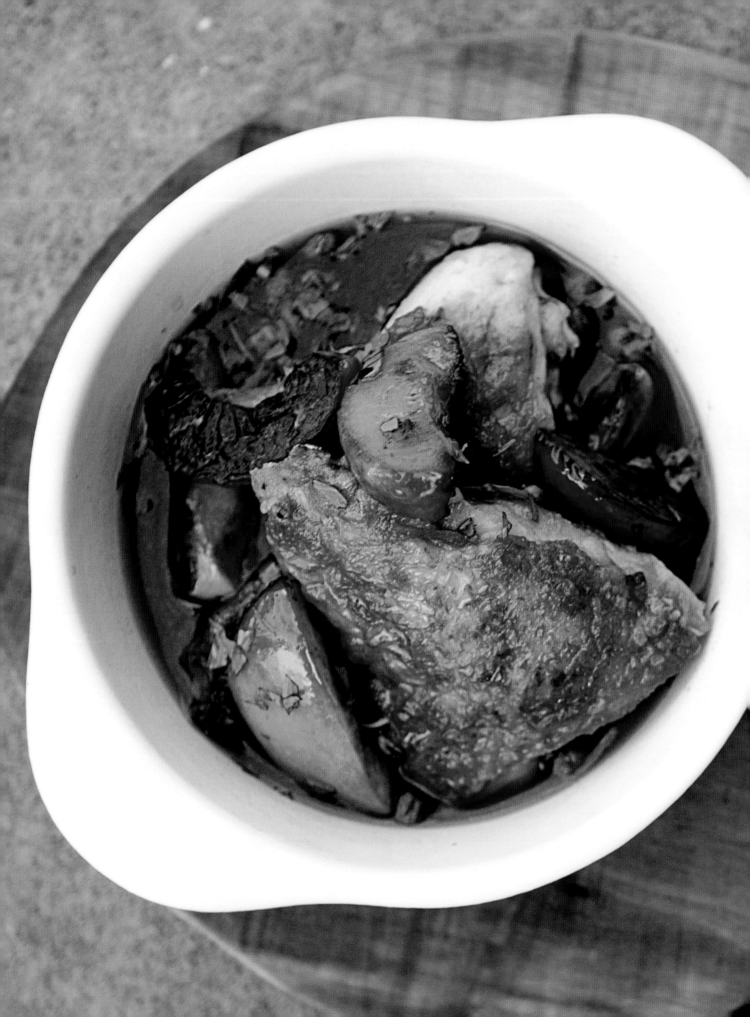

CHICKEN *with*
PEACH, CAPERS AND TARRAGON

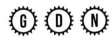

1 CHICKEN (1.4-1.6 KG)
4 PEACHES
2 ONIONS
1 CLOVE GARLIC
50 G CAPERS
200 ML CHICKEN STOCK (SEE PAGE 332)
100 ML CIDER VINEGAR
1 TBSP HONEY
1 STAR ANISE
½ BUNCH OF TARRAGON
SALT AND FRESHLY GROUND
BLACK PEPPER

Clean the chicken. Cut off the wings and tail. Salt the skin, cover the chicken and refrigerate for 30 minutes.

Preheat the oven to 185°C.

Cut the peaches into quarters and remove the stones. Peel the onions and garlic. Quarter the onions and brown them on the cut surfaces in a frying pan with a little olive oil. Place the chicken in an ovenproof pan with the onions, garlic, peaches, capers, vinegar, honey, stock and star anise and cook until the chicken is done – about 40 minutes.

Allow the chicken to rest for a few minutes. Strain the drippings into a saucepan, reduce by half and season with the salt, honey, vinegar and fresh tarragon. Serve the chicken with the peaches and onions and accompany with the quinoa.

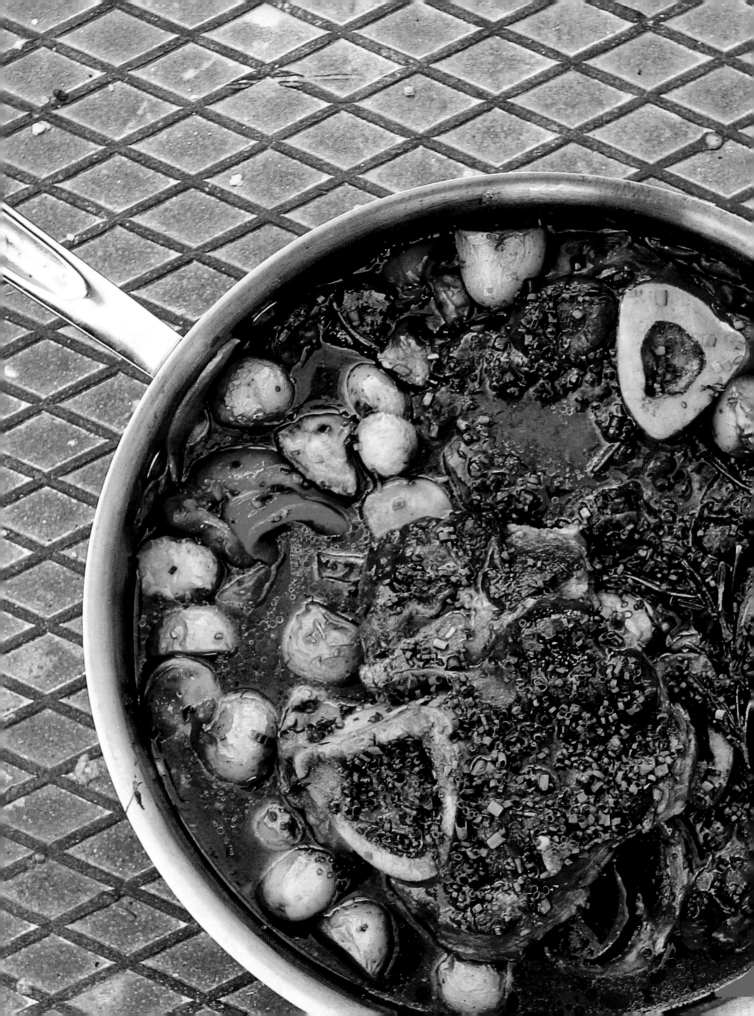

OSSOBUCO

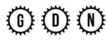

1 KG OSSOBUCO
500 ML RED WINE
100 ML CIDER VINEGAR
½ BUNCH OF THYME, RINSED
6 CLOVES
6 ALLSPICE BERRIES
3 BAY LEAVES
1 CINNAMON STICK
5 STAR ANISE
6 BLACK PEPPERCORNS
3 CARROTS
3 ONIONS
1 WHOLE GARLIC, SPLIT
1 LITRE VEAL STOCK (SEE PAGE 333)
70 G CONCENTRATED TOMATO PURÉE
SALT AND FRESHLY GROUND
BLACK PEPPER

GARNISH

2 COURGETTES
2 RED PEPPERS
2 TBSP OLIVE OIL
SALT
ZEST OF 1 ORGANIC LEMON
½ BUNCH OF PARSLEY,
RINSED AND CHOPPED

Score the silverskin around the edges of the ossobuco, dry well, season with salt and brown in olive oil in a frying pan over high heat. Remove the meat from the pan and pat dry with paper towel.

Pour the red wine, vinegar, thyme, cloves, allspice, bay leaves, cinnamon, star anise and peppercorns into a separate saucepan and reduce by half. Peel the carrots, onion and garlic, cut into large chunks and brown them well in the frying pan in a little olive oil.

Place the ossobuco and the vegetables in an ovenproof pan, pour over the red wine reduction, the stock and tomato purée, cover with tin foil and cook in the oven until the meat is tender and falling off the bone – about 2.5 hours.
Strain the liquid from the ossobuco, pick out all the herbs and spices, reduce by half and season with salt, pepper and vinegar. Pour the sauce back over the meat.

Chop the peppers and courgettes into bite-sized pieces and grill in a grill pan. When the vegetables are cooked, toss them with the olive oil, salt, lemon zest and chopped parsley.

Arrange the ossobuco with the vegetables and serve with roasted potatoes.

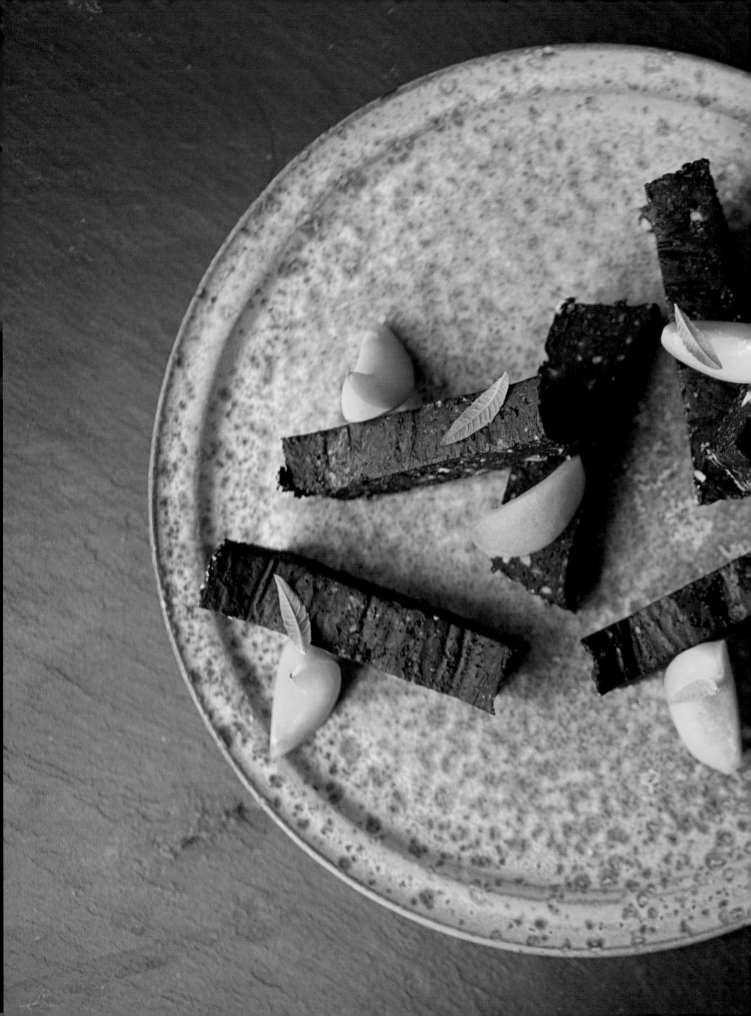

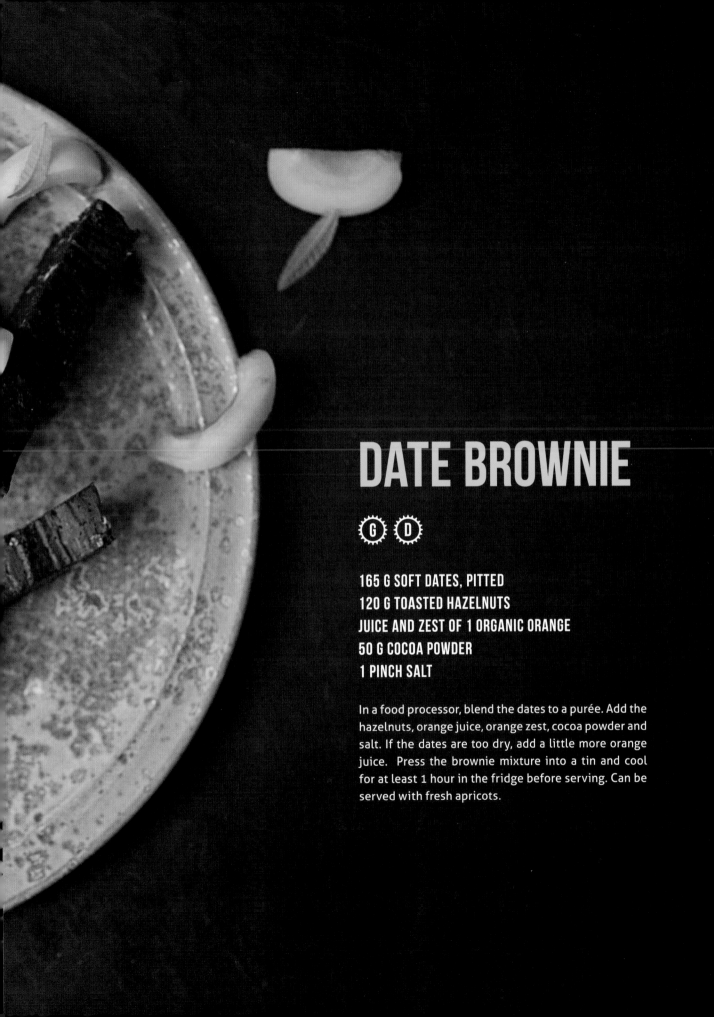

DATE BROWNIE

Ⓖ Ⓓ

165 G SOFT DATES, PITTED
120 G TOASTED HAZELNUTS
JUICE AND ZEST OF 1 ORGANIC ORANGE
50 G COCOA POWDER
1 PINCH SALT

In a food processor, blend the dates to a purée. Add the hazelnuts, orange juice, orange zest, cocoa powder and salt. If the dates are too dry, add a little more orange juice. Press the brownie mixture into a tin and cool for at least 1 hour in the fridge before serving. Can be served with fresh apricots.

ROMAN KREUZIGER

"THE FUTURE OF CYCLING AS A SPORT HAS TO DO WITH THE RIGHT DIET"

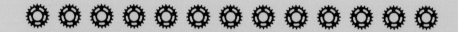

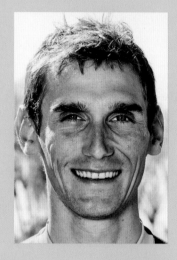

BORN: 6th May 1986
NATIONALITY: Czech
EXPERIENCE: Professional
since 2006
FORMER CYCLING TEAMS:
Astana, Liquigas
FAVOURITE RACES:
Amstel Gold Race,
Liège-Bastogne-Liège
– and the Giro d'Italia
because of the atmosphere

Hannah (H): What difference does food make for you physically and/or mentally during a long season or race?

Roman Kreuziger (RK): Food makes a huge difference both physically and mentally. For many years, my diet consisted of lots of bread and pasta. As a result, my stomach was constantly bloated and I didn't feel very well. I simply had to stuff myself with food to get enough energy to cope with the different stages and races. Now I've changed my diet from a typical cyclist diet with tons of pasta to a gluten-free diet with fewer (and only slow) carbs, more protein and lots of vegetables. For me, it has been an amazing shift.

H: In what way do you think food can change an athlete's performance?

RK: Food can't change a rider but it can help get the best out of any rider and help him stay on top for longer. I believe that the right diet can make a huge difference. It can even mean gaining a few seconds in a race because you have more energy. As I said, my diet now consists mainly of protein, vegetables and far fewer carbohydrates than before and only slow carbohydrates at that. Now, I sleep much better because my blood sugar is stable – not only at night but in general. What's more, I've basically stopped eating carbohydrates out of season, which means I actually lose weight in my free time and so don't have to start over again as soon as the next season starts.

H: What has the proper diet meant for you personally as a cyclist?

RK: I no longer need to eat oceans of pasta and I can generally eat smaller portions and still feel full with tons of energy to do my job.

H: Have you found that food can improve or worsen your condition?

RK: You bet! As I mentioned before, my body simply isn't happy with the wrong food.

H: How do you see the future of cycling in terms of food?
RK: The future of cycling as a sport has to do with the right diet. Optimising your diet, combined with normal training and core exercise means quicker recovery and maybe even a few more wins.

H: What is your favourite food?
RK: Outside the cycling season, steak tartare and pizza. During the cycling season, anything with blue cheese and walnuts.

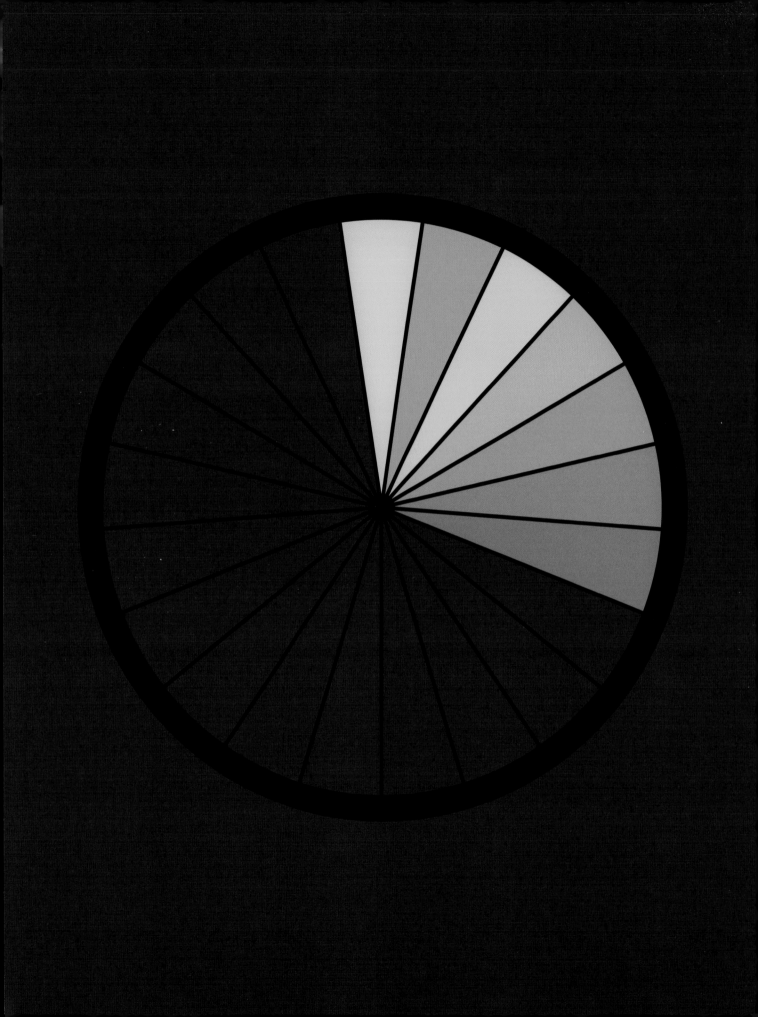

DAY 7

STAGE 6

CHICKEN *and* NOODLES IN LIME AND GINGER BROTH

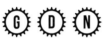

200 G PLUCKED, COOKED CHICKEN
(PERHAPS LEFTOVERS FROM
THE PREVIOUS DAY)
JUICE AND ZEST OF 2 ORGANIC LIMES
100 G FRESH GINGER
2 STALKS OF LEMONGRASS
3 CLOVES GARLIC
1 STAR ANISE
4 TBSP OLIVE OIL
1.5 LITRES CHICKEN STOCK
(SEE PAGE 332)
100 G SHIITAKE MUSHROOMS
100 G CARROTS
JAPANESE SOY SAUCE
200 G RICE NOODLES
3 SPRING ONIONS

Cut half the ginger into slices. Chop the lemon grass and garlic. In a mortar or spice grinder, crush the finely grated lime zest, the ginger slices, lemongrass, garlic and star anise with the olive oil. Sauté in a saucepan over a medium heat for 2 minutes, stirring constantly. Add the stock, bring to a boil and skim off any impurities. Turn down the heat and let the soup simmer for 15 minutes.

Clean and slice the mushrooms. Julienne the carrots with a mandolin. Rinse and chop the spring onions. Grate the remaining ginger.

Strain the soup and season with the lime juice, soy sauce and grated ginger. Prepare the noodles according to the directions on the package. Add the chicken, mushrooms, carrots, spring onions and noodles to the soup. Warm everything through before serving. Can be topped with toasted sesame seeds and fresh coriander.

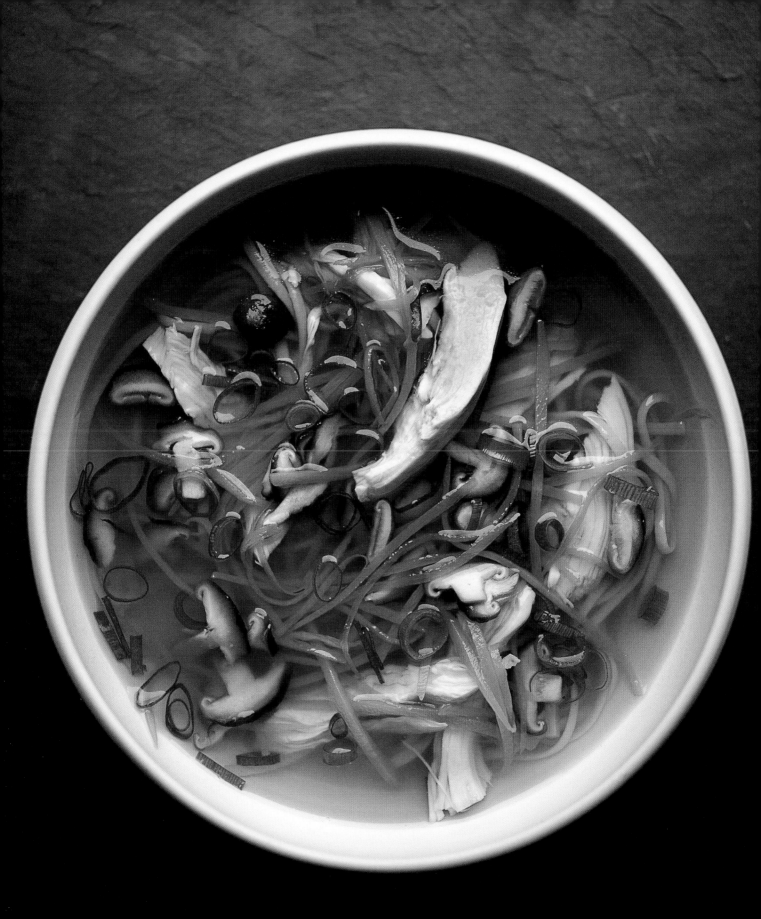

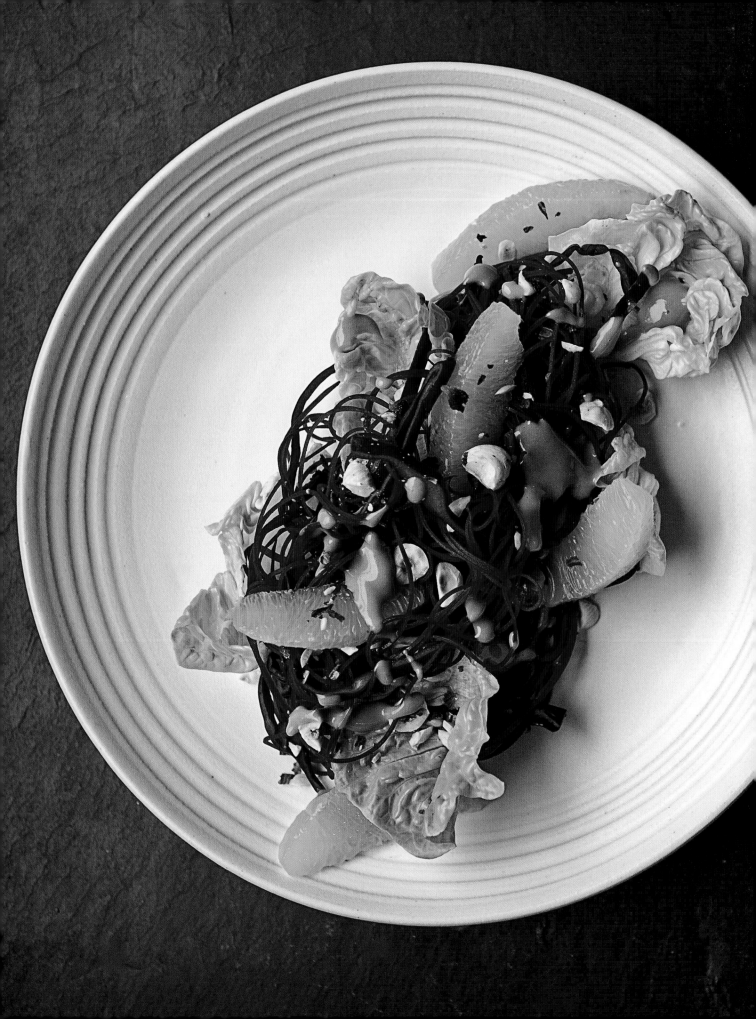

BEETROOT, *orange* AND TOASTED HAZELNUTS

(G) (D)

500 G BEETROOT
2 BLOOD ORANGES
2 HEADS ROMAINE LETTUCES
50 G HAZELNUTS
100 ML BALSAMIC VINAIGRETTE
(SEE PAGE 324)

Peel the beetroot and grate them using a grater or a food processor. Toast the hazelnuts in a preheated oven until golden – about 8 minutes – and chop coarsely. Peel and slice the oranges. Separate the romaine lettuce into leaves, rinse and spin. Mix the grated beetroot with the dressing and serve with the orange segments, romaine lettuce and chopped hazelnuts.

CHICKEN BAKED *in* CASHEW AND SAGE WITH LEMON-STEAMED CABBAGE

1 CHICKEN (1.4-1.6 KG)
1 TBSP CORIANDER SEEDS
4 BLACK PEPPERCORNS
¼ BUNCH SAGE
200 G CASHEWS
½ TSP SALT
4 TBSP COCONUT OIL

LEMON-STEAMED CABBAGE

1 POINTED CABBAGE
2 LEMONS
SALT
2 TBSP OLIVE OIL

Preheat the oven to 170°C.

Cut the chicken into 8 pieces (2 thighs, 2 drumsticks and 2 halved breasts) and remove the skin. Grind the coriander seeds and peppercorns in a mortar or spice grinder. Rinse and chop the sage leaves. Finely chop the cashews and mix them with the coriander-pepper mixture, chopped sage, salt and coconut oil.

Rub each piece of the chicken with 1 tbsp of the nut mixture. Place the chicken pieces on a baking tray covered with baking paper and roast in the preheated oven for about 35-40 minutes until the chicken juices run clear. While the chicken is roasting, prepare the garnish.

Remove the outer leaves from the cabbage and trim the bottom. Cut the cabbage into 8 wedges and place them in a sauté pan with olive oil, 50 ml water and a pinch of salt.

Wash the lemons and zest them over the cabbage. Cover the pan and steam the cabbage over medium heat until the cabbage is cooked through but still has a bite and a nice green colour – about 2-3 minutes.

Serve the cabbage immediately. Drizzle the cabbage and chicken with olive oil and freshly squeezed lemon juice. Serve with roast potatoes.

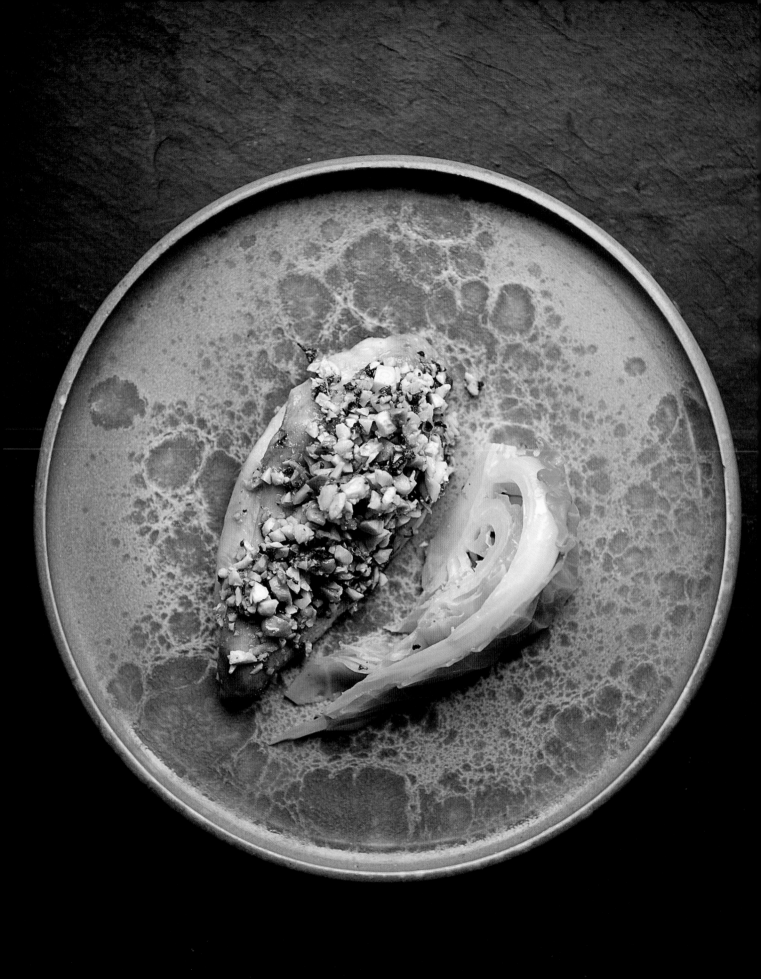

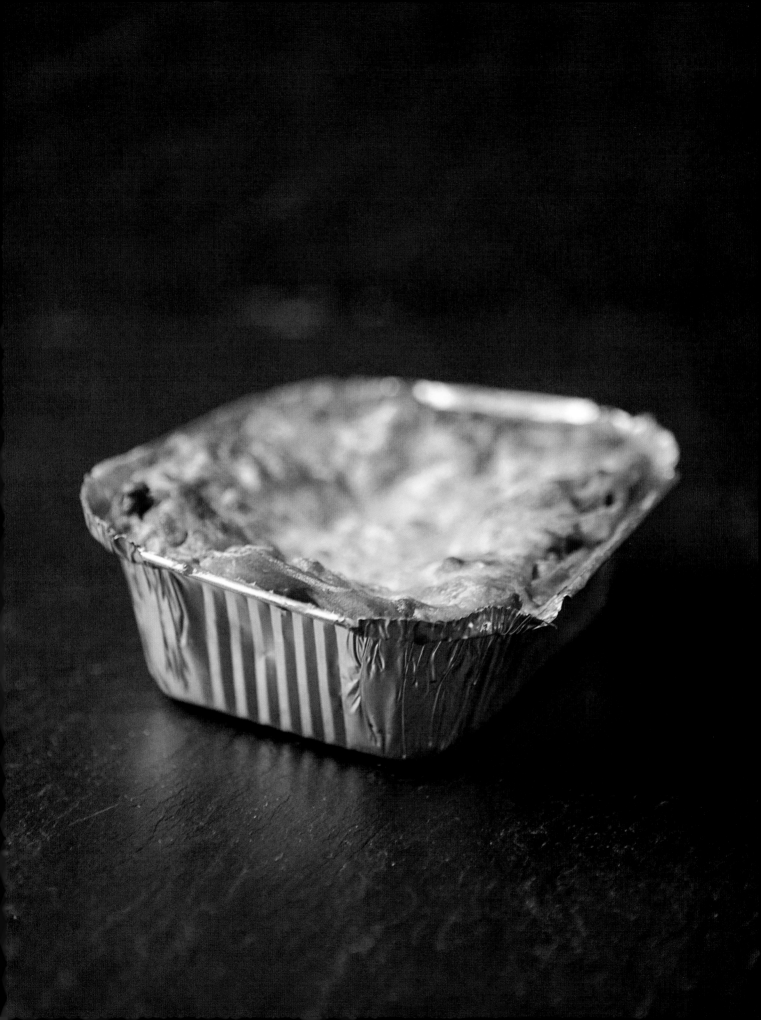

LASAGNE

500 G MINCED BEEF
1 LITRE TOMATO SAUCE OF YOUR
OWN CHOICE (SEE PAGES 330-331)
1 LITRE MILK
1 STAR ANISE
3 CLOVES
2 BAY LEAVES
4 TBSP CORN FLOUR
50 ML COLD WATER
SALT AND FRESHLY GROUND
BLACK PEPPER
1 TSP GROUND NUTMEG
150 G GRATED PARMESAN
500 G LASAGNE SHEETS

Preheat the oven to 160°C.

Brown the beef in a hot frying pan with olive oil and season with salt. Pour the tomato sauce into a saucepan and add the meat. Let it simmer until it comes together – about 30 minutes over low heat. Bring the milk to a boil with the star anise, cloves and bay leaves. Whisk the cornflour with the water and whisk into the milk. Bring the milk to a boil again, turn down the heat and simmer for 5 minutes. Season the sauce with salt, pepper and nutmeg. Strain the sauce and add 100 g parmesan.

Assemble the lasagne in an ovenproof dish in the following order: first white sauce, then a lasagne sheet and then meat sauce. Repeat until you run out of the meat sauce and sheets. Top with a layer of white sauce sprinkled with the rest of the parmesan.

Bake the lasagne until the lasagne sheets are soft throughout – about 50-60 minutes.

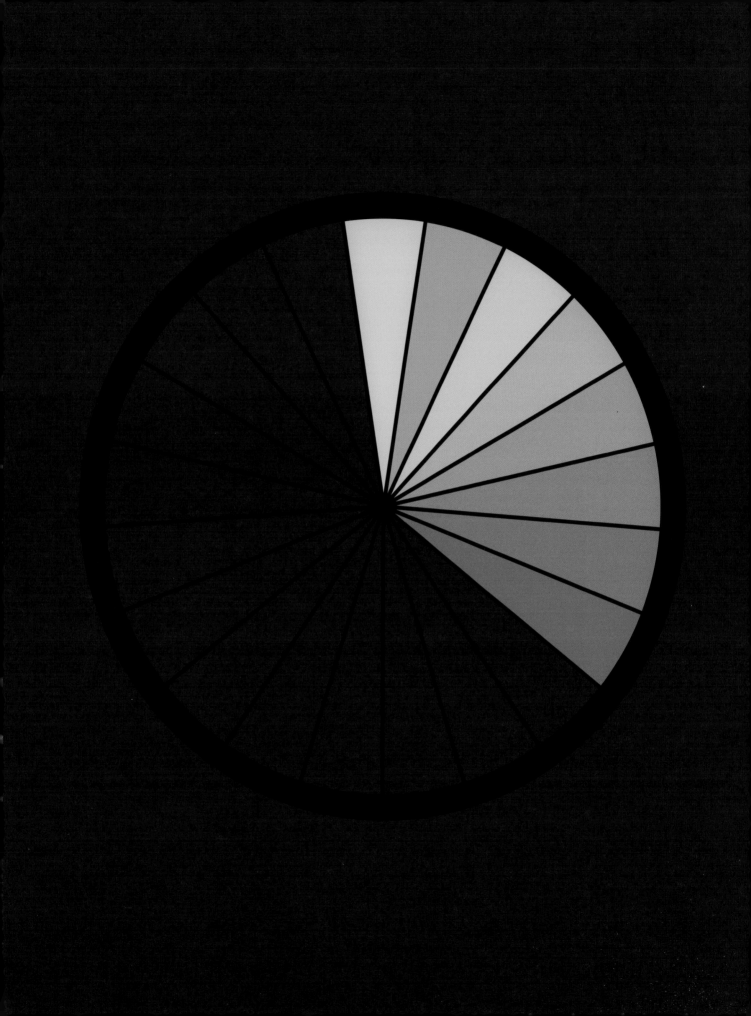

DAY

STAGE 7

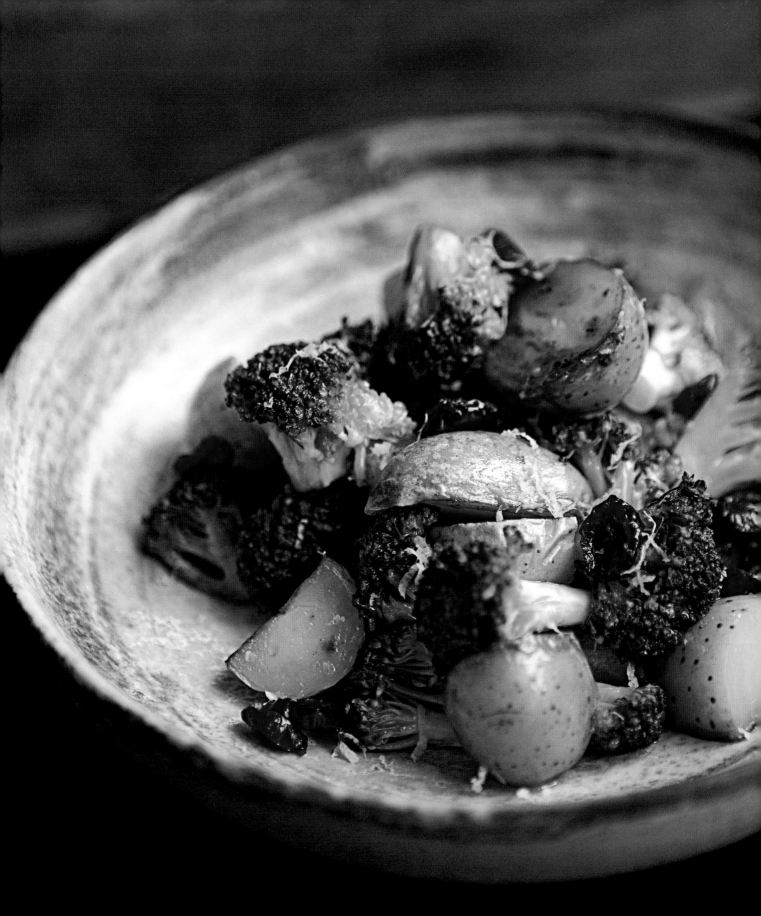

WARM POTATO SALAD
with BROCCOLI AND CRANBERRIES

500 G NEW POTATOES
1 HEAD OF BROCCOLI
2 TBSP COCONUT OIL
SALT
50 G DRIED CRANBERRIES
ZEST OF 1 ORGANIC LEMON
100 ML ORANGE VINAIGRETTE
(SEE PAGE 325)

Scrub the potatoes and cut them into bite-sized pieces. Pan-roast in a frying pan over medium heat in the coconut oil and season with salt. Remove the potatoes from the pan. Separate the broccoli into small florets. Rinse, drain and pan-roast with coconut oil until the florets are nicely browned but still have a bite and a vibrant green colour. Season with salt.

Mix the potatoes, broccoli and cranberries. Rinse the lemon and zest onto the salad. Toss with the dressing.

CELERIAC,
SAVOY CABBAGE, APRICOT
and ## SUNFLOWER SEEDS

(G) (D) (N)

50 G SUNFLOWER SEEDS
½ HEAD OF CELERIAC, PEELED
2 CARROTS
½ SAVOY CABBAGE
10 DRIED APRICOTS
50 ML MUSTARD VINAIGRETTE
(SEE PAGE 322)

Preheat the oven to 170°C.

Toast the sunflower seeds in the oven until golden – about 7 minutes – then cool down. Julienne the celeriac and carrots in a food processor or grate with a grater. Remove the outer leaves of the savoy cabbage and cut off the stalk. Slice the leaves into ½ cm strips. Cut each dry apricot into 4 strips. Toss all the ingredients in the vinaigrette at least 10 minutes before serving.

If you wish, substitute 3 fresh apricots for the dry apricots for a lighter salad.

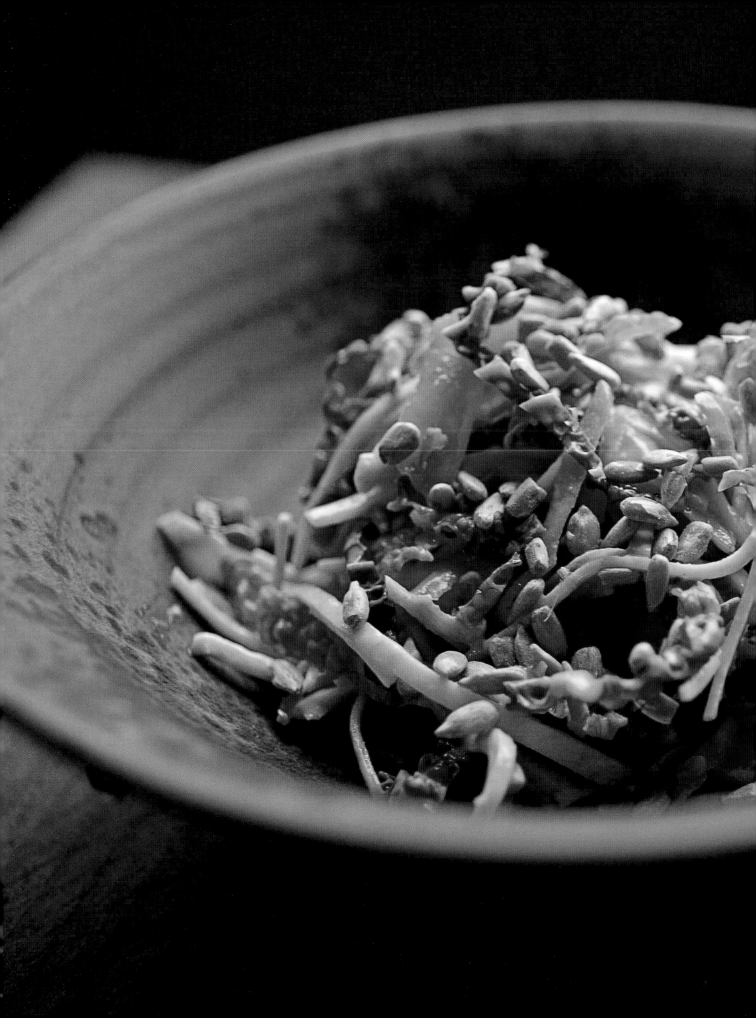

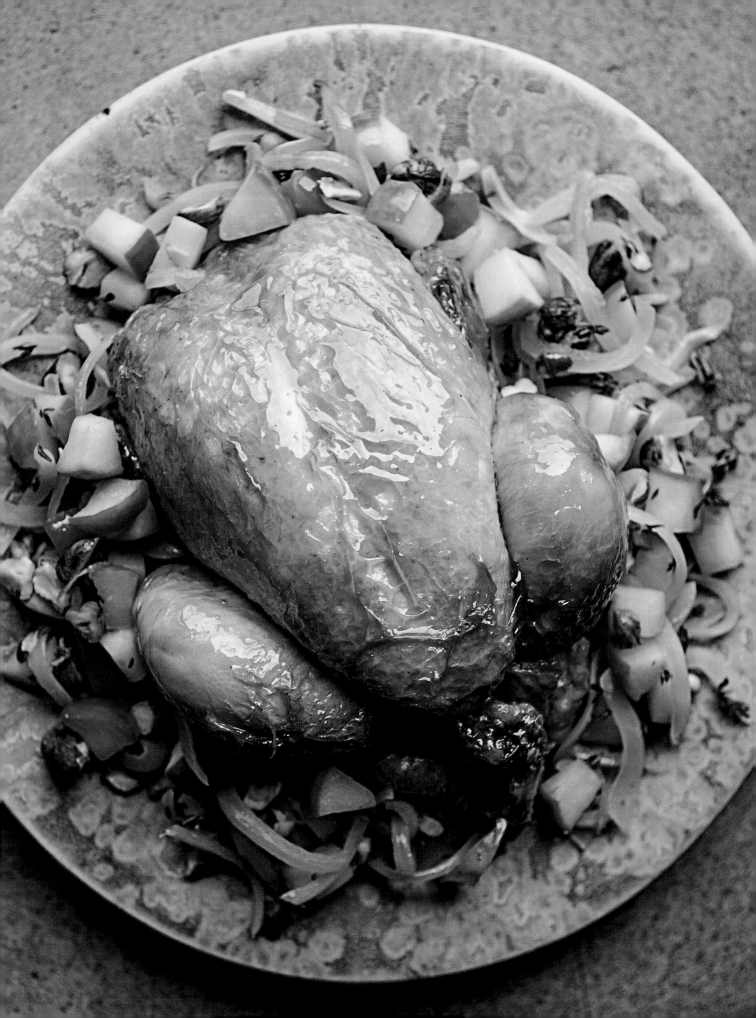

WHOLE ROAST
CHICKEN WITH APPLE AND HAZELNUT STUFFING

1 CHICKEN (1.4-1.6 KG)
100 G HAZELNUTS
3 TART APPLES (E.G. BELLE DE BOSKOOP,
COX'S ORANGE OR INGRID MARIE)
OLIVE OIL
2 ONIONS
2 STAR ANISE
ZEST OF 2 ORGANIC LEMONS
SALT

Preheat the oven to 175°C.

Toast the hazelnuts in the oven until nicely golden brown – about 7-8 minutes – and chop coarsely.

Clean the chicken. Cut off the wings and the tail and rub the chicken with salt. Cover and refrigerate.

Rinse the apples, quarter and remove the cores. Cut the apple into wedges and then into chunks. Fry them in a frying pan over medium heat with a little olive oil and salt. Leave the apples in the pan until they have a lovely, caramelised surface.

When the apples are ready, transfer to a bowl. Wipe the pan with a paper towel. Peel the onions, slice them and caramelise in the same pan with a little olive oil, star anise and salt. Mix the apples with the onions, hazelnuts, grated lemon zest and 2 tbsp olive oil. Season with a little salt.

Stuff the chicken with the apple mixture, tie up the chicken legs with meat string and put any extra stuffing in a baking pan underneath the chicken. Brush the chicken with a little olive oil and roast for about 50 minutes until the juices run clear and the legs separate easily from the carcass. Let the chicken rest for 10-15 minutes before serving.

Remove the stuffing from the chicken, part the chicken into 8 pieces and serve on top of the mixture with crushed potatoes, seasoned with salt, fresh herbs and olive oil.

FLOUNDER *with* STEAMED CAULIFLOWER AND NEW POTATOES

4 FRESH WHOLE FLAUNDERS, SKINNED,
CLEANED AND HEADS REMOVED
1 CAULIFLOWER
1 TBSP LAVENDER
100 G RYE FLOUR OR WHOLE GRAIN
SPELT FLOUR (RICEFLOUR FOR
A GLUTEN-FREE VERSION)
OLIVE OIL FOR FRYING
1 LEMON
SALT AND FRESHLY GROUND
BLACK PEPPER

Preheat the oven to 180°C.

Separate the cauliflower into golf ball sized florets, rinse and steam until tender in a colander placed over boiling water with the lavender. Cool the cauliflower, halve the florets lengthwise and sear the cutting face.

Rinse the flounders and pat dry with paper towel. Between and along the thickest part of both sides of the fillets, cut a slit 1/3 of the length of the fillet from the top towards the tail. Sprinkle with salt and freshly ground black pepper and press the flounders into the rye flour so it sticks to both sides.

Brown the fish on both sides in olive oil in a frying pan over medium heat until golden. Turn only once, otherwise the fish will flake and fall to pieces.

When the surfaces are golden, place the fish on a baking tray covered with baking paper and bake until the meat can be lifted from the bone easily – about 6-7 minutes.

Serve the fish with the roasted cauliflower, lemon and new potatoes dressed with butter or olive oil.

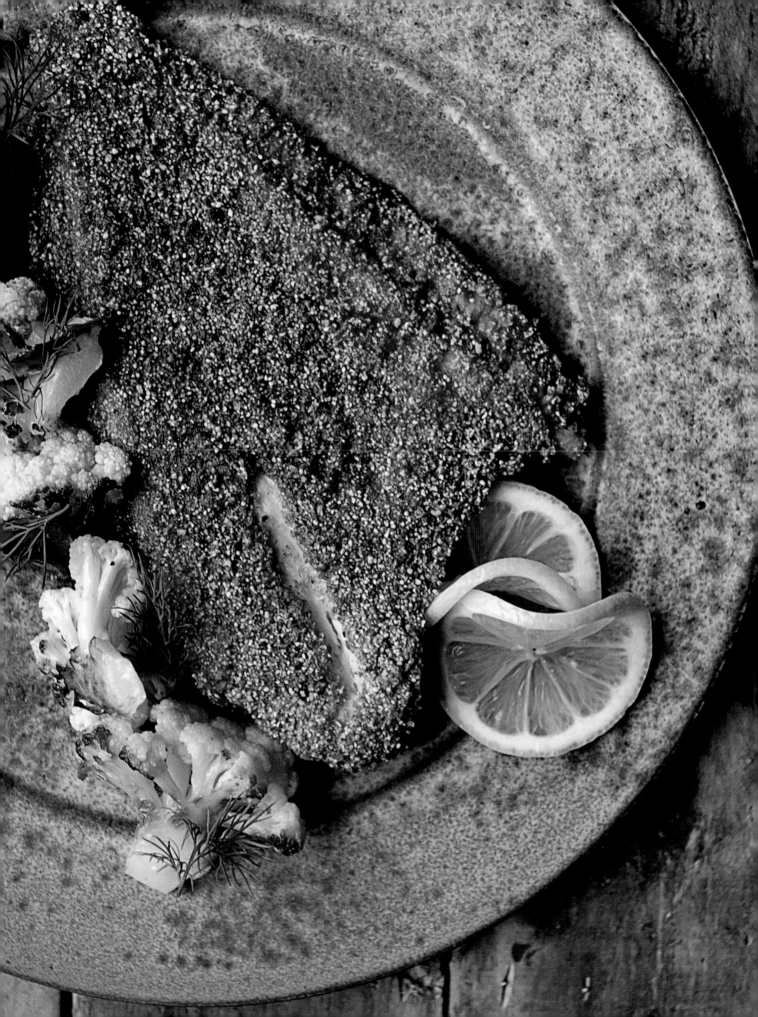

NICOLAS ROCHE

"THE PROPER DIET HAS HELPED ME BECOME A BETTER CYCLIST"

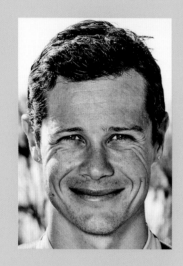

BORN: 3rd July 1984
NATIONALITY: Irish
EXPERIENCE: Professional
since 2005
FORMER CYCLING TEAMS:
Cofidis, Crédit Agricole, AG2R
La Mondiale, Tinkoff-Saxo
FAVOURITE RACES: Tour de
France and Vuelta a España

Hannah (H): What difference does food make for you physically during a long season or race?
Nicolas Roche (NR): Food is a key element. If you don't get the right energy in your food, you can't expect the best results.

H: In what way do you think food can change an athlete's performance?
NR: Food can do an awful lot. Firstly, the right diet means that you can easily get rid of extra kilos. But it also takes care of your vitamin and mineral requirements.

H: What has the proper diet meant for you personally as a rider?
NR: It has helped me become a better rider. That isn't necessarily as easy as it sounds, especially if you like to eat. But it makes a big difference in the long run.

H: Have you found that food can improve or worsen your condition?
NR: If I overeat during a race, I sleep badly and don't recover properly. When I sit in the saddle again the following day, it takes me ages to properly get into gear.

H: In what way has your opinion on food for athletes changed over the past year?
NR: To begin with, I thought it was hard to follow a healthy diet. The only thing I thought about was pasta and chicken! But now that I've tried to follow a specific diet, I have to admit that I'm in better shape and perform better.

H: How do you see the future of cycling in terms of food?
NR: There are already many teams that have adopted a gluten-free diet or other kinds of diets. I also think that there are many riders who follow one

diet or another, but mostly because it seems modern to do so and because someone has told them to do it. There are probably loads of different trends and I'm sure that more will come. There are also more and more cycling teams who have hired a private chef because it's not possible to stick to a diet when you eat in different hotels and restaurants every day.

H: What is your favourite food?
NR: Probably lasagne or pizza – if I am allowed...

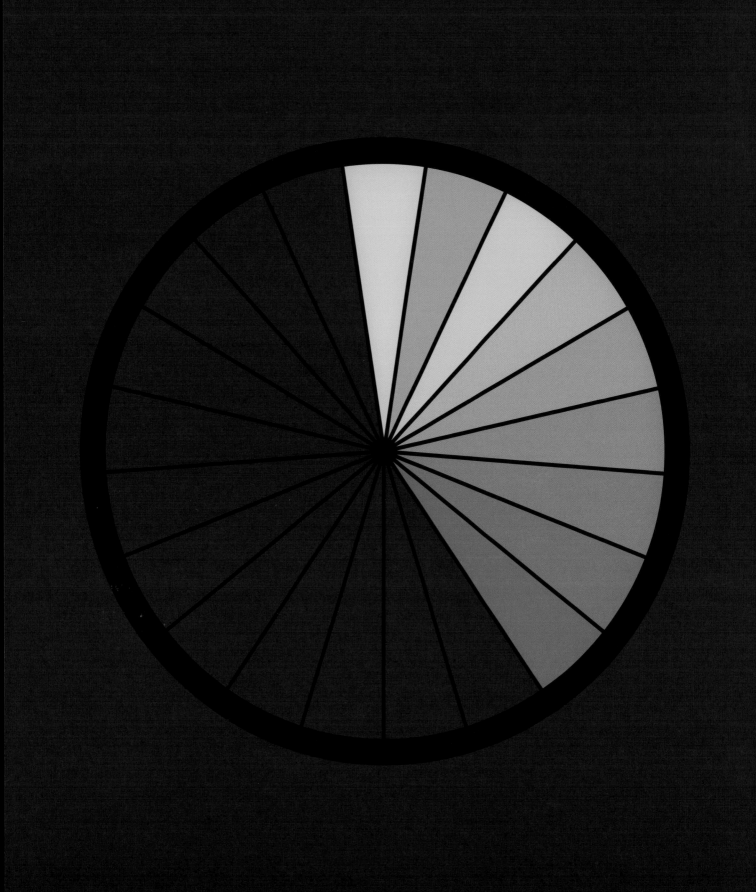

DAY 9

STAGE 8

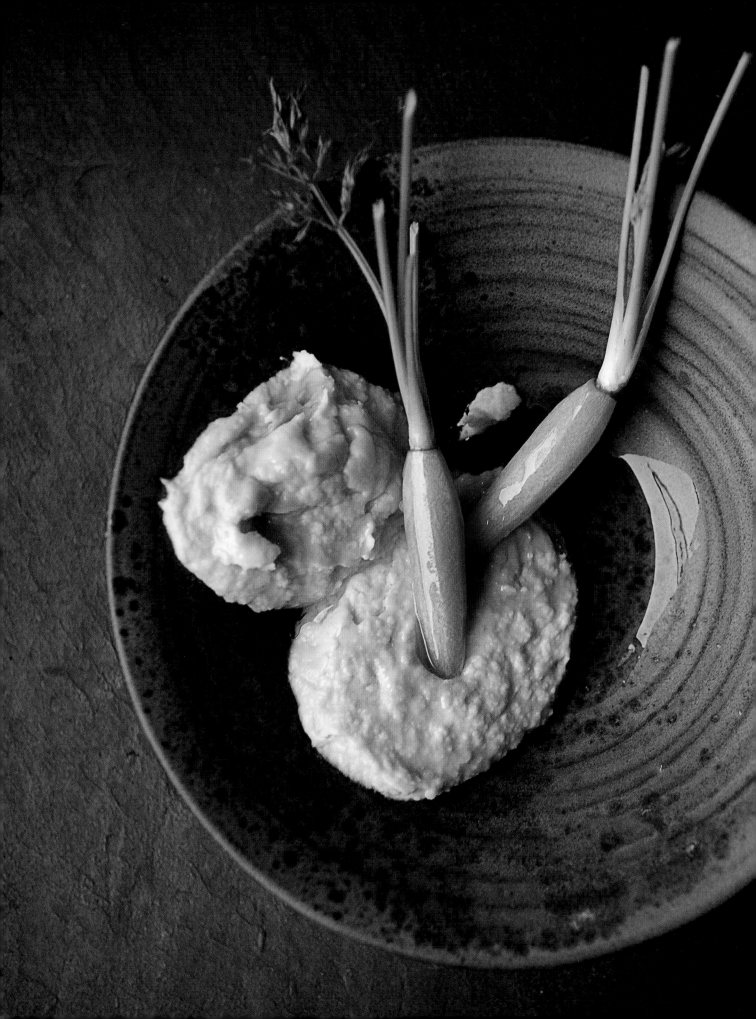

WHITE BEAN DIP *with* BABY VEGETABLES

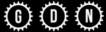

250 G WHITE BEANS
3 SPRIGS THYME
2 STAR ANISE
2 BAY LEAVES
1 TSP SALT
1 PIECE KOMBU SEAWEED
200 ML MINERAL WATER
3 TBSP TAHINI
1 CLOVE GARLIC
¼ BUNCH TARRAGON
100 ML OLIVE OIL
SALT
1 TBSP HONEY
JUICE OF 1 LEMON

ACCOMPANIMENT:
BABY CARROTS,
CELERY STALKS,
CUCUMBER ETC.

Soak the beans in cold water overnight.

Drain and rinse the beans. Bring to a boil in unsalted water with the thyme, star anise, bay leaves, salt and kombu. Reduce the heat and simmer until the beans are ready – about 40 minutes.

Drain the beans and blend them with the water, tahini, grated garlic and tarragon. While blending, slowly pour in the olive oil. Season with salt, honey and lemon juice. If necessary, adjust the consistency with water.

Serve with raw, clean baby vegetables and freshly baked bread.

CHICKPEAS, *fennel,* PINEAPPLE AND MINT

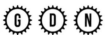

250 G DRIED CHICKPEAS
2 STAR ANISE
2 BAY LEAVES
SALT
1 PIECE KOMBU SEAWEED
1 FENNEL BULB
JUICE OF 1 LEMON
2 YELLOW PEPPERS
1 PINEAPPLE
½ BUNCH MINT
100 ML LIME VINAIGRETTE
(SEE PAGE 325)

Soak the chickpeas in cold water overnight.

Drain, rinse and bring the chickpeas to a boil in unsalted water with the star anise, bay leaves, salt and kombu. Reduce the heat and simmer for about 40 minutes until the chickpeas are tender. Remove from the heat and let cool in the liquid.

Rinse the fennel and cut thinly across the grain on a mandolin. Submerge in cold water with lemon juice. Wash the peppers and dice them.

Cut off the top, bottom and peel of the pineapple. Quarter, cut out the core and dice the wedges into roughly 1x1 cm cubes. Rinse the mint leaves and slice them thinly. Drain the chickpeas and fennel. Toss together with the peppers, pineapple, mint and lime vinaigrette.

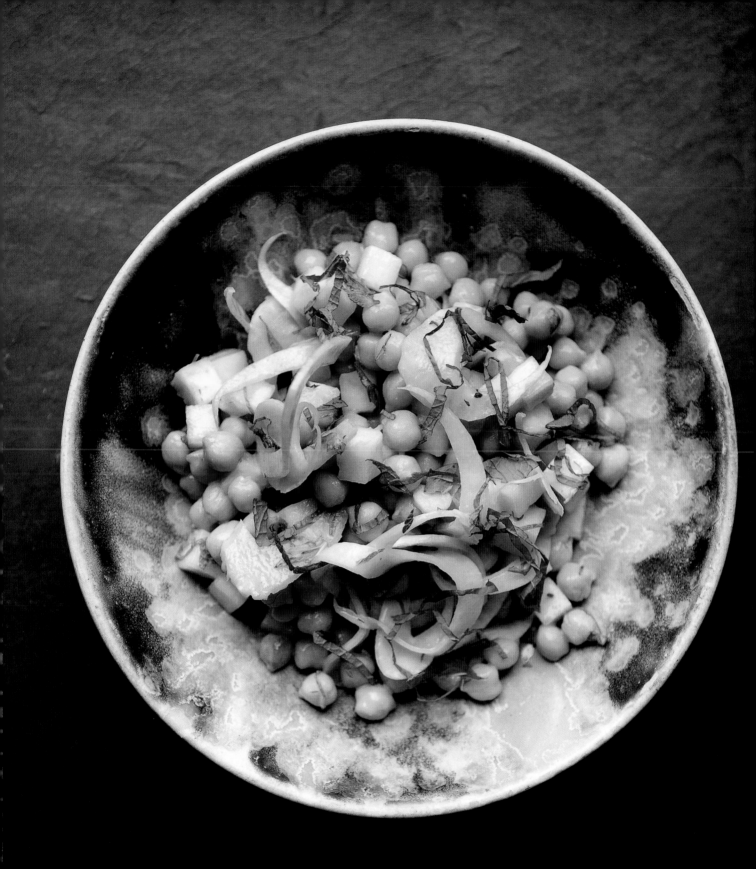

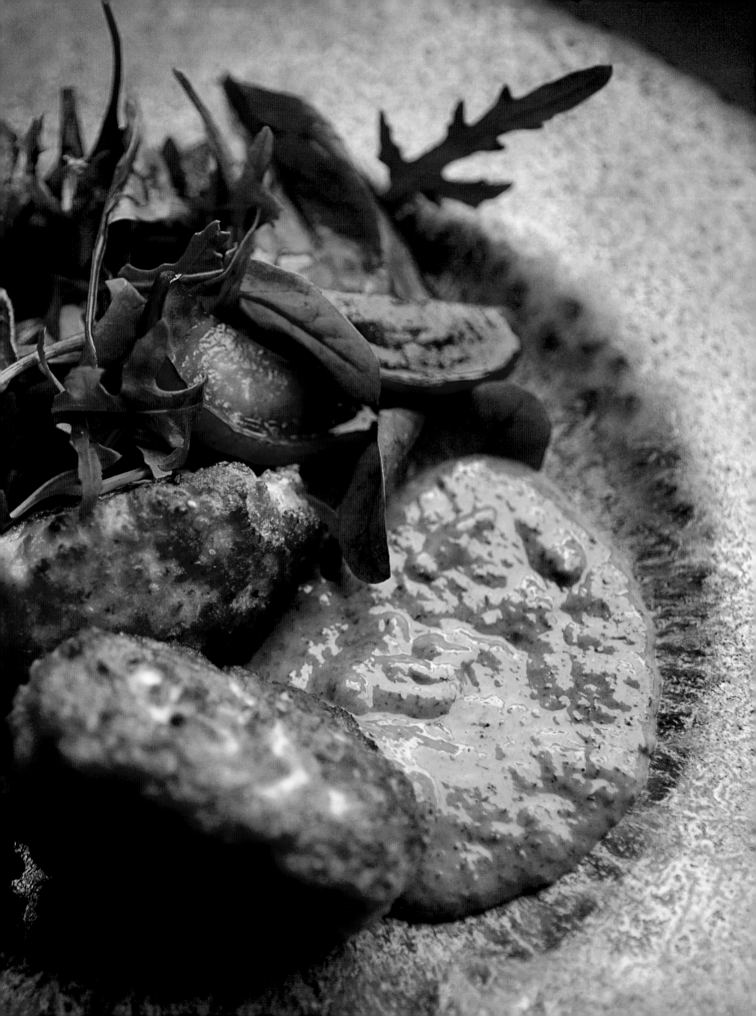

CHICKEN *meatballs*
WITH ROCKET SAUCE

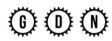

500 G MINCED CHICKEN

2 EGGS

100 G GLUTEN-FREE OATMEAL

100 ML RICE MILK OR WHOLE MILK

1 RED ONION

1 CLOVE GARLIC

1 TBSP DIJON MUSTARD

1 TSP GROUND CORIANDER

ZEST OF 1 ORGANIC LEMON

SALT AND FRESHLY GROUND
BLACK PEPPER

300 ML ROCKET SAUCE (SEE PAGE 328)

Preheat the oven to 200°C.

Thoroughly mix the chicken mince with salt, then eggs and oatmeal. Warm the milk to bathwater temperature and slowly pour into the mince, stirring until homogenised. Peel and mince the onions and garlic, mix with the mustard, coriander and lemon zest and stir into the chicken mince. To test the seasoning, fry a teaspoon of the mince in a pan with a little olive oil. If necessary, season the rest of the mixture with salt and pepper. Refrigerate for 30 minutes.

Scoop out the mince mixture with a tablespoon and place each spoonful on a baking tray covered with baking paper leaving 3-4 cm around each one. Drizzle with olive oil and bake until the meatballs are firm and cooked through – about 8 minutes.

Serve with the rocket sauce, roasted plums and fresh rocket.

SEA BREAM *with* SWEETCORN AND TARRAGON

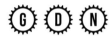

4 SEA BREAM, SCALED AND CLEANED
4 BANANA SHALLOTS
200 ML PICKLING LIQUID #2
(SEE PAGE 334)
2 CLOVES GARLIC
50 ML OLIVE OIL
2 LEMONS
4 FRESH CORN COBS
1 BUNCH TARRAGON
OLIVE OIL
SALT AND FRESHLY GROUND
BLACK PEPPER

Preheat the oven to 175°C.

Peel the shallots and slice them into rings about 2 cm thick. In a frying pan over high heat, fry the cut surface of each ring in a little olive oil until one side is well caramelised and the shallot is cooked through. Transfer to a bowl and cover with hot pickling liquid. Set aside.

Rinse the bream and pat dry with a paper towel. Score the skin diagonally on both sides with a knife. Peel the garlic and crush it in a mortar with olive oil, zest and juice of one lemon and salt. Rub the fish with the mixture, season with salt and pepper and place on a baking tray covered with baking paper. Cook the fish for about 15 minutes until the flesh easily can be lifted off the bone.

Remove the husk and silk from the corn and cut off the kernels. Drain the pickled shallots. Rinse the tarragon, pick off the leaves and chop them. Sauté the corn in a frying pan with a little olive oil and salt. Add the shallots and tarragon and cook until evenly heated.

Serve the fish topped with the corn and onion garnish and the lemon slices and couscous on the side.

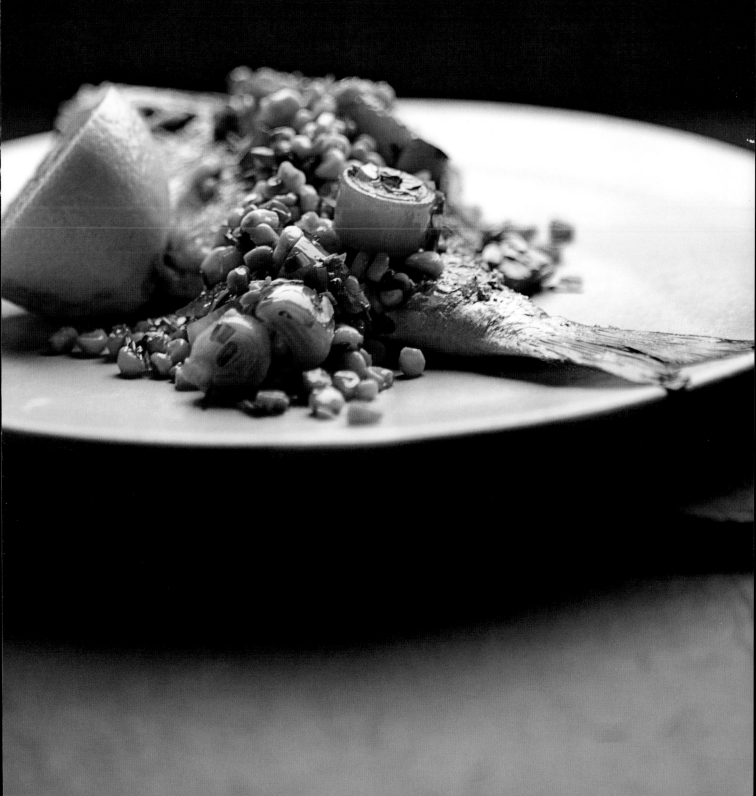

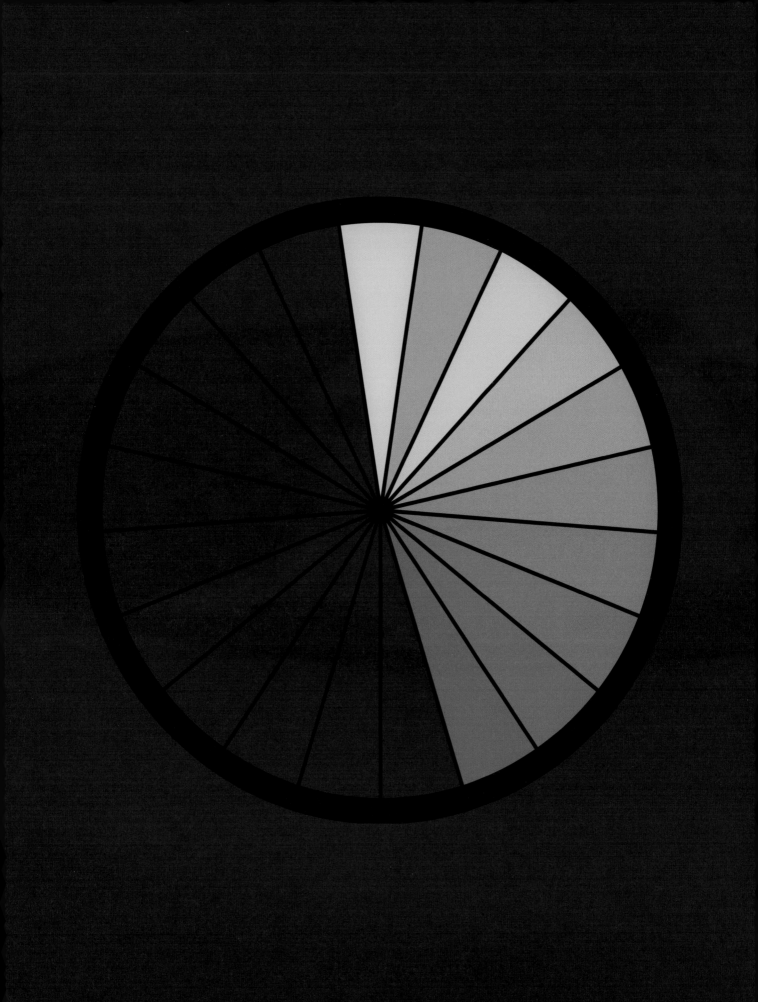

DAY 10

STAGE 9

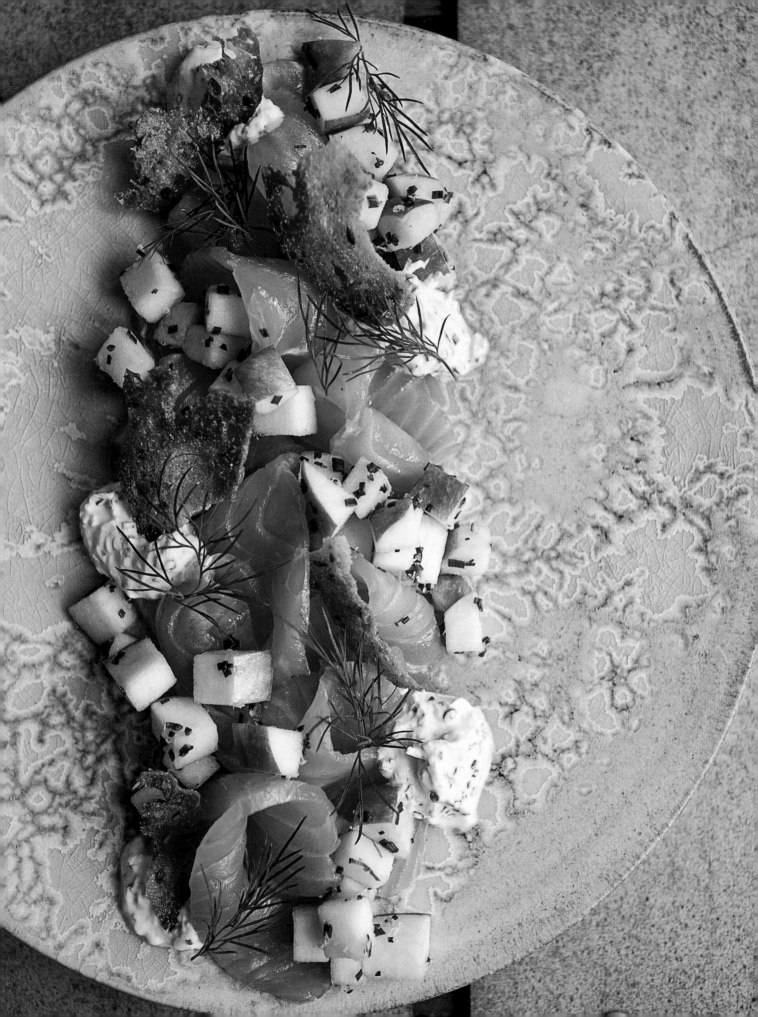

CURED SALMON,
DILL, APPLE *and*
SHEEP'S YOGHURT

500 G SALMON FILLET, DEBONED
3 TSP SALT
1 TBSP CLEAR HONEY
16 THIN SLICES OF DAY OLD BREAD
2 APPLES
JUICE AND ZEST OF 2 ORGANIC LEMONS
100 ML SHEEP'S YOGHURT
½ BUNCH CHIVES
½ BUNCH DILL
2 TBSP OLIVE OIL
SALT AND FRESHLY GROUND
BLACK PEPPER

Trim the salmon and lay it skin-side down. Sprinkle the flesh side with salt and drizzle with honey. Cover the salmon with cling film and refrigerate overnight.

Preheat the oven to 170°C.

Lay the bread slices on a baking tray covered with baking paper, drizzle with olive oil and sprinkle with salt. Bake for about 7-8 minutes until golden and crisp.

Rinse the apples, quarter, remove the cores and dice. Zest both lemons. Finely chop the chives.

Marinate the apple in the juice and the zest of one lemon. Stir the zest from the other lemon and a little more than half of the chives into the yoghurt. Season to taste with freshly ground pepper and the remaining lemon juice.

Drain the apple cubes. Toss with the remainder of the finely sliced chives and a little olive oil.

Rinse and drain the dill.

Cut the salmon into thin slices and plate with the apple, yoghurt and croutons. Garnish with dill.

ROAST VEAL, SWEET POTATO COMPOTE AND COOKED ONION

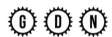

1 KG VEAL SIRLOIN, TRIMMED
¼ BUNCH THYME
2 TBSP OLIVE OIL
SALT AND FRESHLY GROUND
BLACK PEPPER
4 RED ONIONS
1 KG SWEET POTATOES
½ BUNCH CHIVES
2 LEMONS
2 BANANA SHALLOTS
50 ML OLIVE OIL

Preheat the oven to 200°C.

Wrap the sirloin in thyme and tie it up with meat string. Rub the veal with olive oil and season with salt and pepper. Place the meat on a rack in the oven above a roasting tin. Roast for 15 minutes and rest for 15 minutes, then roast for another 10 minutes. When the sirloin feels firm and no longer soft in the centre, it's done. Take it out and let it rest for 10 minutes before slicing it. The core temperature should be between 54 to 56°C. Depending on the thickness, increase or decrease the final interval.

Rinse, but do not peel, the red onions. Bring the onions to a boil in lightly salted water, reduce the heat and simmer for 5 minutes. Remove the pan from the heat and let it rest for 10 minutes. Peel off the outer skin and halve the onions.

Peel the sweet potatoes, chop them into large chunks and boil until tender. Rinse and finely cut the chives. Rinse and zest the lemons. Peel the shallots and cut into thin rings.

Drain the potatoes and let them steam dry over low heat in the pan. Using a whisk, crush the potatoes and add olive oil to make a coarse compote. Season with salt, pepper, lemon juice. Add the chives, lemon zest and shallots just before serving.

Serve the veal, compote and onions with olive oil and lemon juice.

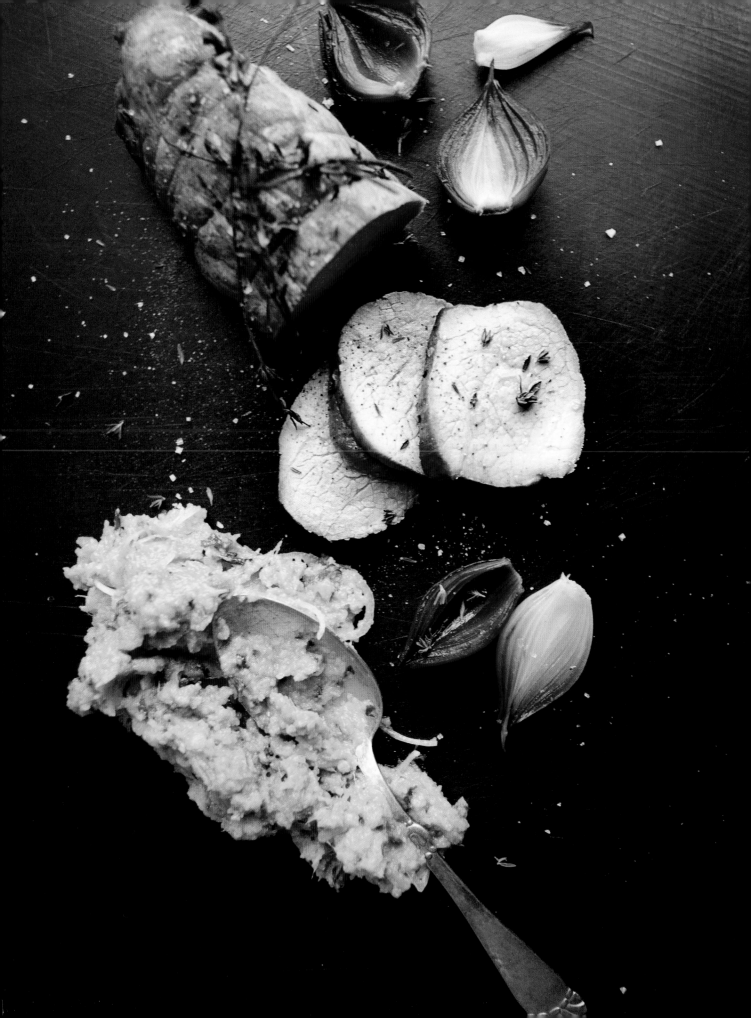

CHOCOLATE MOUSSE
70%

300 G 70% DARK CHOCOLATE
200 ML EGG WHITE, PASTEURISED
80 G LIGHT CANE SUGAR
1 PINCH FINE SALT
100 ML EGG YOLK, PASTEURISED
500 ML WHIPPING CREAM

Melt the chocolate in a double boiler.

Whisk at medium speed, in a mixer, the egg whites with 40 g of sugar, adding it a little at a time until you can make soft peaks and it's firm enough to stick to the bowl when turned upside down. In a clean bowl, whisk the egg yolks with the remaining 40 g of sugar until white and fluffy. Lightly whisk the cream to a soft consistency – the cream should not be straight out of the fridge.

Folding the mousse needs care and attention. Fold with a rubber spatula by cutting through the mixture and then twisting the bowl around a quarter, counter clockwise. Use this technique throughout all the stages of folding. Work fast and efficiently once you start folding or else it will split or set.

Fold the egg yolks into the melted chocolate with a rubber spatula, then fold in the egg whites and finally, gently fold in the cream. Spoon the mousse into cups or bowls and chill for at least 3 hours before serving. Serve with fresh fruit of your choice.

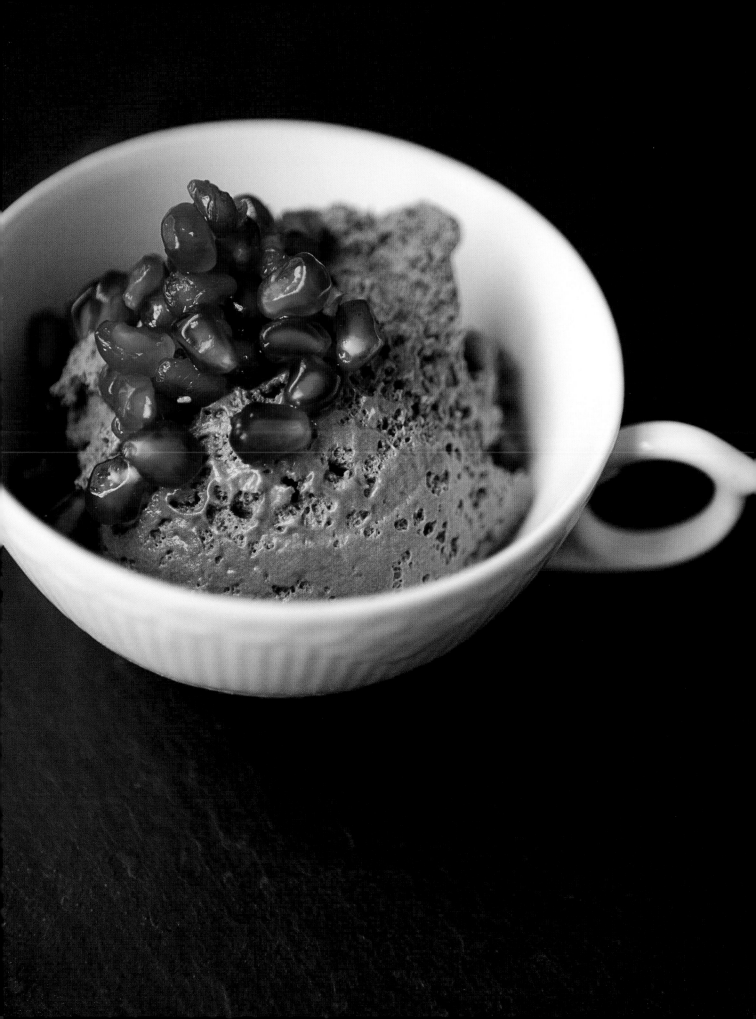

ALBERTO CONTADOR

"IT'S DURING THE MEAL THAT THE STRENGTH OF THE TEAM IS BUILT UP"

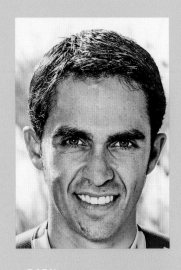

BORN: 6th December 1982
NATIONALITY: Spanish
EXPERIENCE: Professional since 2003
FORMER CYCLING TEAMS: Once, Discovery Channel and Astana
FAVOURITE RACE: Giro d'Italia – partly because of the wonderful "tifosi"

Hannah (H): Why is it important for you to sit at a table and eat together with your teammates at the end of a day's stage or race?

Alberto Contador (AC): It's probably the most important time of the day because we are able to sit still, calm down and talk about the day's race and about our private lives. And of course it's important to have a bit of time to relax after a hard day's work. This is where we, as a team, bond.

H: What difference does the meal make for you as a rider?

AC: The first thing, of course, is refuelling. We know what is waiting ahead of us and it's crucial that we eat a nutritious meal so we can be well prepared for the next day. Also it's during the meal that the strength of the team is built up. Suddenly our relationships aren't just professional but also personal. Not just with the riders, but also with the other team members.

H: What do you think of the fact that the team employs a chef who makes sure that the food you eat is healthy and properly prepared?

AC: It's great. As professional riders, we are under a lot of pressure both physically and mentally. This means it's important that we, with a team chef, can trust that all the food is fresh and prepared with care and good hygiene so we can stay well, fresh and strong. The timing is also very important. We don't have to sit and wait for a long time to get the food served. It's always there on time and that is important when, for example, you are doing a time trial. Also, there's the benefit that you can request something special like your favourite dish or, for example, we can have dishes prepared from the tomatoes grown in my dad's garden served for dinner. It's little special things like this that also make a big difference. Then of course, when there is a celebration or a birthday, there is always something made especially for that.

H: What is your opinion on healthy food for athletes in general?

AC: My motto is: the simpler, the better. The best ingredients and a gifted and accomplished chef in the kitchen make for the best results. The food is prepared with care and thought and you know that all the products are of high quality. For the well being of the riders, this is for sure the way to go.

H: What is your favourite food?

AC: *Tortilla de patatas* (potato tortilla)! And I love the Paella from my hometown.

MICHAEL MØRKØV

"I CAN FEEL MY BODY WORKING BETTER"

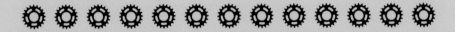

Hannah (H): What difference does food make for you physically and/or mentally during a long season or race?

Michael Mørkøv (MM): As far as I'm concerned, during a cycle race, breakfast and dinner are the highlights of the day. Getting the right food is extremely important. But it is equally important to keep up the morale and enjoy meals.

H: In what way do you think food can change an athlete's performance?

MM: The right diet is crucial for a cyclist. You should preferably be loaded with the right energy, which not only lasts a long time, but also helps your recovery.

H: What has the proper diet meant for you personally as a cyclist?

MM: When I eat healthy, nutritious food, I can feel my body working better and find it easier to recover, and everybody knows that good recovery is the key to a successful race.

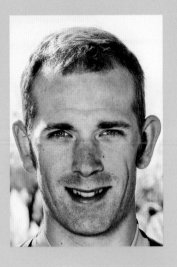

H: In what way has your opinion on food for athletes changed over the past year?

MM: I've always paid great attention to what I eat. In particular, I noticed that my pollen allergy was much less severe when last year I stopped eating dairy and wheat products for three months.

H: Have you found that food can improve or worsen your condition?

MM: There's no doubt that I've become aware that there are some foods which I find more difficult to digest and which I have an allergic reaction to, and when I avoid these types of food, I can breathe better, it's easier for me to lose weight and I have more energy in general.

H: How do you see the future of cycling in terms of food?

MM: It's getting more and more common for teams to have a chef and a kitchen truck, so it looks like an area that's getting a lot of attention and that teams are trying to make the most of it.

H: What is your favourite food?

MM: Spare ribs!

BORN: 30th April 1985
NATIONALITY: Danish
EXPERIENCE: Professional since 2005
FORMER CYCLING TEAMS: Team GLS
FAVOURITE RACE: The Tour of Flanders

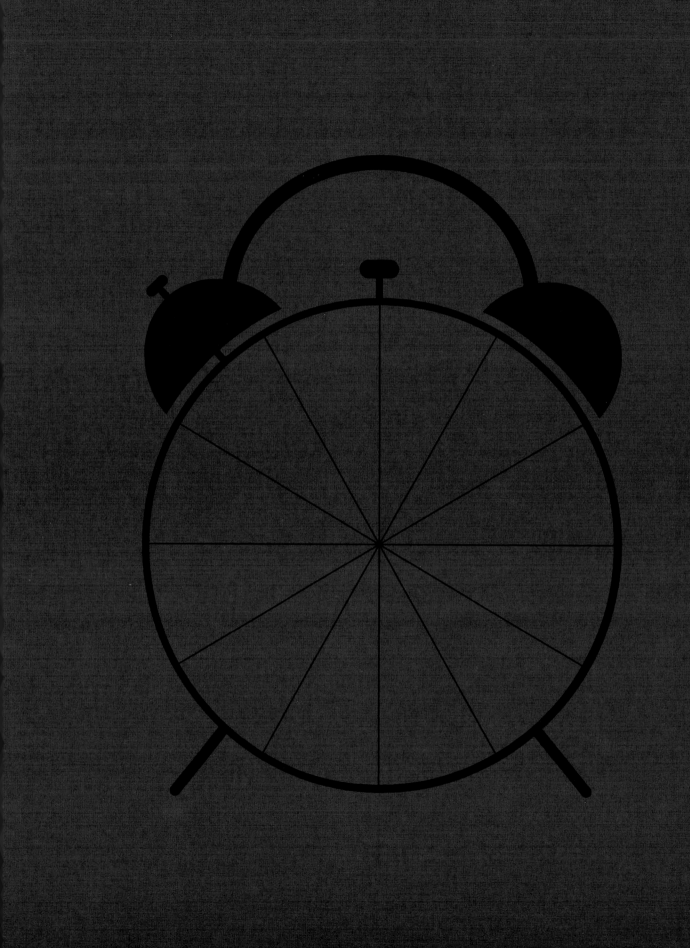

1

REST DAY

LUNCH

EGGS, TOMATO *and* BAKED SALMON

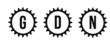

600 G SALMON
6 EGGS
6 TOMATOES
1 BUNCH CHIVES
SALT AND FRESHLY GROUND
BLACK PEPPER

Preheat the oven to 170°C.

Clean and trim off the fat and small bones from the salmon, season with salt and bake for about 8 minutes until you can slide a carving fork through the flesh without resistance. Let the salmon rest and cool down before serving.

Bring a pot of salted water to a boil, submerge the eggs and boil for 8 minutes. Cool the eggs under cold, running water. Peel and halve. Rinse the tomatoes, slice into wedges. Finely cut the chives.

Carefully flake the fish onto a serving platter and top with the tomato and egg. Garnish with the chives, salt and pepper.

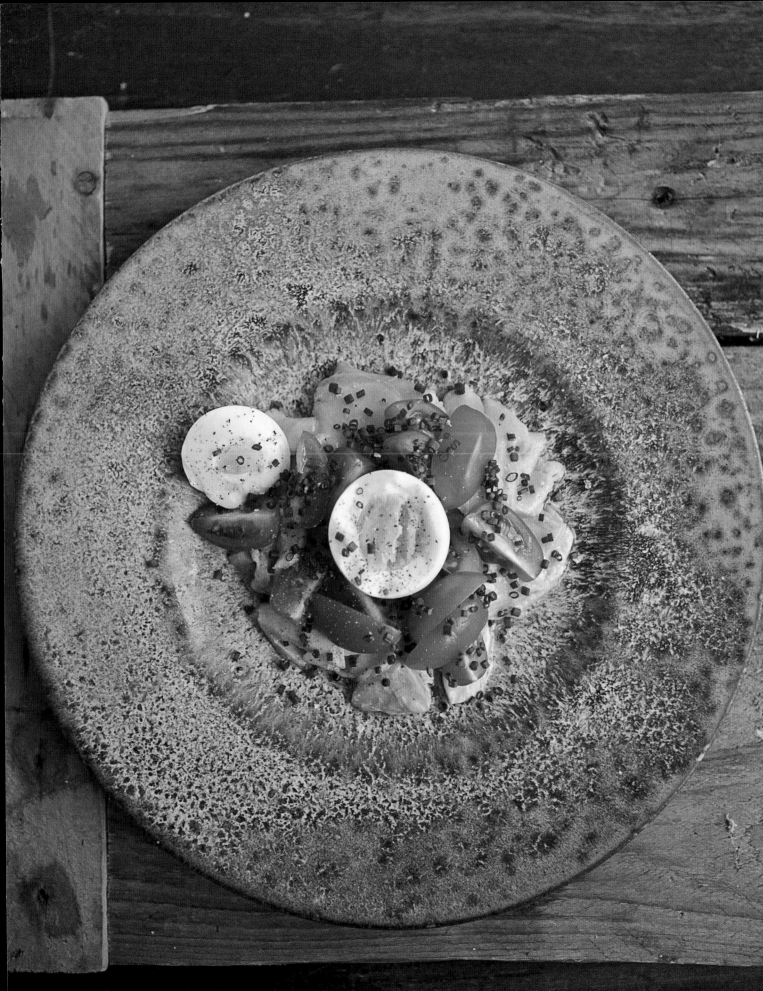

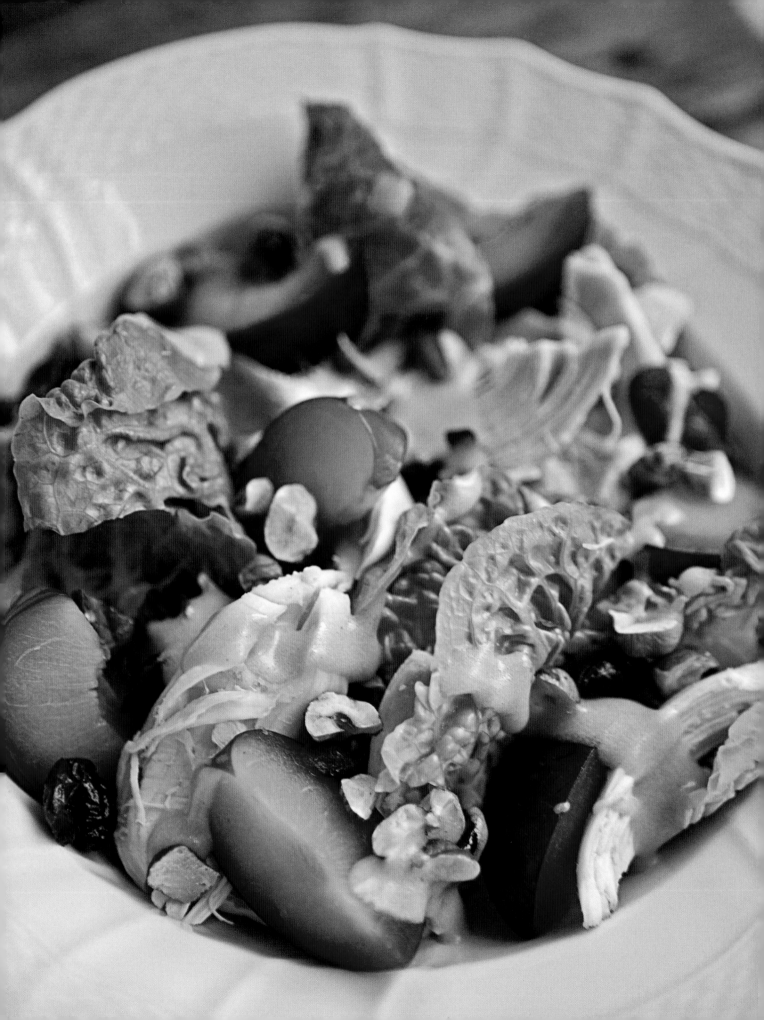

LUNCH

SALAD *with*
CHICKEN, FRESH PLUMS, CRANBERRIES AND HAZELNUTS

1 COLD, COOKED CHICKEN
3 PLUMS
50 G DRIED CRANBERRIES
50 G HAZELNUTS
2 HEADS ROMAINE LETTUCE
100 ML ELDERFLOWER VINAIGRETTE
(SEE PAGE 323)

Preheat the oven to 170°C.

Pull the chicken into bite-sized pieces. Rinse and halve the plums. Remove the pits and slice into thin wedges. Tear, rinse and spin the romaine lettuce. Roast the hazelnuts in the oven for 6-7 minutes. Let them cool and chop coarsely.

Toss the chicken, plums, romaine lettuce and vinaigrette together and top with cranberries and hazelnuts.

LUNCH

CHARCUTERIE, FENNEL, RED ONION AND CAPERBERRIES

80 G EACH OF A SELECTION OF
CHARCUTERIE, E.G. COPPA, PARMA HAM,
BRESAOLA, CURED SAUSAGE
1 FENNEL BULB
2 TBSP OLIVE OIL
3 TBSP BALSAMIC VINEGAR
1 RED ONION
50 ML PICKLING LIQUID #1
(SEE PAGE 334)
1 BUNCH CHERVIL
½ FRISÉE LETTUCE
50 G CAPERBERRIES

Cut the top off the fennel bulb. Halve the bulb lengthwise and cut into 1 cm thick wedges. Rinse well and drain on paper towels. Sear the cut surfaces on a pan with olive oil and salt until they are well caramelised. Add the balsamic vinegar and reduce.

Peel and finely slice the red onion. Place in a bowl and pour over the cold pickling liquid. Rinse and pick the chervil. Tear the frisée lettuce into bite-size pieces, rinse well and spin dry.

Arrange the charcuterie with the fennel, top with caperberries, lettuce and the pickled onion. Serve with bread and Dijon mustard.

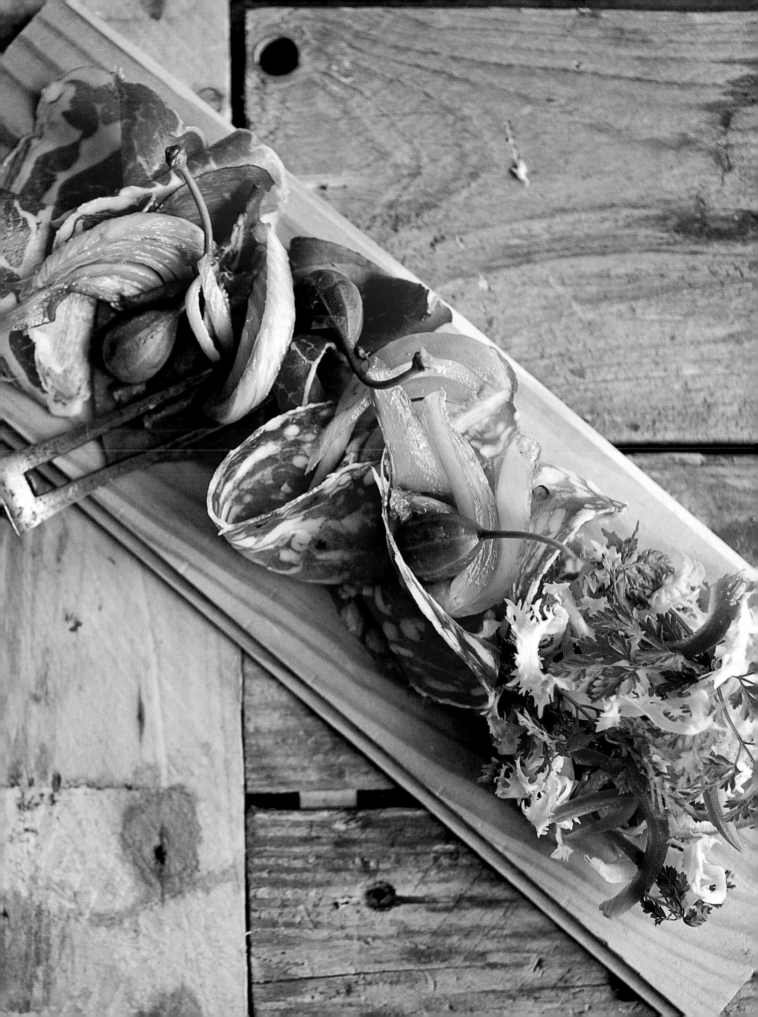

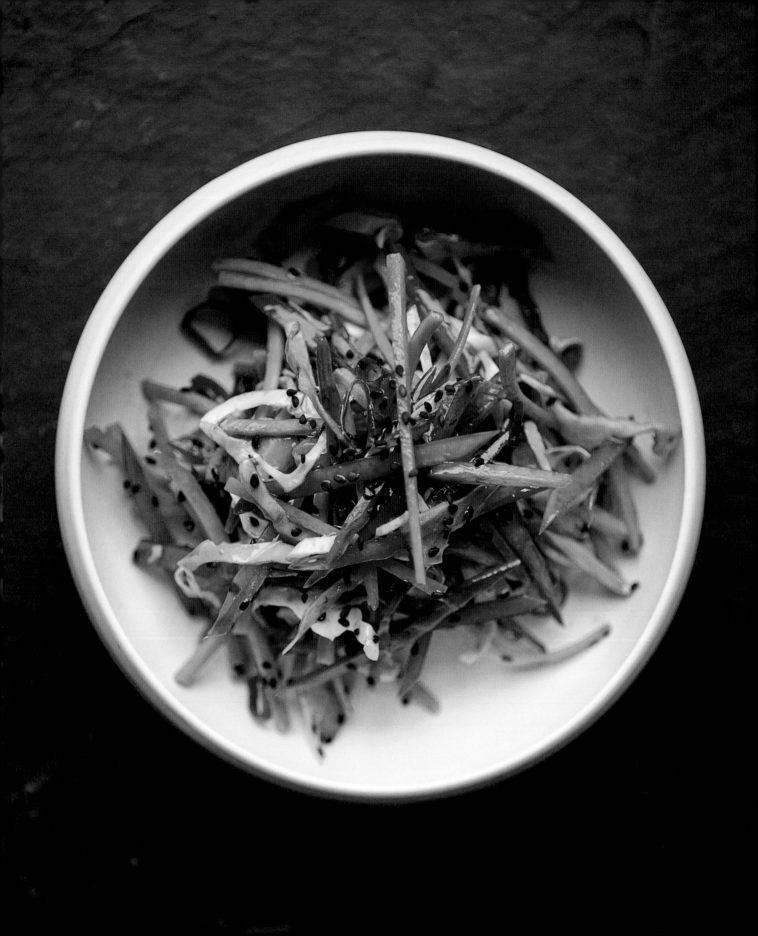

SUGAR SNAP PEA
AND CABBAGE SALAD

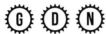

100 G SUGAR SNAP PEAS
1 LITRE WATER
1 TSP SALT
3 CARROTS
¼ HEAD OF WHITE CABBAGE
1 TBSP GRATED GINGER
50 ML SOY SAUCE AND SESAME
DRESSING (SEE PAGE 326)

Rinse the sugar snap peas and pinch off the ends. Blanch in salted boiling water for 7-8 seconds and immediately immerse them in a bowl of iced water. Slice diagonally.

Peel the carrots and grate them in a food processor or julienne with a mandolin. Slice the white cabbage finely with a mandolin or by hand. Toss the white cabbage, carrot, sugar snap peas and ginger in the soy sauce and sesame dressing. Finish off with a sprinkle of black sesame seeds.

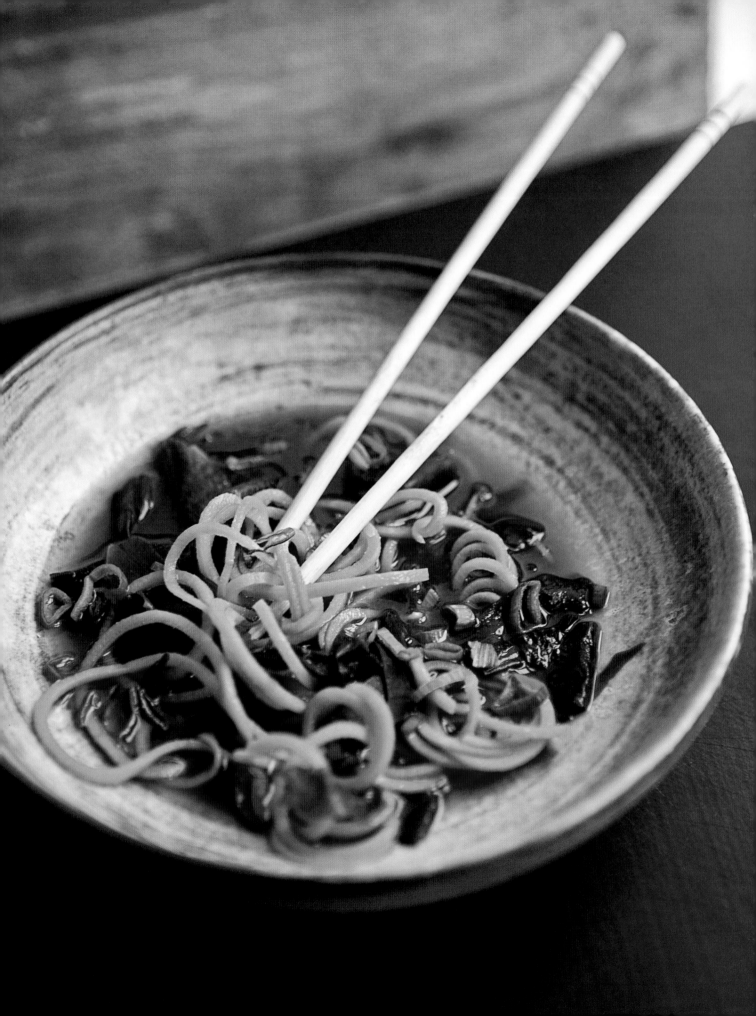

DINNER

MISO SOUP,
CARROT NOODLES *and*
WAKAME SEAWEED

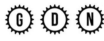

**1 LITRE MISO SOUP,
FROM PASTE OR INSTANT
4 CARROTS
1 BUNCH SPRING ONIONS
50 G WAKAME SEAWEED**

Start by making the miso soup according to the instructions on the packet. Peel the carrots and create spaghetti-like noodles using a spiralizer. Alternatively, you can slice thinly with a mandolin and cut into spaghetti with a sharp knife. Peel off the outer skin of the spring onions, cut off the top and cut finely. Bring the soup to a boil, season with salt, add the carrots, wakame and spring onions and then simmer for 2 minutes.

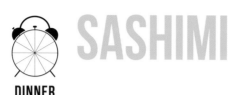

SASHIMI

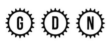

DINNER

200 G SALMON FILLET
200 G TUNA FILLET
200 G WHITE FISH FILLET
250 G BROWN SUSHI RICE
1 TSP SALT
1 CUCUMBER
100 G PICKLED GINGER
SOY SAUCE
WASABI

Go to your fishmonger and get fresh fish ideal for eating raw. Slice into thin slices and refrigerate.

Prepare the sushi rice according to the instructions on the packet and allow to cool.

Peel the cucumber and shave it into long ribbons using a peeler. Let the cucumber ribbons crisp up in iced water for 30 min.

Plate the fish on top of the rice, top with cucumber ribbons and serve with soy sauce, pickled ginger and wasabi.

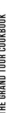

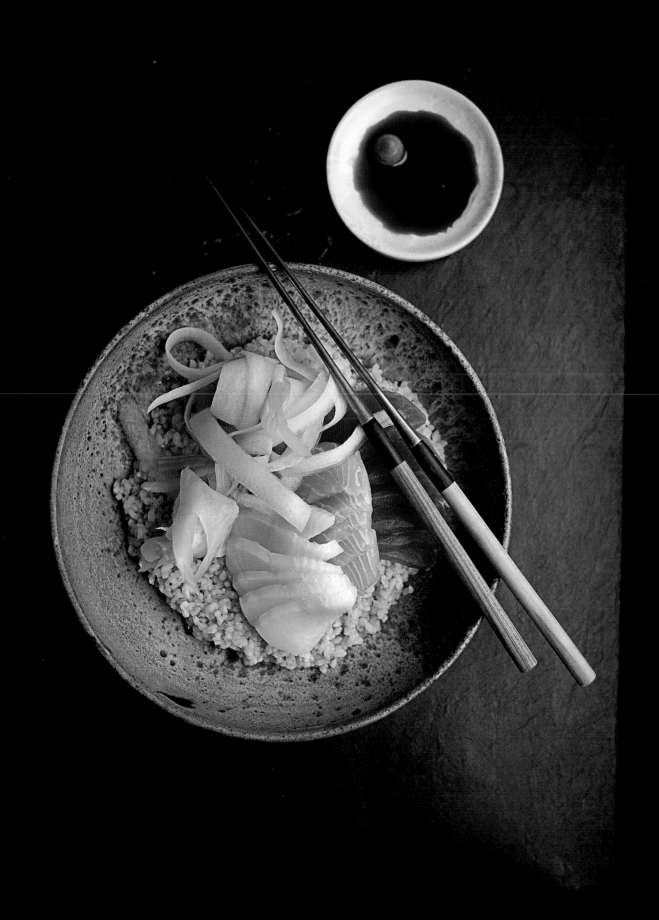

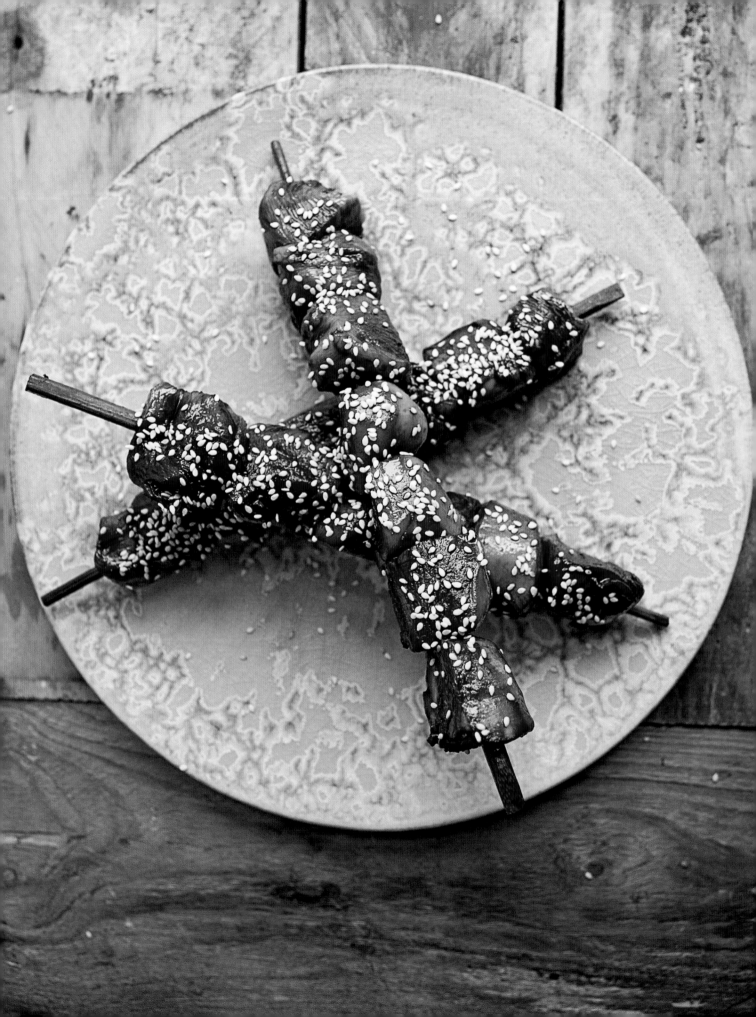

CHICKEN TERIYAKI
SKEWERS

DINNER

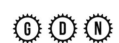

600 G BONELESS CHICKEN LEGS
4 TBSP SAKE
100 ML SOY SAUCE
50 ML MIRIN
2 TBSP HONEY
1 TBSP OLIVE OIL
WHITE SESAME
WOODEN SKEWERS

Cut the chicken into bite-sized pieces. Mix the sake, soy sauce, mirin, honey and olive oil. Marinate the chicken in the mixture for at least 20 minutes or preferably overnight.

Preheat the oven to 175°C.

Place the wooden skewers in water for 5-10 minutes to prevent them from burning during cooking. Spear 5-6 pieces of chicken on each wooden skewer and roast them in the oven for about 10-12 minutes until the chicken is firm and but still juicy. In a saucepan, reduce the leftover marinade to a thick sauce and pour over the chicken pieces before serving. Sprinkle with sesame seeds.

A DAY
IN THE KITCHEN TRUCK

A NORMAL WORKING DAY FOR ME LASTS BETWEEN 14 AND 18 HOURS SPREAD OVER THE DAY, INCLUDING COOKING, DRIVING, SHOPPING, CLEANING AND PREPARATION.

6.00 am – I get up two hours before the riders eat breakfast and cook the breakfast buffet so everyone can get what they need in order to get through the day's stage.

8.00 am – The food's ready and the riders eat. Meanwhile, my colleague and I pack up the kitchen truck so it's ready for the 200 km long transfer to the next hotel.

9.00 am – The riders have finished eating. We pack up the coffee machine and buffet, hop into a team car and drive to the next hotel.

12.00 noon – We arrive at the hotel, park the cars and trucks, introduce ourselves to the kitchen staff, eat lunch and take a small break before we have to go shopping.

1.30 pm – When we shop, we fill up for about four days at a time, so we have more time on a daily basis to create new dishes in the kitchen. An efficient shopping trip takes 2-2.5 hours and fills up two shopping carts to the top.

3.30 pm – We return to the hotel and the kitchen truck, organise everything and immediately start cooking. We plan the menu from day to day according to the stages, the weather, the ingredients available and the occasion.

The riders' meal time changes depending on the stages and how long it takes to get back to the hotel. But, generally speaking, I plan on 8.00 pm and always get things going in the kitchen four hours before dinnertime.

6.00 pm – The riders arrive at the hotel and just over two hours later, dinner has to be on the table.

8.00 pm – While the hungry riders eat, we thoroughly clean the kitchen truck, all the surfaces, cabinets and drawers are washed down and the floor is scrubbed so the kitchen's ready for a new day.

9.00 pm – The riders have usually finished eating by now so my colleague and I grab a bite to eat before we clear the buffet.

9.30 pm – The last task on the agenda is to pack the following day's after-race food boxes, which the riders eat on the bus after the next day's stage.

10.00 pm – I close up the kitchen truck and update my Instagram and Twitter profile (@dailystews) with the menu of the day for all the fans to see.

11.00 pm – Zzzzz...

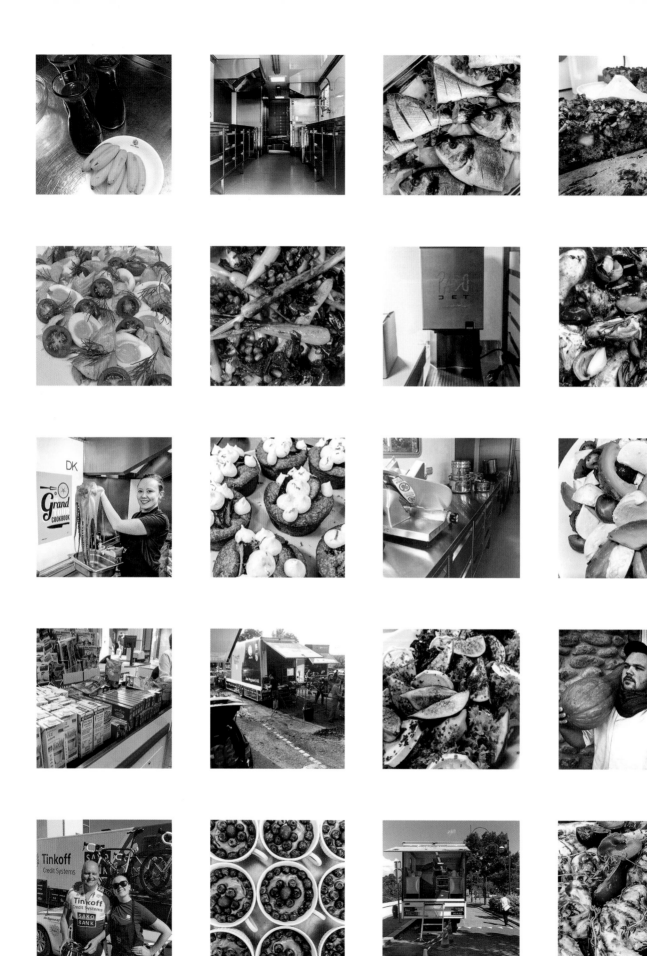

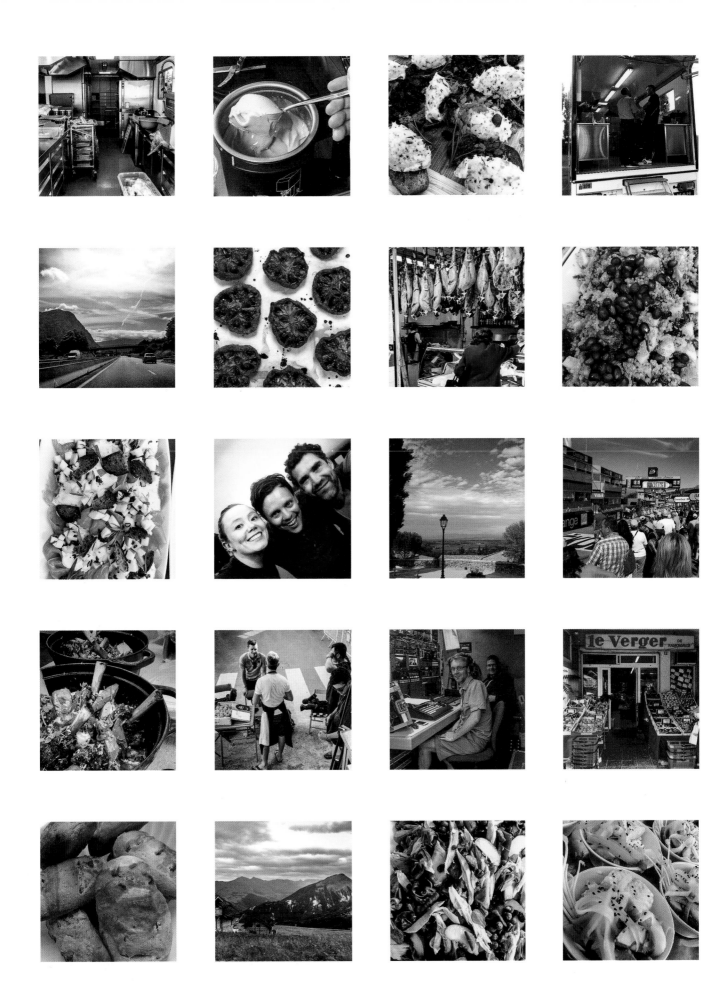

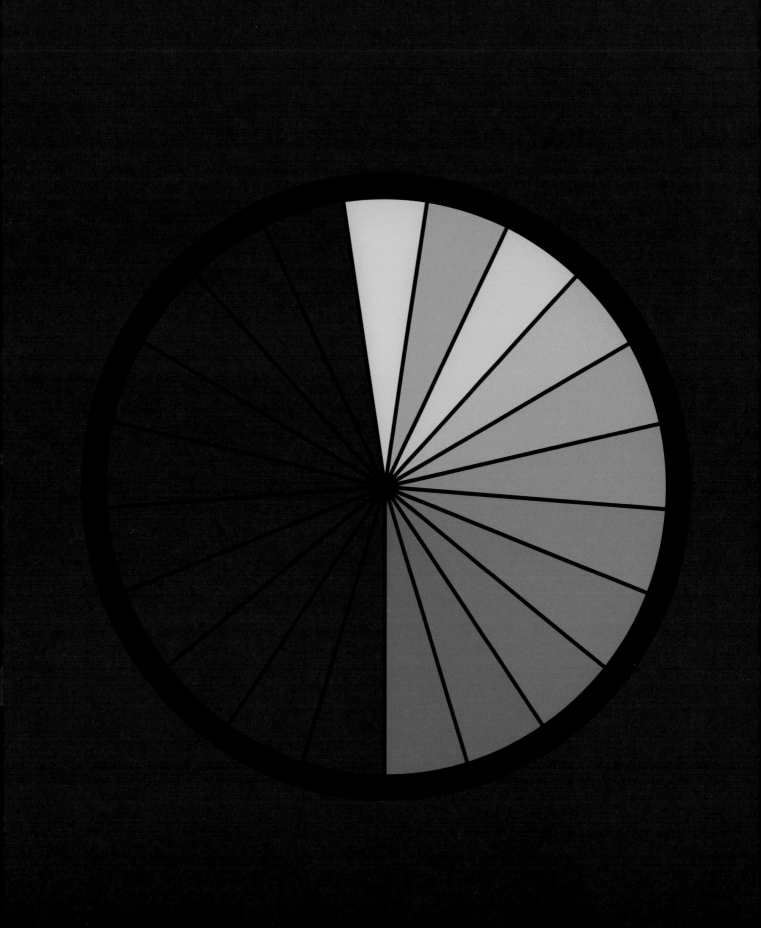

11

DAY

STAGE 10

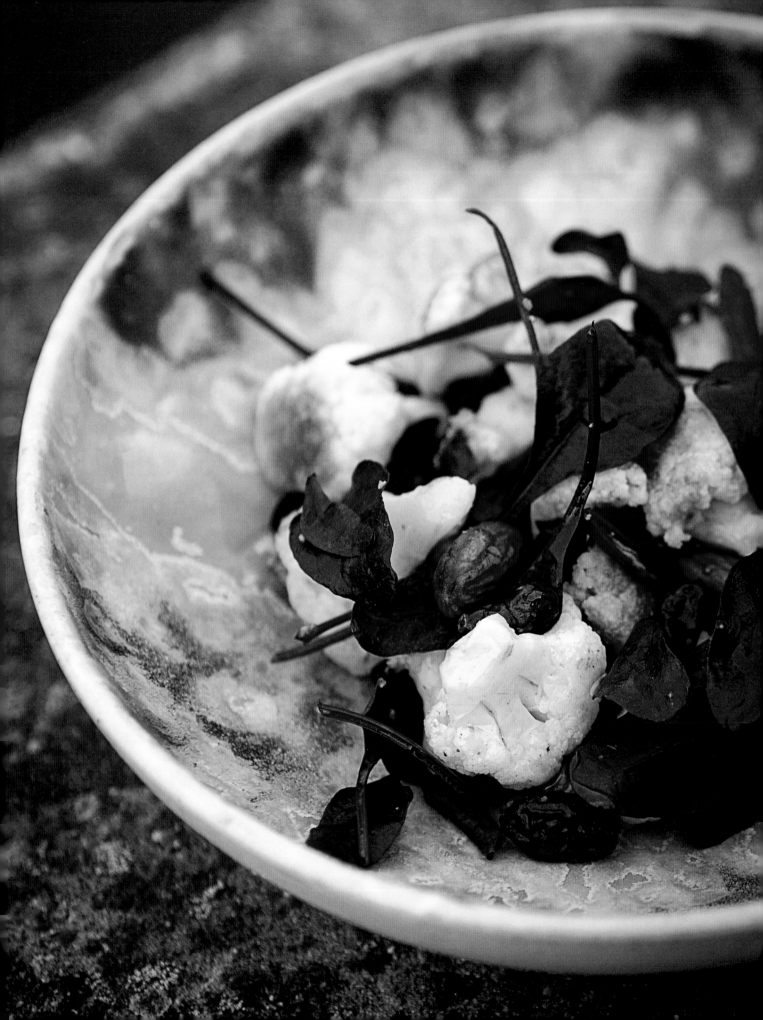

CARAMELISED
CAULIFLOWER *and*
ALMOND SALAD

1 CAULIFLOWER
3 TBSP OLIVE OIL
100 G ALMONDS
200 G BULLS BLOOD LEAFS OR OTHER
BABY LETTUCE
50 G GOJI BERRIES
50 ML CIDER VINEGAR VINAIGRETTE
(SEE PAGE 323)

Preheat the oven to 170°C.

Separate the cauliflower into bite-sized florets and chop the stalk into chunks of the same size. Pan-roast the cauliflower in a splash of olive oil until nicely caramelised, sweet and tender with a bit of bite. Cool to room temperature before serving.

Toast the almonds in the oven until golden – about 7-8 minutes – let them cool down. Rinse the salad leaves and drain.

Toss the cauliflower with the almonds, salad leaves, goji berries and vinaigrette.

PEARL BARLEY,
ROASTED FENNEL, MANGO AND MINT

1 LARGE MANGO
2 FENNEL BULBS
1 CLOVE GARLIC
JUICE AND ZEST OF 1 ORGANIC LEMON
½ BUNCH PARSLEY
200 G PEARL BARLEY, BOILED
5 TBSP OLIVE OIL
SALT AND FRESHLY GROUND
BLACK PEPPER

Cut the mango lengthwise along the stone and separate the halves. Cut the two halves into wedges, peel and cut into cubes.

Cut the tops off the fennel bulbs, rinse and dice. In a pan over medium heat caramelise in olive oil and salt until the fennel is tender. Grate the garlic and zest the lemon over the warm fennel and mix well. Pick the parsley off the stalk, rinse well, dry and chop.

Toss the pearl barley, mango, fennel and parsley together. Season with olive oil, lemon juice, salt and pepper.

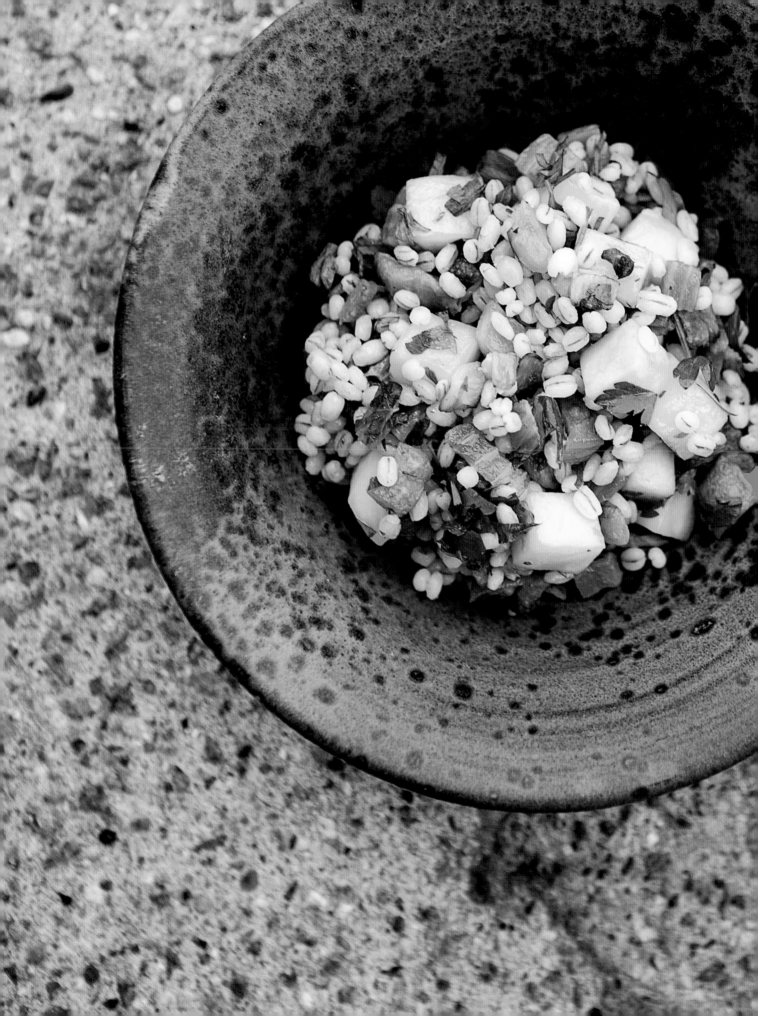

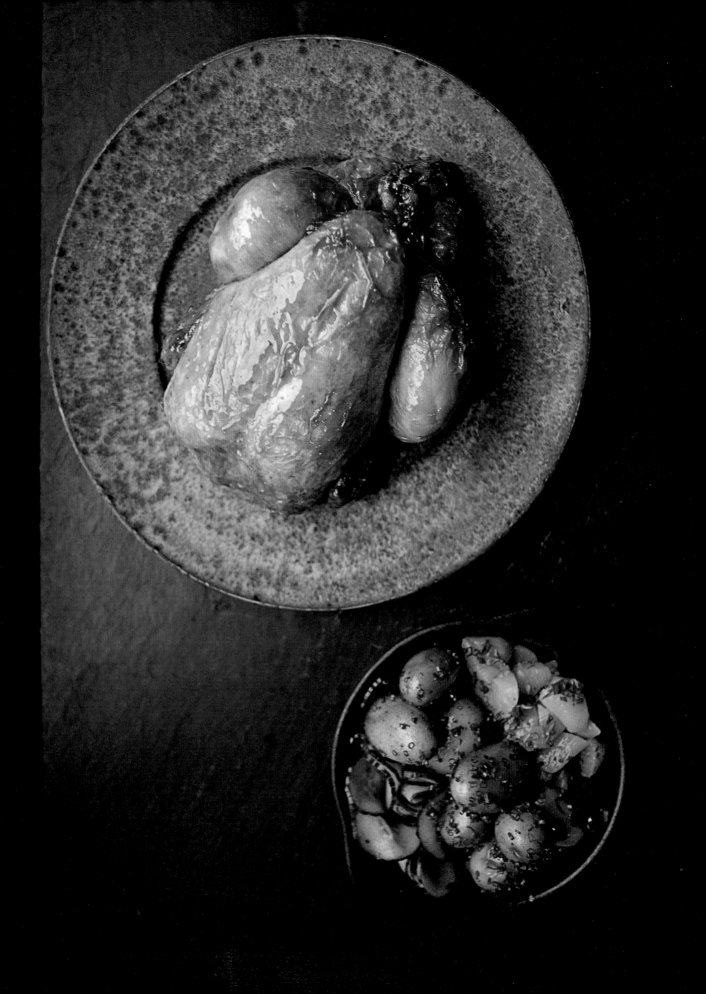

DANISH STYLE
WHOLE ROAST CHICKEN, PEAR COMPOTE AND NEW POTATOES

1 CHICKEN (1.4-1.6 KG)
SALT
2 CUCUMBERS
1 TSP SALT
200 ML PICKLING LIQUID #1
(SEE PAGE 334)
1 KG PEARS
2 STAR ANISE
1 CINNAMON STICK
100 ML APPLE JUICE
3 TBSP ACACIA HONEY
JUICE AND ZEST OF 1 ORGANIC LEMON
½ BUNCH TARRAGON

ACCOMPANIMENT
1 KG NEW POTATOES
SALT AND FRESHLY GROUND
BLACK PEPPER
OLIVE OIL
½ BUNCH CHIVES

Preheat the oven to 200°C.

Clean the chicken and cut off the tail and wings. Sprinkle with salt, cover with cling film and refrigerate.

Wash the cucumbers, slice thinly on a mandolin and put into a strainer. Sprinkle with salt and let them sit for half an hour or more to drain out the water. Transfer to a bowl and pour over the cool pickling liquid. Set aside.

Peel the pears, quarter, remove the cores, dice and add to a saucepan with the star anise, cinnamon stick, apple juice and acacia honey. Cover and cook the pears slowly over medium heat until tender. Stir occasionally. If there is a lot of liquid, remove the lid from the saucepan and let it evaporate. Season to taste with honey, lemon zest and lemon juice. Let the pears cool and stir in the chopped tarragon.

Roast the chicken for 15 minutes at 200°C and reduce the oven temperature to 165°C. Cook until the juices run clear and the leg joints separate easily – about 45 minutes. Rest for 10-15 minutes and carve.

While the chicken is in the oven, scrub or peel the potatoes and boil in salted water until tender. Drain and season with salt, pepper, olive oil and chives.

Serve the chicken with the pear compote, pickled cucumber and boiled potatoes.

PORK CHEEKS,
SALT-BAKED CELERIAC, BEETROOT AND SAVOY CABBAGE

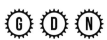

1 KG PORK CHEEKS, TRIMMED
3 ONIONS
1 WHOLE GARLIC
2 HEADS OF CELERIAC
1 BUNCH THYME, RINSED
3 STAR ANISE
3 CARDAMOM PODS
3 BAY LEAVES
1 LITRE VEAL STOCK (SEE PAGE 333)
50 ML CIDER VINEGAR
200 ML RED WINE
500 G BEETROOT
1 SAVOY CABBAGE
2 LEMONS
OLIVE OIL
SALT AND FRESHLY GROUND BLACK PEPPER

Preheat the oven to 150°C.

Peel and halve the onions and garlic. Peel one of the heads of celeriac and chop into large chunks. Brown the celeriac and onions in olive oil.

Sear the pork cheeks in a little olive oil and salt.
Place them in a deep, ovenproof dish with the celeriac, onion, garlic, half the thyme and the dried spices. Pour the stock, vinegar and red wine over the cheeks and cover the dish with foil. Roast for 2.5-3 hours until the meat easily separates. Check the cheeks regularly to avoid overcooking.

Cut off the root part of the second celeriac and wash thoroughly. Place two layers of foil on the counter and wrap the celeriac – drizzled with olive oil and seasoned with salt – in it. Bake in the oven until tender – about 1.5-2 hours. Before serving, peel the baked celeriac, cut into bite-sized pieces and sear in a frying pan with olive oil and salt.

Remove the cheeks from the braising liquid, strain it and reduce to a quarter of the volume. Season with salt and vinegar.
Before serving, warm the cheeks in the sauce.

Wash the beetroot and boil in salted water until tender. Squeeze off the skin and cut into bite-sized pieces. Remove the outer leaves of the savoy cabbage, trim the bottom and slice the cabbage into 10-12 wedges. Place in a sauté pan, season with salt and cover the bottom with water. Zest a lemon over the cabbage, cover, bring to a boil and steam for 2 minutes. Serve immediately.

Serve the cheeks, celeriac, beetroot and cabbage with soft polenta or crushed potatoes with olive oil and herbs.

If you wish, garnish with freshly grated horseradish.

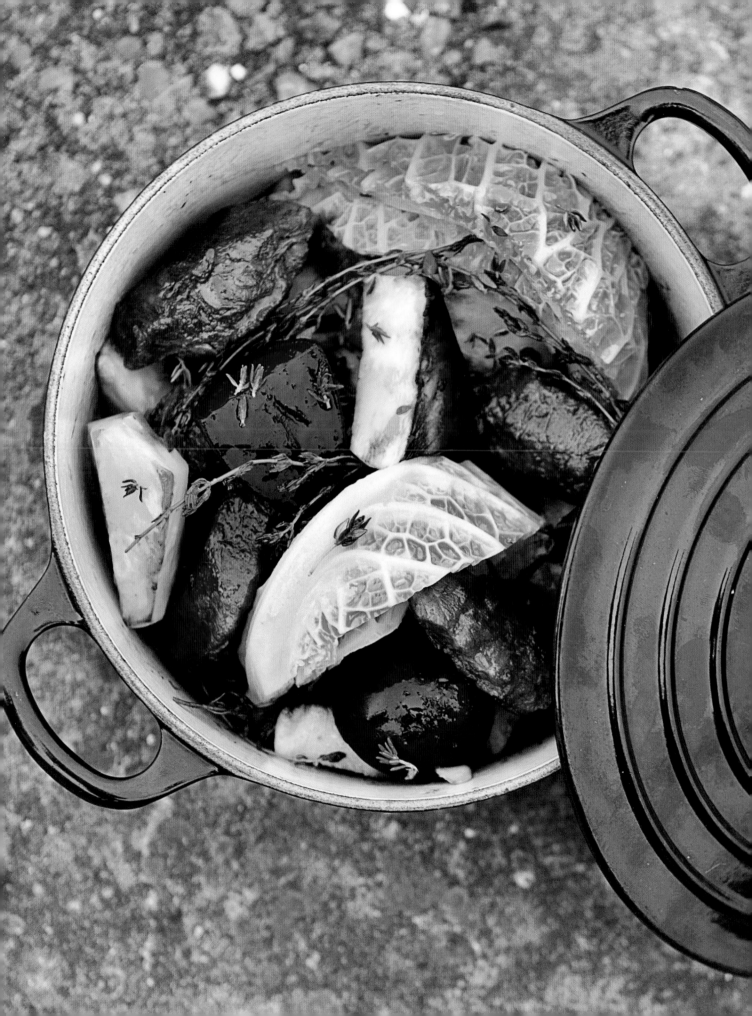

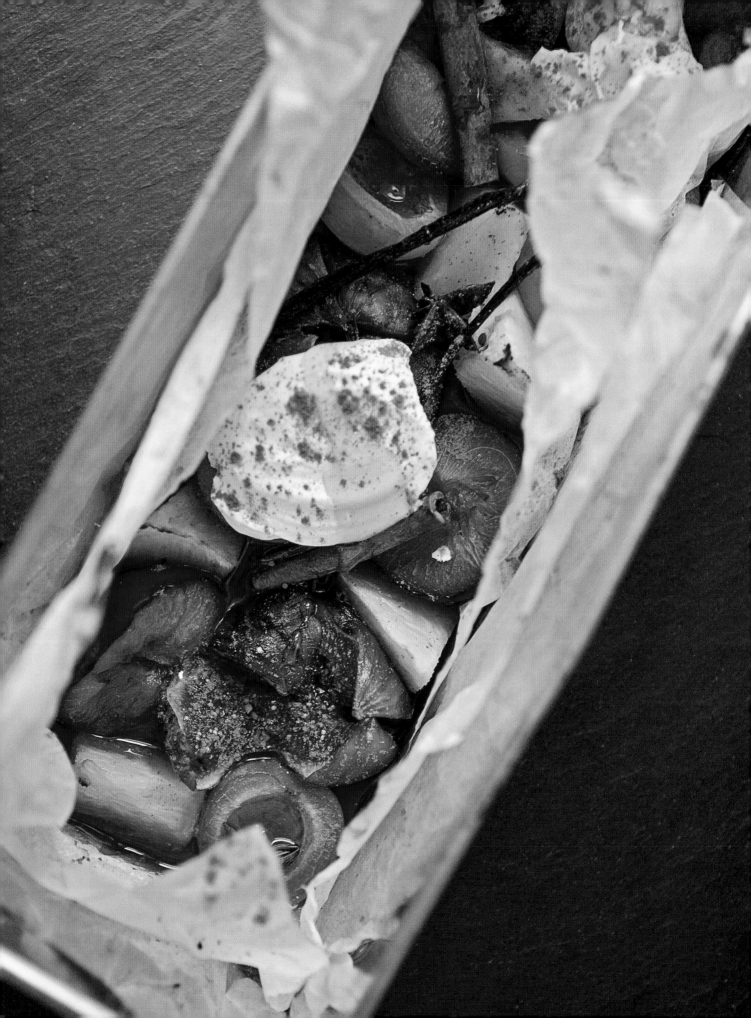

BAKED FRUIT *with*
VANILLA SKYR

4 FIGS
4 APRICOTS
2 PLUMS
½ PINEAPPLE
2 TBSP BALSAMIC VINEGAR
100 ML WHITE WINE
1 CINNAMON STICK
2 STAR ANISE
4 TBSP SKYR OR GREEK YOGHURT
SEEDS OF 1 VANILLA POD
JUICE AND ZEST OF 1 ORGANIC LEMON
2 TBSP CLEAR HONEY

Preheat the oven to 175°C.

Wash the fruits and peel the pineapple. Cut into large chunks, halve the apricots and plums and remove the stones. Cut a cross in the top of each fig and open carefully. Arrange all the fruits in an ovenproof dish, drizzle with the white wine and vinegar and add the cinnamon stick, star anise. Bake for 15-20 minutes.

Mix the skyr/yoghurt with the vanilla seeds and lemon zest. Stir in the honey and lemon juice to taste.

Serve the baked fruits with the vanilla skyr and the rest of the honey.

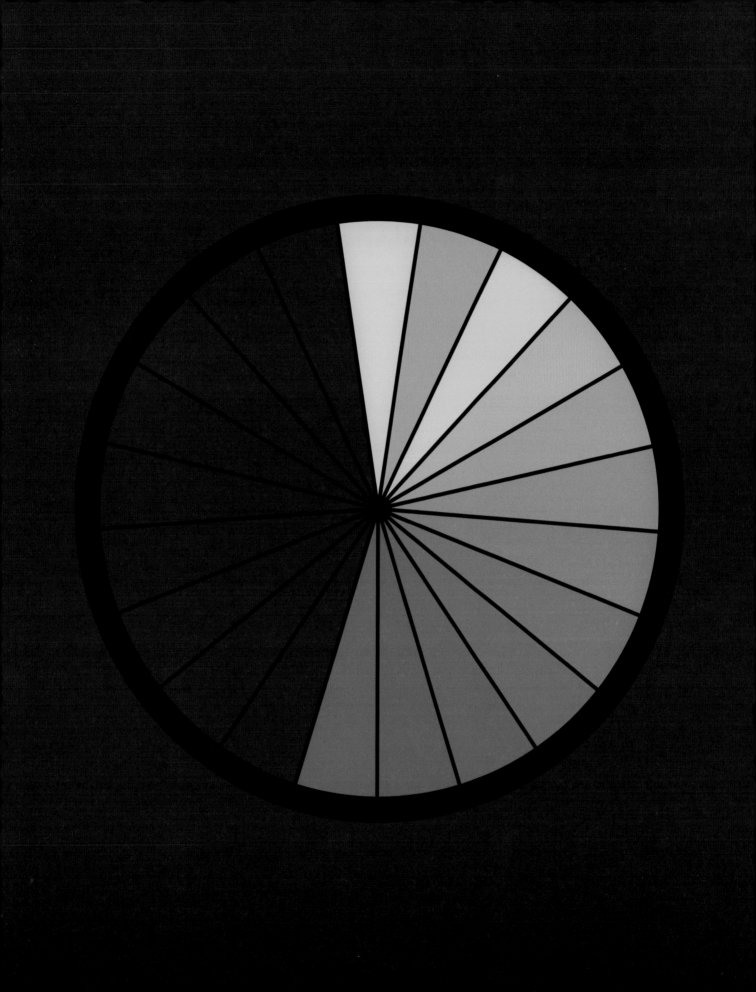

DAY

STAGE 11

COUSCOUS *with*
MELON AND ORANGE

250 G COUSCOUS
JUICE AND ZEST OF 2 ORGANIC ORANGES
3 TBSP OLIVE OIL
½ TSP FINE SALT
1 TSP WHOLE CLOVES
1 CINNAMON STICK
1 CANTALOUPE
250 G CARROTS
200 G YELLOW CHERRY TOMATOES
½ BUNCH PARSLEY
50 G RAISINS
200 ML ORANGE VINAIGRETTE
(SEE PAGE 325)

Rinse the oranges and zest over the dry couscous. Add olive oil and salt. Rub everything together with your fingers. Lay the cinnamon and cloves on top. Boil 250 ml water, pour over the couscous, cover with cling film and steep for at least 5 minutes.

Remove the seeds from the melon and cut off the rind then cut the melon into cubes. Peel the carrots and grate or shave them into long strips. Rinse and quarter the cherry tomatoes. Rinse, spin and finely chop the parsley.

Remove the cloves and the cinnamon stick from the couscous. Stir lightly with a fork and toss with the raisins, carrots, melon, parsley and vinaigrette. Season with salt and orange juice.

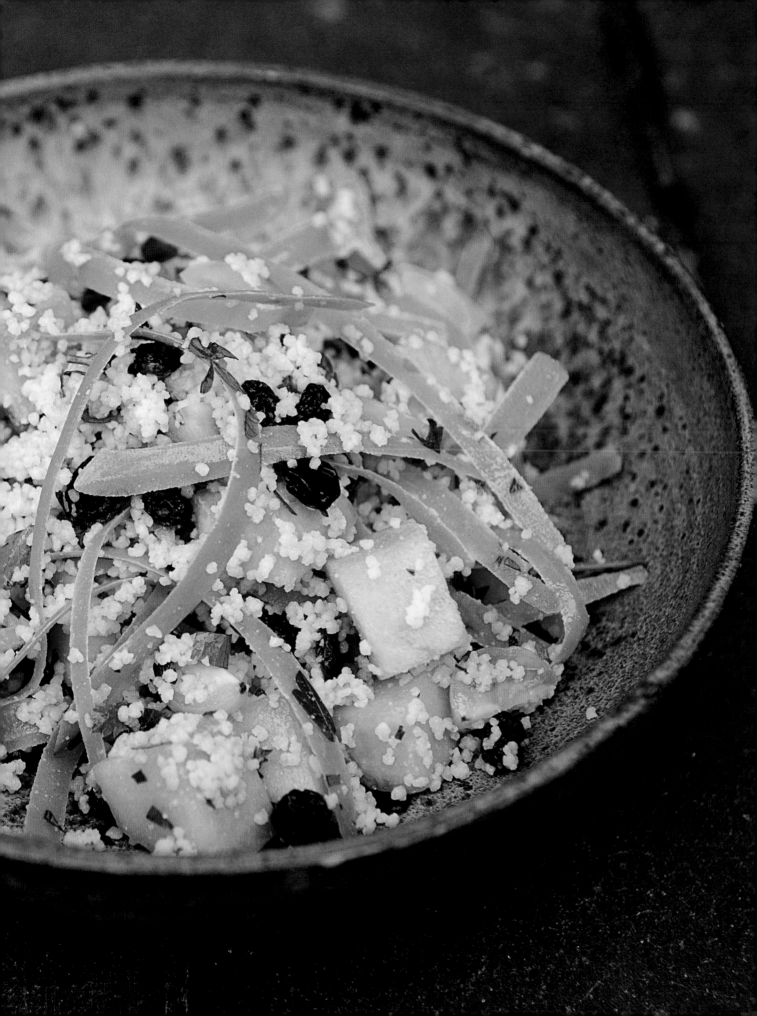

KALE, RED CABBAGE,
APPLE AND PISTACHIOS

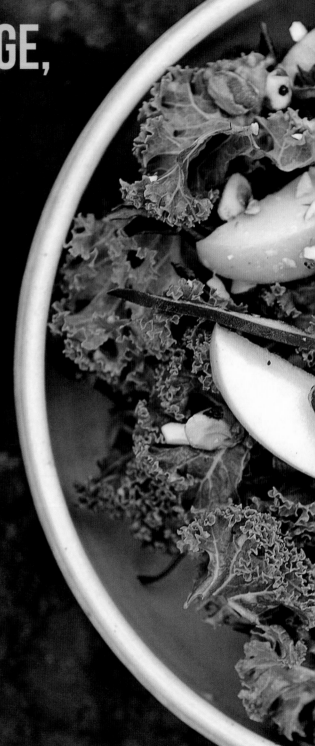

(G) (D)

200 G KALE
2 APPLES
3 TBSP CIDER VINEGAR
¼ RED CABBAGE
50 G PISTACHIOS
50 ML HAZELNUT VINAIGRETTE (SEE PAGE 322)

Divide the kale into small pieces, rinse and spin thoroughly. Rinse, quarter and core the apples. Slice the quarters into thin slices and marinate in vinegar. Peel off the outer layers of the cabbage, remove the stalk and shred finely on a mandolin. Toss with the hazelnut vinaigrette. Drain the apples and gently mix with the kale and cabbage. Top with the chopped pistachios.

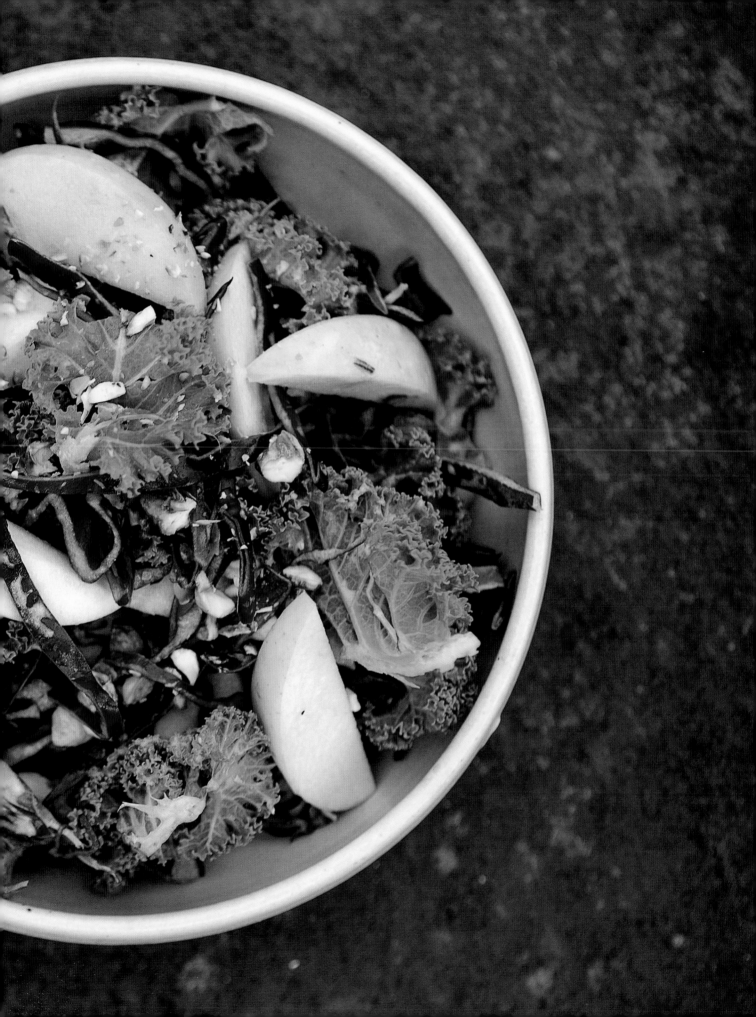

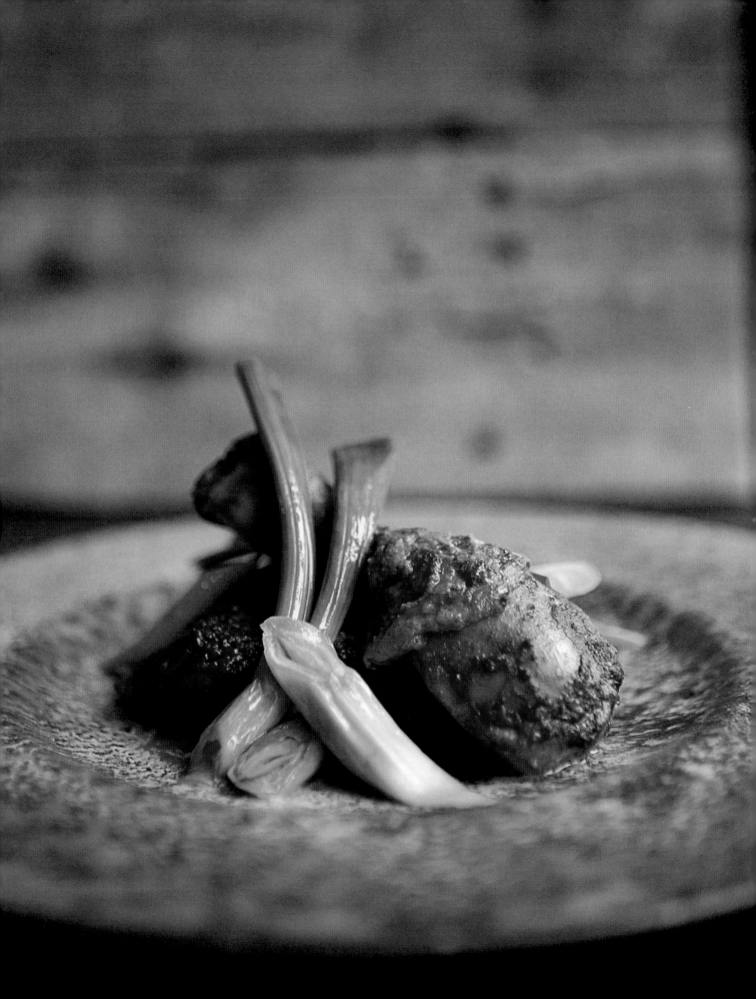

CHICKEN *in*
TURMERIC AND LEMON

**4 WHOLE CHICKEN LEGS
WITH DRUM AND THIGH
2 LEMONS
3 TBSP COCONUT OIL
3 TBSP GROUND CORIANDER
2 TBSP GROUND CUMIN
2 TBSP TURMERIC
4 CLOVES GARLIC
1 TSP SALT
200 ML CHICKEN STOCK (SEE PAGE 332)
12 SPRING ONIONS**

Trim off any surplus fat from the chicken legs and divide each leg at the joint for a total of 8 pieces. Peel and chop the garlic. Squeeze the lemon juice over the chicken portions and rub into the meat. Mix the spices, salt and chopped garlic with the coconut oil and rub firmly into the meat. Cover the chicken and refrigerate for at least 30 minutes.

Preheat the oven to 170°C.

Brown the chicken portions skin side down over medium heat. Transfer to an ovenproof dish, pour the stock over the chicken, cover with foil and roast for 20 minutes. Remove the foil from the dish and roast the chicken for a further 10 minutes. When the meat is falling off the bone, the chicken is ready.

Clean the spring onions and cut off the top and roots. Slice each spring onion diagonally into 3 parts and blanch for a couple of minutes in lightly salted water. Serve the chicken with the spring onions and bulgur wheat, rice, or lentils.

BRAISED
LAMB SHANK

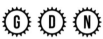

4 X 300-400 G LAMB SHANKS
750 ML RED WINE (1 BOTTLE)
4 STAR ANISE
4 BAY LEAVES
1 TSP CORIANDER SEEDS
½ TSP BLACK PEPPERCORNS
4 CLOVES
4 SPRIGS ROSEMARY
2 CARROTS
6 ONIONS
1 LITRE VEAL STOCK (SEE PAGE 333)
100 ML CIDER VINEGAR
2 TBSP HONEY
1 WHOLE GARLIC
LEMON JUICE
SALT AND FRESHLY GROUND
BLACK PEPPER
4 CLOVES GARLIC
100 ML OLIVE OIL
1 TSP CUMIN
1 TSP GROUND CORIANDER
1 TBSP CLEAR HONEY
½ TSP SALT
1 BUNCH PARSLEY
½ BUNCH THYME
ZEST OF 1 ORGANIC LEMON

Preheat the oven to 180°C.

In a saucepan, add the star anise, bay leaves, coriander seeds, peppercorns, cloves and rosemary to the red wine and reduce by half.

Trim the lamb shanks, season with salt and sear them in a hot pan with olive oil. Peel the carrots and cut off the tops and bottoms. Split lengthwise. Halve, peel and trim the ends off two onions. Brown the cut surfaces of the onions and carrots in a hot pan and put them in a deep ovenproof dish with the lamb shanks. Pour over the stock, red wine reduction and vinegar. Add honey and one whole garlic head split in half horizontally.

The liquid should cover half of the shanks. Cover and braise until the meat falls from the bone – about 2.5 hours. Turn the shanks occasionaly so they do not dry out.

Finely grate four cloves of garlic and place in a bowl with the olive oil, cumin, ground coriander, honey and salt. Blend with a hand blender. Rinse the parsley and thyme, tear off the leaves and chop separately. Zest the lemon.

When the shanks are tender, carefully transfer them to a large plate and cover with foil. Strain the remaining liquid and reduce it by two thirds. Season with salt, pepper and lemon juice. If you want a thicker sauce, whisk 1 tbsp corn flour in 250 ml water and bring to a boil with the sauce.

Serve the shanks in a dish with freshly boiled green puy lentils and roasted celeriac cubes. Add the chopped parsley, thyme and lemon zest to the stock reduction and pour over the lamb and lentils. Just before serving, pour the cumin mixture through a sieve over the shanks.

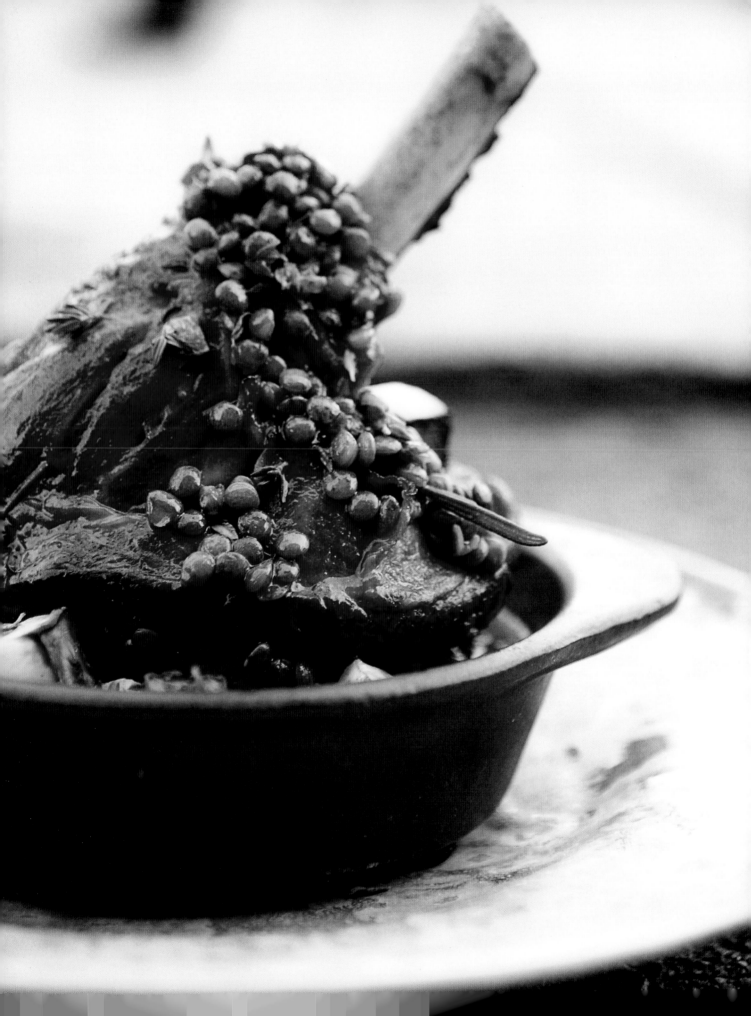

NICKI SØRENSEN

"I HAVE MORE STAMINA DURING RACES"

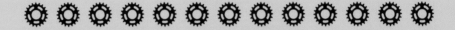

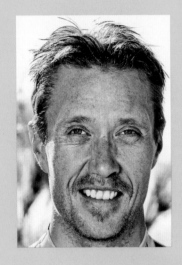

BORN: 14th May 1975
NATIONALITY: Danish
EXPERIENCE: Professional
from 1999-2014 – now retired
FORMER CYCLING TEAMS:
**Team Fakta, Team Chicky
World, Tinkoff-Saxo**
FAVOURITE RACE:
Tour de France

Hannah (H): What difference does food make for you physically and/or mentally during a long season or race?

Nicki Sørensen (NS): It helps me to perform at my best every day and cuts down on the recovery period after a race. And often, after a tough day on the bike, dinner is the highlight of the day – but only if it's a delicious meal!

H: In what way do you think food can change an athlete's performance?

NS: For me personally, the changes to my diet mean that I have more stamina during races. I very rarely hit the wall.

H: What has the proper diet meant for you personally as a rider?

NS: I think it's important to eat easily digestible food. In other words, large quantities of foods that don't cause any stomach problems when racing, like high quality protein such as fish and chicken, which is both easy to digest and low in fat. There also needs to be the right amount of dietary fibre in the food – not too little and not too much – because that can also have a negative effect.

H: In what way has your opinion on food for athletes changed over the past year?

NS: It turns out that the food the body can tolerate differs a lot from one cyclist to another. For example, some riders function really well on large quantities of eggs, while others prefer other forms of protein. Until just a few years ago, we simply weren't aware of that and it was all pasta and ketchup.

H: Have you found that food can improve or worsen your condition?

NS: Again, I think that digestion is important. Because of the huge amounts of food a rider eats, it's important not to eat anything that causes bad digestion and which then hurts you when riding. So, yes, food can worsen, but also improve your condition.

H: How do you see the future of cycling in terms of food?

NS: Hannah's food is the future!

H: What is your favourite food?
NS: Homemade burgers, a big steak and old-fashioned, Danish apple pie with whipped cream.

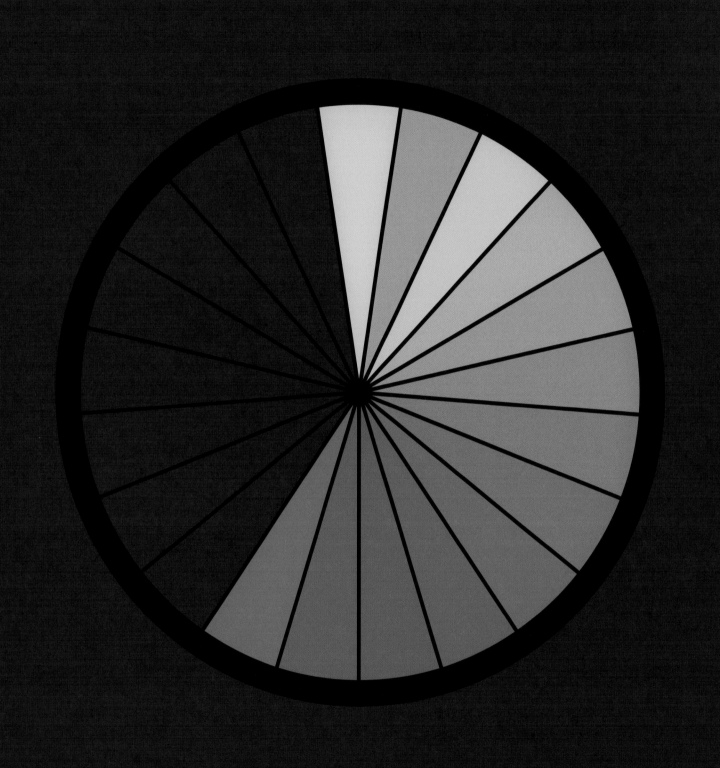

DAY 13

STAGE 12

RUBY GRAPEFRUIT,
AVOCADO AND PINE NUTS

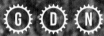

2 RUBY GRAPEFRUITS
4 AVOCADOS
50 G PINE NUTS
50 ML OLIVE OIL
SALT AND FRESHLY GROUND BLACK PEPPER

Cut the tops and bottoms off the ruby grapefruits, carefully cut off the peel and slice between the segments so they separate from the membrane and fall into a bowl. After cutting out all the segments, squeeze the juice from the membranes over them.

Halve the avocados and remove the stones. Scoop out the flesh with a spoon and cut into chunks. Strain the grapefruit juice and lightly toss the avocado in it. Whisk the olive oil and grapefruit juice together, season with salt and pepper and spoon over the salad. Top with the pine nuts.

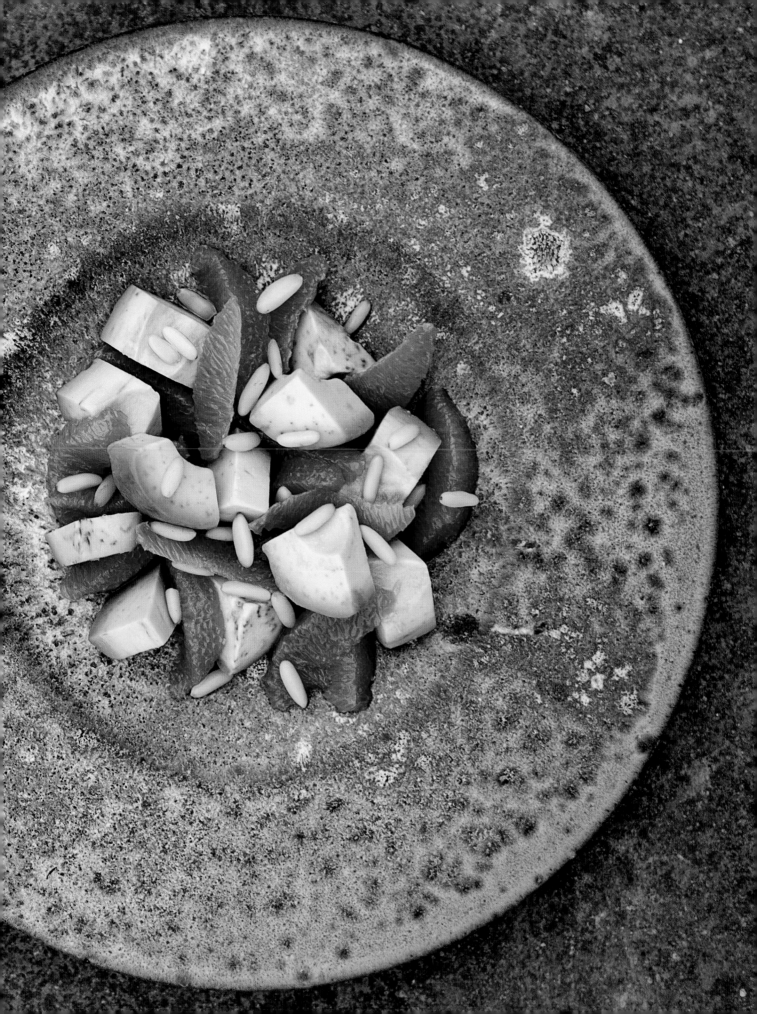

CARAMELISED
ONION SOUP

8 ONIONS
4 CLOVES GARLIC
3 TBSP OLIVE OIL
4 STAR ANISE
200 ML WHITE WINE
1.5 LITRES VEAL STOCK (SEE PAGE 333)
½ TSP SALT
FRESHLY GROUND BLACK PEPPER
4 TBSP SHERRY VINEGAR
50 G GRATED GRUYÈRE

Peel and finely slice the onions and garlic. Heat the oil in a thick-bottomed pan over medium heat and sauté the onions, garlic and star anise until completely caramelised. Stir frequently with a wooden spoon to keep from burning. When the onions are soft, sweet and caramel-coloured, pour in the white wine and reduce by a little more than half. Add the stock and bring to the boil. Reduce the heat slightly and let the soup simmer for 15-20 minutes. Pick out the star anise and season with salt, pepper and sherry vinegar.

Serve in ovenproof bowls topped with cheese and grill in the oven or burn with a gas torch.

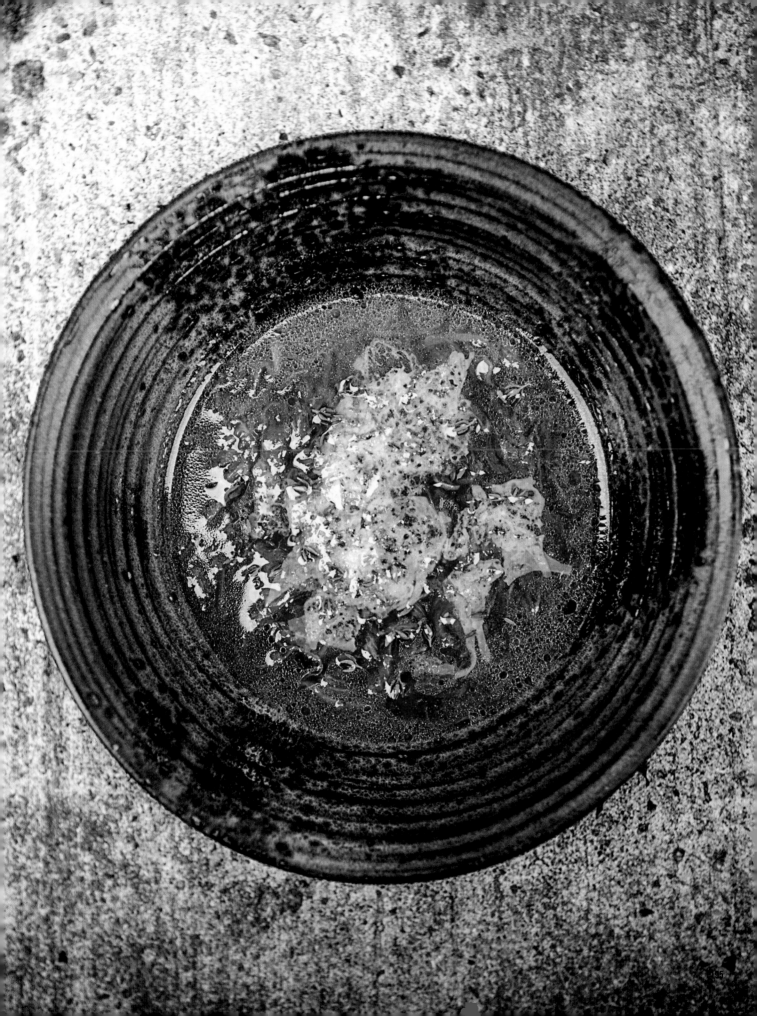

CHICKEN,
RED PEPPER SALSA *and*
PEARL BARLEY RISOTTO

RED PEPPER SALSA

4 RED PEPPERS
100 ML OLIVE OIL
100 G ALMONDS
70 G CONCENTRATED TOMATO PURÉE
1 TSP EDELSÜSS PAPRIKA
4 CLOVES GARLIC
JUICE AND ZEST OF 2 ORGANIC LEMONS
SALT

CHICKEN

8 CHICKEN LEGS
¼ BUNCH PARSLEY
3 CLOVES GARLIC
4 TBSP OLIVE OIL
¼ TSP SALT

RED PEPPER SALSA
Preheat the oven to 220°C.

Wash the peppers, halve and scrape out the seeds. Grease the outside of the peppers with olive oil and grill them until the skin is blackened – about 8-10 minutes. Move the peppers to a dish and cover with foil to retain the steam. Rest for 10-15 minutes.

Turn the oven down to 170°C and roast the almonds for 7-8 minutes until golden.

Roast the tomato purée with the paprika for 2-3 minutes. Peel the blackened skin off the peppers and peel the garlic cloves. Blend the peppers, almonds, garlic and olive oil to a paste. Season with lemon zest, juice, salt and adjust the consistency to your liking with more olive oil.

CHICKEN LEGS
Turn the oven up to 180°C. Cut the chicken legs at the joint, separating the drumsticks from the thighs.

Tear the parsley leaves off the stalk, rinse and chop. Peel and chop the garlic. Mix the olive oil with the chopped parsley, garlic and salt and rub it under the skin of the chicken. Roast the chicken legs in the oven until the skin is crisp and the chicken is cooked through – about 30 minutes.

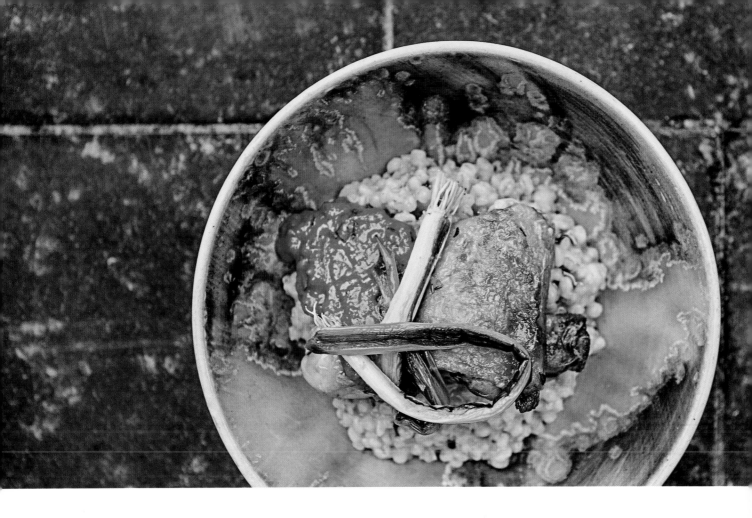

PEARL BARLEY RISOTTO

200 G PEARL BARLEY
2 SHALLOTS
2 CLOVES GARLIC
3 TBSP OLIVE OIL
3 SPRIGS ROSEMARY
300 ML DRY WHITE WINE
500 ML CHICKEN STOCK (SEE PAGE 332)
4 TBSP SHEEP'S YOGHURT
100 G GRATED PARMESAN
SALT AND FRESHLY GROUND BLACK PEPPER
LEMON

FRIED SPRING ONIONS

10 SPRING ONIONS
OLIVE OIL
SALT

PEARL BARLEY RISOTTO

Peel and chop the shallots and garlic. Rinse the rosemary. Heat the olive oil over a medium heat and sauté the onions and garlic with the rosemary. Add the pearl barley and sauté until glossy. Add the white wine and bring to a boil while stirring with a wooden spoon. Remove the sprigs of rosemary, pour in 1/3 of the chicken stock and cook until the liquid thickens. Repeat with the rest of the stock.

When the pearl barley is tender but still has bite, reduce the heat and stir in the sheep's yoghurt. Add the parmesan and lemon zest left over from the salsa and season to taste with salt, pepper and lemon juice.

FRIED SPRING ONIONS

Rinse the spring onions and roast them in a hot pan with olive oil and salt until nicely caramelised and tender.

Serve the pearl barley risotto with chicken legs and a spoonful of red pepper salsa topped with spring onions. Drizzle with a little olive oil and top with tarragon leaves.

DUCK BREAST, PAN-ROASTED CARROTS, ORANGE AND RADICCHIO

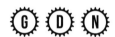

4 DUCK BREASTS
200 G BABY CARROTS
3 ORANGES
50 ML OLIVE OIL
2 TBSP SHERRY VINEGAR
SALT AND FRESHLY GROUND
BLACK PEPPER
200 G ROCKET
1 HEAD RADICCHIO
¼ BUNCH PARSLEY

Preheat the oven to 200°C.

Trim the duck breasts. Score the skin with a knife and sprinkle with salt. Place the duck breasts skin side down in a medium/hot pan and let them slowly brown until the skin is caramelised and most of the fat has rendered. Transfer to an ovenproof dish and roast for about 8 minutes until the duck breasts are firm and the juice runs red. Let them rest for 8 minutes.

Scrub or peel the carrots, cut off the tops and slice into 3 cm pieces. Sauté the carrots in olive oil and salt. They should still have a bite. Zest 1 orange into a bowl. Cut the tops and bottoms off all 3 oranges, cut off the peel and slice out the segments along the inside of the membranes. When all the segments have been cut out, squeeze the juice from the membranes into the bowl with the grated orange zest. Whisk the juice with the olive oil and season with salt, honey, sherry vinegar and pepper.

Slice the radicchio finely. Rinse with the rocket and spin dry. Rinse and chop the parsley. Toss the parsley and roasted carrots together. Slice the duck breasts diagonally and drain on a paper towel. Season with salt and pepper. Arrange the duck breast slices with the salad, orange segments, vinaigrette and carrots.

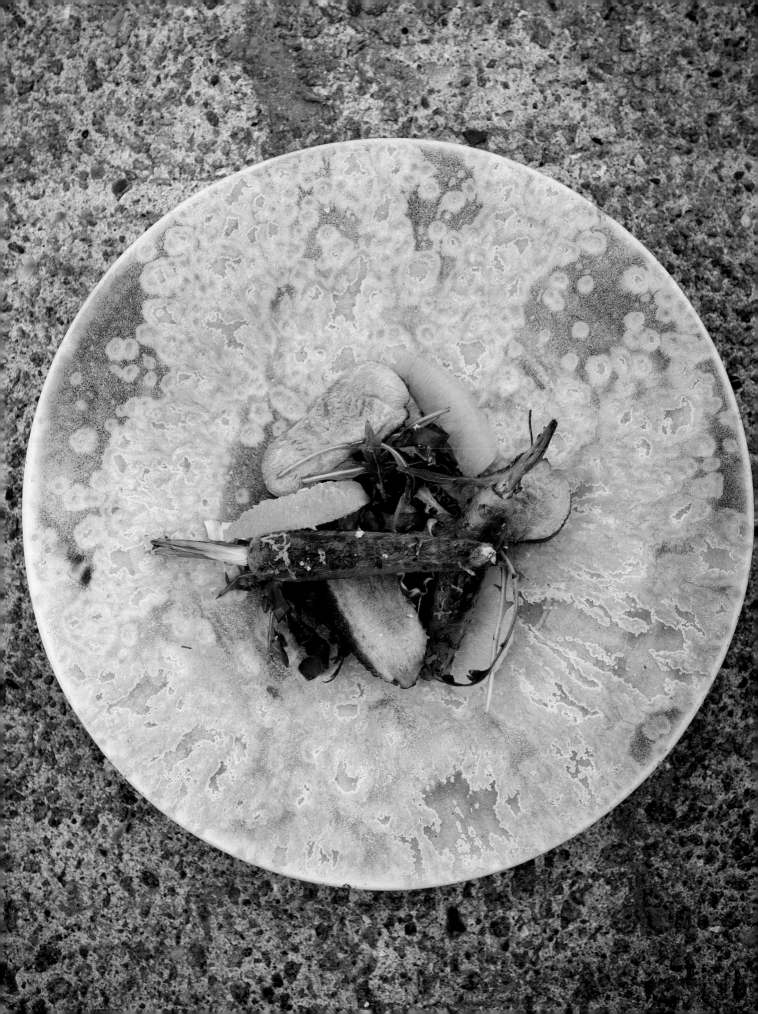

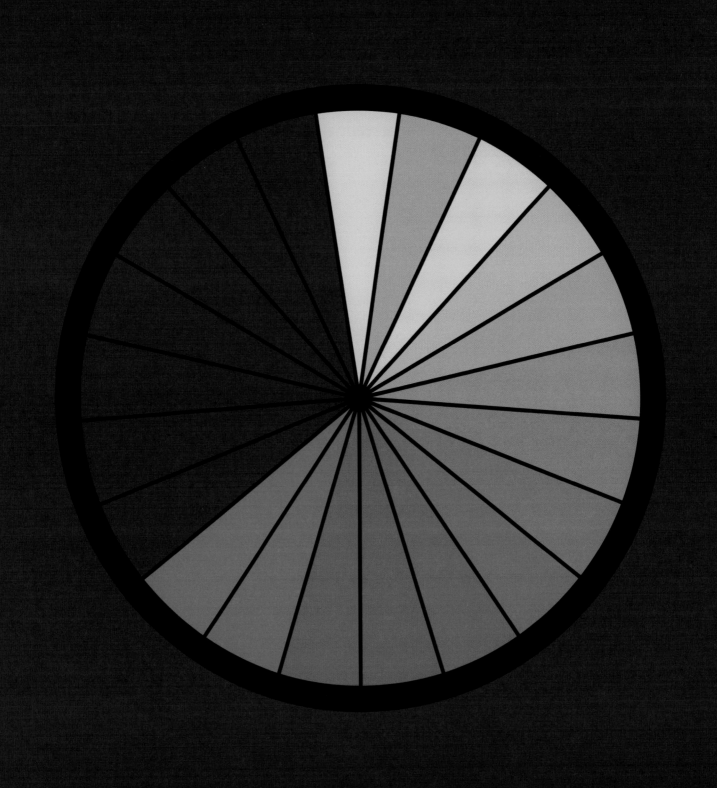

DAY

STAGE 13

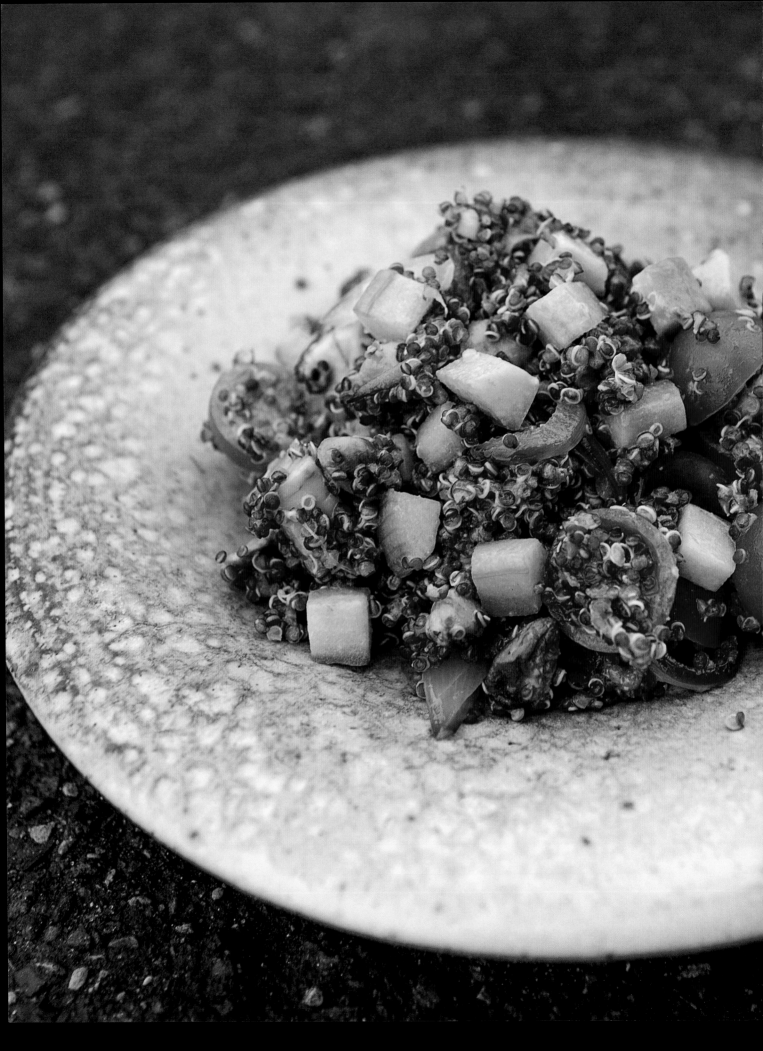

RED QUINOA
TABBOULEH

500 G RED QUINOA
1 STAR ANISE
2 BAY LEAVES
½ BUNCH ROSEMARY
2 RED ONIONS
250 G CHERRY TOMATOES
2 CUCUMBERS
50 G PISTACHIOS
50 ML LEMON VINAIGRETTE
(SEE PAGE 325)
2 TBSP OLIVE OIL
SALT AND FRESHLY GROUND
BLACK PEPPER

Rinse the quinoa and boil for 10 minutes in lightly salted water with the star anise, bay leaves and rosemary. Strain and cool. Peel and slice the onions and sauté them in olive oil and salt until tender. Rinse and halve the cherry tomatoes. Peel the cucumber, quarter lengthwise, cut out the seeds and dice.

Toss the quinoa with the tomato, cucumber, onions, pistachios and the lemon vinaigrette.

BROWN RICE,
CELERIAC AND FIGS

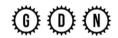

250 G BROWN RICE
½ HEAD OF CELERIAC
3 CARROTS
2 RED ONIONS
150 G DRIED FIGS
100 ML SOY SAUCE AND SESAME
DRESSING (SEE PAGE 326)
4 TBSP OLIVE OIL
JUICE OF 1 LIME

Boil the brown rice in lightly salted water until tender – about 40 minutes. Drain and toss with 1 tbsp olive oil. Peel the celeriac and carrots. Julienne or grate them. Peel and slice the onions, then sauté them in olive oil and salt. Halve the figs.

Mix the rice, carrots, celeriac, onions and figs with the dressing. Season with salt and lime juice.

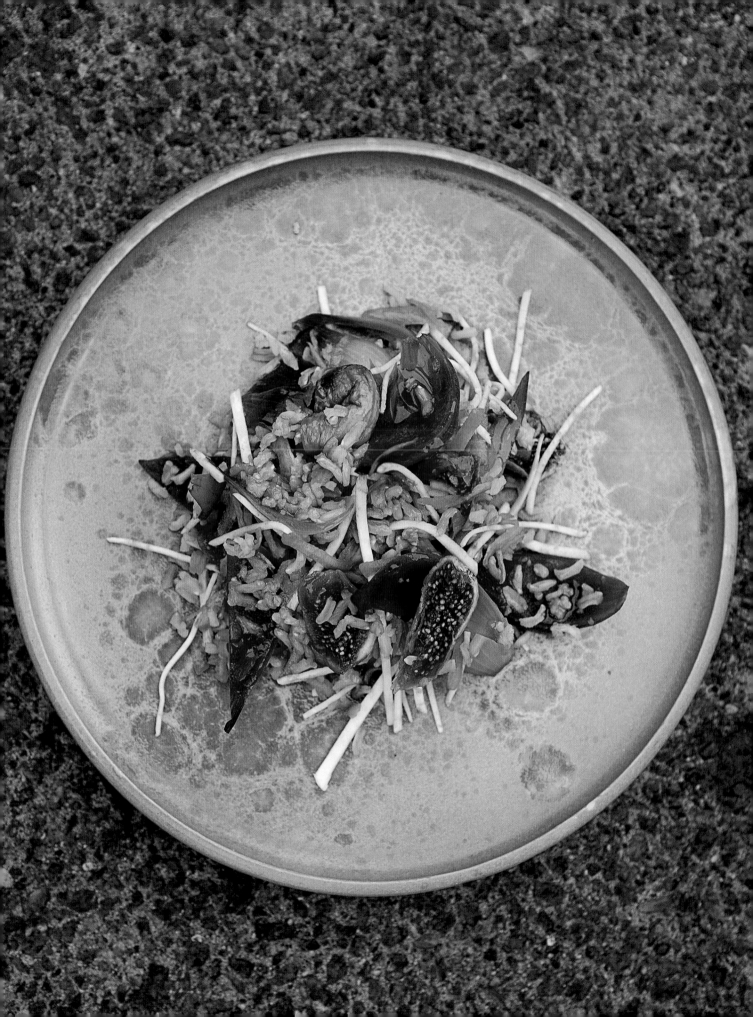

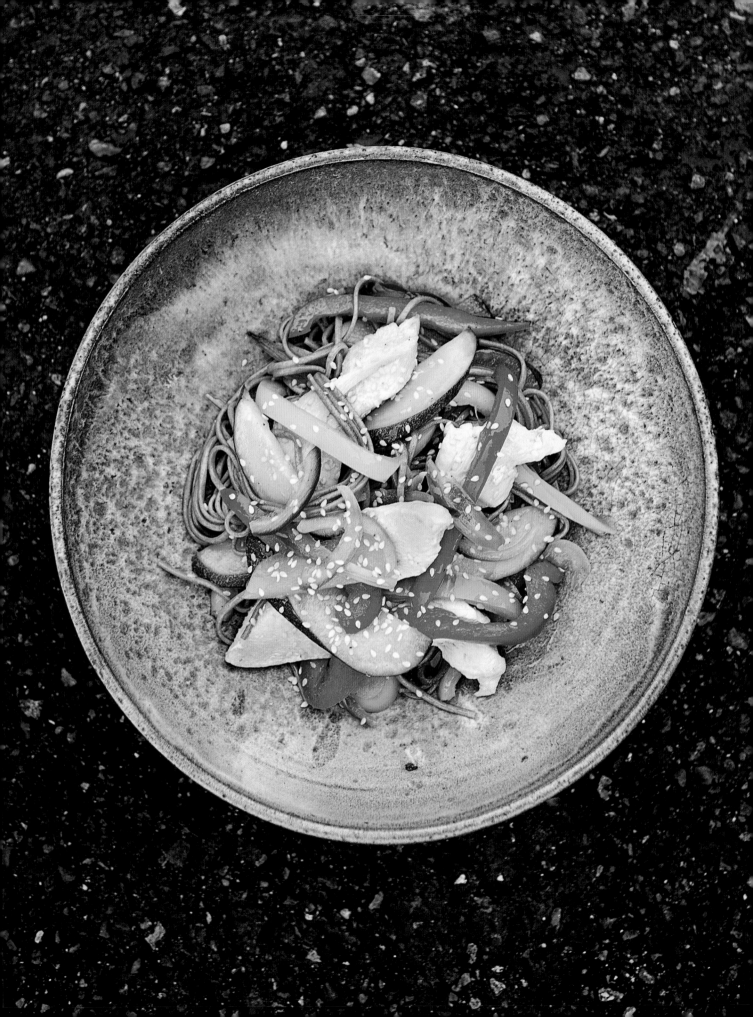

SOY-SESAME *chicken* WITH BUCKWHEAT NOODLES

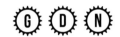

400 G CHICKEN BREAST
2 YELLOW PEPPERS
1 COURGETTE
2 RED ONIONS
4 TBSP SOY SAUCE
2 TBSP SESAME OIL
1 TBSP WHITE SESAME
4 TBSP OLIVE OIL
500 G BUCKWHEAT NOODLES,
COOKED ACCORDING TO THE
INSTRUCTIONS ON THE PACKET

Cut the chicken breast diagonally into roughly 1 cm strips. Rinse, halve and scoop out the seeds from the peppers. Slice into strips. Halve the courgette lengthwise, then cut into diagonal 1 cm slices. Peel the red onion and slice finely.

Heat the oil in a large frying pan or wok. Stir fry the chicken until cooked through and add the vegetables. Stir fry until the vegetables are tender but still have a bite. Add the soy sauce and sesame oil and remove the pan from the heat. Sprinkle with the sesame seeds just before serving. Serve with the buckwheat noodles.

MANGO,
JUNKET PANNA COTTA AND POMEGRANATE

6 SERVINGS

2 POMEGRANATES
2 LEAVES GELATINE
800 ML JUNKET OR YOGHURT
3 TBSP HONEY
100 ML WHIPPING CREAM
½ BUNCH MINT
2 MANGOS
JUICE OF 1 LEMON

Knock the seeds out of the pomegranates by banging the skin of the halved fruit while holding over a paper towel. Remove any rests of the white membrane and divide the pomegranate seeds into 6 glasses.

Soak the gelatine in cold water for 5 minutes. Mix the junket and honey in a bowl and season to taste with lemon juice. Warm the whipping cream. Squeeze the water from the gelatine and dissolve it in the warm cream. Let it sit for 2 minutes and then slowly mix with the junket. Pour the mixture over the pomegranate and place the glasses in the fridge for 4 hours before serving.

Rinse the mint, tear the leaves off the stalks and chop finely. Halve the mango, remove the stone and peel. Chop the flesh into cubes and toss with the chopped mint. Serve with the junket panna cottas.

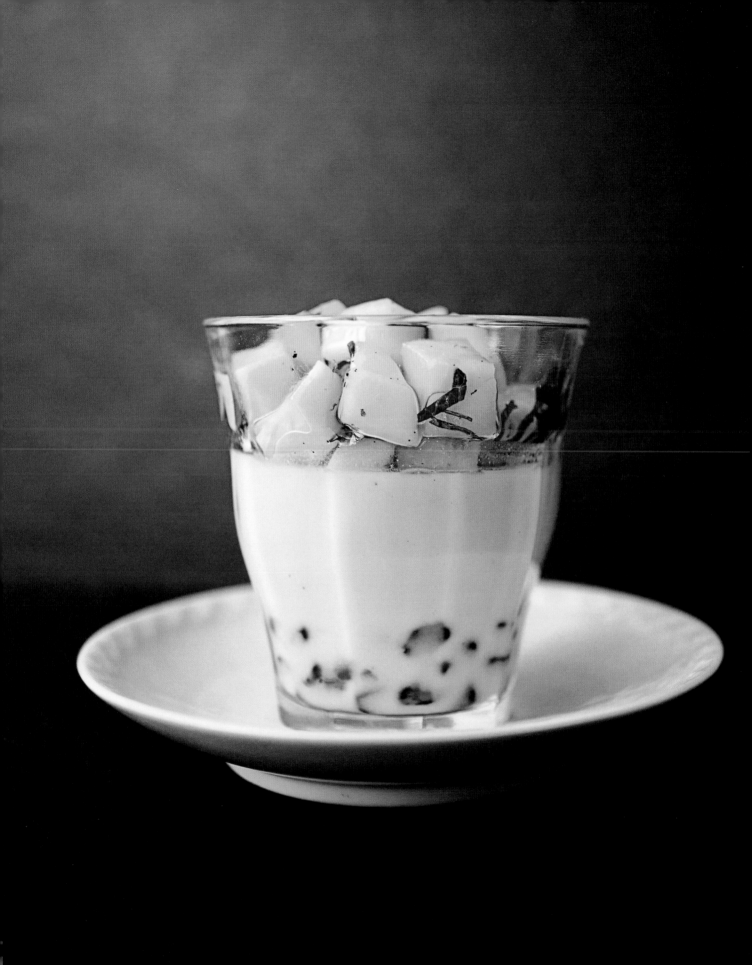

MICHAEL ROGERS

"I'VE NEVER BEEN FASTER"

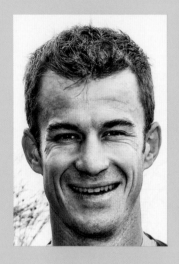

BORN: 20th December 1979
NATIONALITY: Australian
EXPERIENCE: Professional
since 2001
FORMER CYCLING TEAMS:
TeamSky, HTC, Team Mobile,
Quickstep, Mapei
FAVOURITE RACES:
Milano-San Remo and
Tour Down Under

Hannah (H): What difference does food make for you physically and/or mentally during a long season or race?
Michael Rogers (MR): Food makes a world of difference. Before the 2012 Tour de France, I had changed my eating habits and during the Tour my body fat percentage was the lowest ever. I've never been faster.

H: In what way do you think food can change an athlete's performance?
MR: It can change quite a lot! In 2012 I made radical changes to my diet. I switched from a diet consisting of fast carbs and no fat to a ketogenic diet: lots of fats, proteins and vegetables, slow carbohydrates and virtually no sugar. I decided to change my diet because I had previously had stomach problems. I completely stopped eating sugar unless I was sitting on the bike or when I really needed it, but never when I was "just" craving some. It took me just over a month to get used to my new diet but all of a sudden I felt better and had loads more energy than before. I did it outside of the cycling season so I could pay attention to how my body reacted to the changes. Of course, the reaction differs from person to person, but for me it was a key factor. During the 2012 Tour, I started every morning with fresh berries, protein powder and cream. It gave me the right amount of energy to get through the day's stage. The average human body can store 2000 kcal of muscle glycogen and that is not enough for completing an average stage. But the thinnest cyclists, who have only 4-5% body fat, can store up to 50,000 kcal of fat and this can actually keep you going for a really long time if you know how. In theory, it's only the brain that needs glycogen to function while the body can easily operate exclusively on fat and protein.

H: What has the proper diet meant for you personally as a cyclist?
MR: It has been a key factor.

H: In what way has your opinion on food for athletes changed over the past year?
MR: It has changed radically. As I said, I have changed my eating habits completely and, during the 2012 Tour, I decided to stop eating gels and bars at all during the race. Just 10 years ago, this would have been unthinkable. Instead, I ate rice cakes and little sandwiches.

H: How do you see the future of cycling in terms of food?
MR: As a professional cyclist, my body is the tool I work with and I'm obliged to look after it the best I can so it can continue as long as possible. The amount of energy we need to consume for this to happen is huge and, if we just continue to fill our bodies with sugar year in year out, we'll end up with type 2 diabetes. With a healthy and balanced diet, not only do we end up performing better, we also avoid a lot of health-related complications which result from too high an intake of energy. If I had to give some advice to beginners, it would be: train your body to store glycogen for when you need it. And be aware that, though the industry will doubtlessly pressure you to eat more sugar, this is not necessarily the right thing for you. Learn to listen to your body, to the way it teaches you what works best for you.

H: What is your favourite food?
MR: Outside the cycling season, my favourite is lamb shank followed by a big dollop of tiramisu. During the cycling season, it's anything involving salmon and eggs.

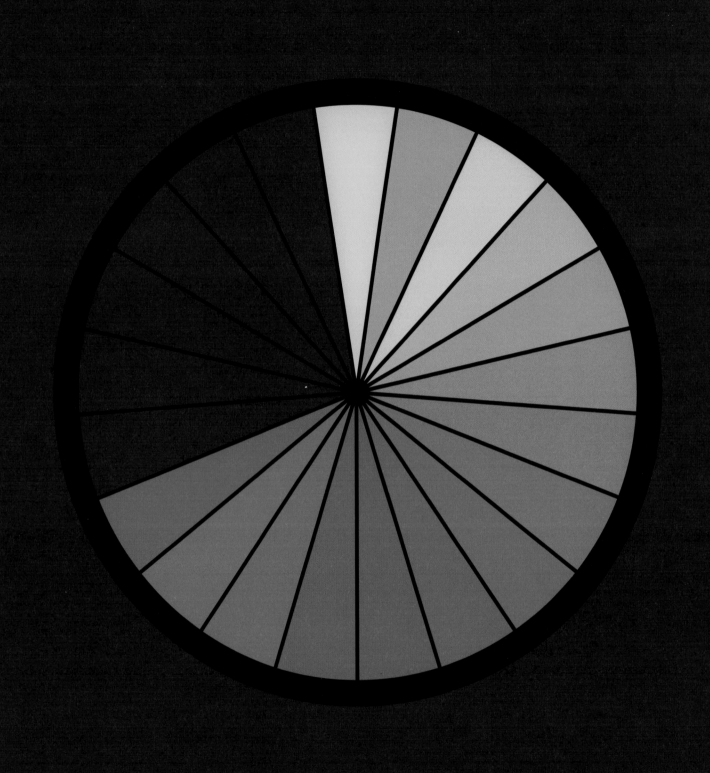

DAY 15

STAGE 14

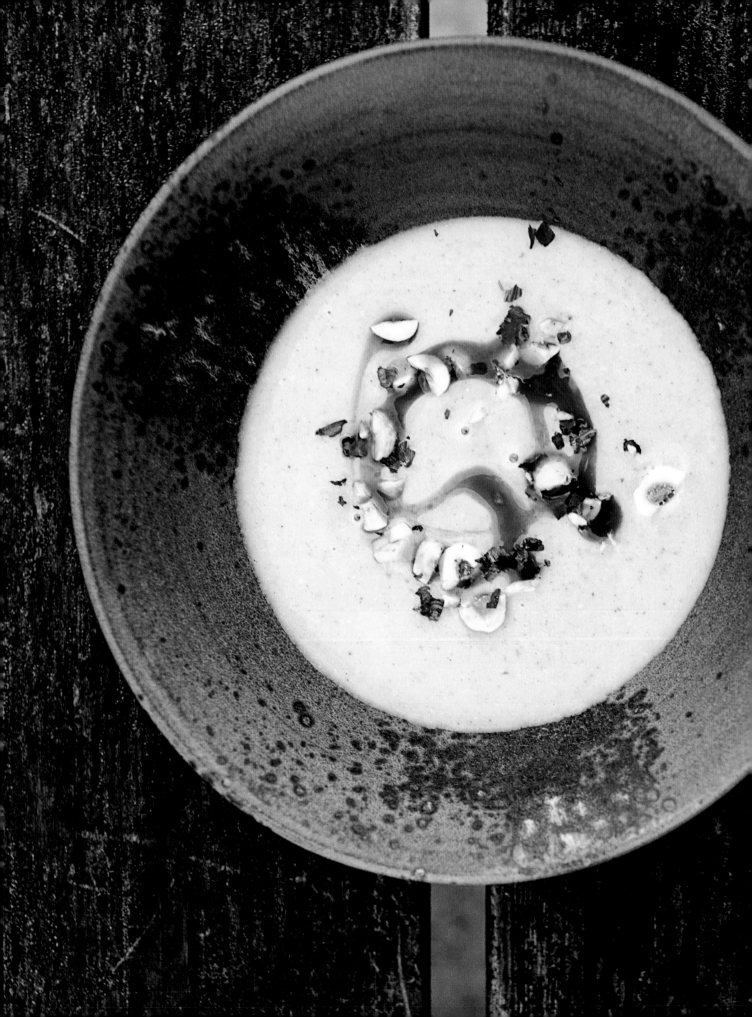

CAULIFLOWER *and* CELERIAC SOUP

1 HEAD OF CELERIAC
½ CAULIFLOWER
2 ONIONS
2 CLOVES GARLIC
¼ BUNCH THYME
500 ML CHICKEN STOCK (SEE PAGE 332)
500 ML RICE MILK OR MILK
3 TBSP OLIVE OIL
SHERRY VINEGAR
SALT AND FRESHLY GROUND
BLACK PEPPER
50 G HAZELNUTS

PARSLEY OIL
¼ BDT BUNCH PARSLEY
100 ML OLIVE OIL
1 LEMON
1 CLOVE GARLIC

Pre-heat the oven to 175°C.

Peel the celeriac and dice into 1x1 cm cubes. Cut the cauliflower into small florets, rinse and drain. Peel and finely slice the onions and garlic. Rinse the thyme. Heat some olive oil in a thick-bottomed pan and sauté the cauliflower, half of the celeriac plus the onion and garlic until it's tender. Pour in the milk and stock, bring to a boil and reduce the heat to low. Simmer until the cauliflower and celeriac are completely tender – about 15-20 minutes. Remove the thyme stalks.

For the parsley oil, rinse and pick the parsley leaves, blend with olive oil, lemon zest, lemon juice and garlic. Season with salt.

Roast the hazelnuts in the oven for 7-8 minutes.

Pan-roast the rest of the celeriac until caramelised and tender. Blend the soup to a purée. Thin down with milk for the desired consistency. Season with salt, pepper and sherry vinegar.

Serve the soup with the pan-roasted celeriac, parsley oil and roasted hazelnuts.

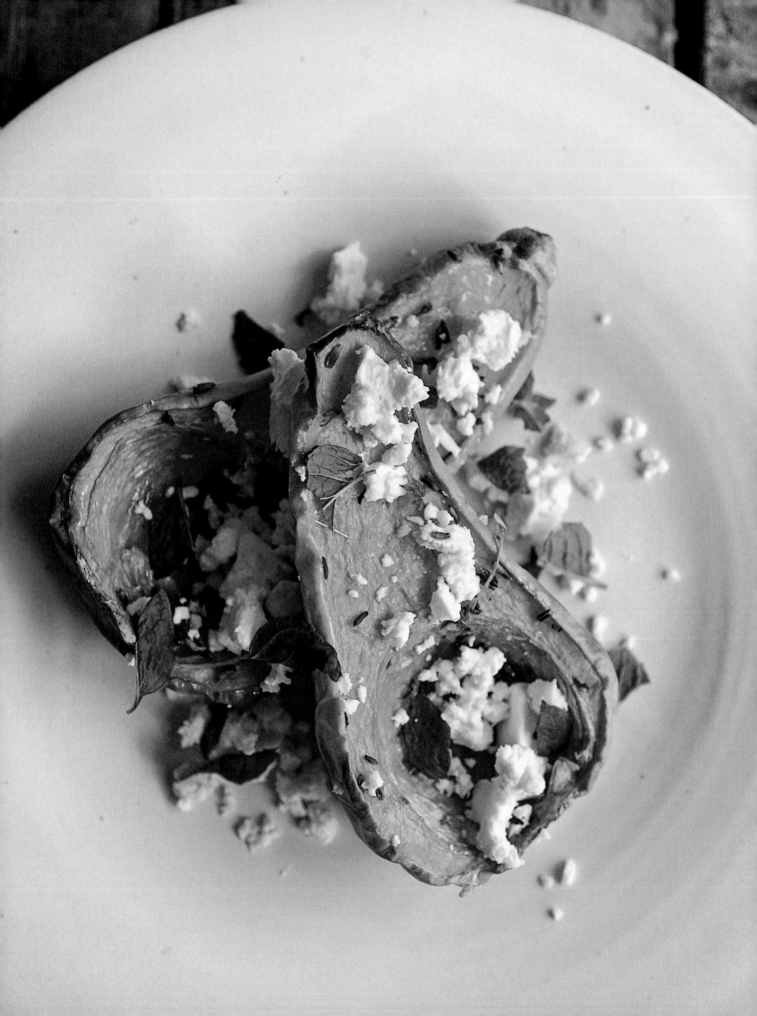

BAKED BUTTERNUT
SQUASH, FETA AND MINT

2 SMALL (300 G) BUTTERNUT SQUASH
1 TSP DRIED LAVENDER
½ BUNCH MINT
200 G FETA
100 ML OLIVE OIL
SALT

Preheat the oven to 160°C.

Halve the squash and scrape out the seeds. Place the squash on a baking tray covered with baking paper. Sprinkle with salt and lavender and drizzle with a little olive oil. Bake in the oven until the flesh is very tender – about 1 hour. Rinse the mint and tear the leaves off the stems. Serve the baked butternut squash with the mint leaves, crumbled feta and olive oil.

PASTA *puttanesca*

1 LITRE TOMATO SAUCE OF YOUR OWN CHOICE (SEE PAGES 330-331)
2 RED ONIONS
½ BUNCH OREGANO
50 G CAPERS
100 G KALAMATA OLIVES, PITTED
½ BUNCH CHERVIL
500 G PASTA
4 TBSP OLIVE OIL
SALT AND FRESHLY GROUND BLACK PEPPER
100 G PARMESAN

Peel the onions and cut into ½ cm rings. Sauté in olive oil and salt until tender. Rinse and chop the oregano. Mix the onion, capers, olives and oregano with the tomato sauce, bring to a boil and reduce the heat. Let simmer for 15-20 minutes.

Meanwhile, boil the pasta in a large pot of salted water. Serve the pasta with the sauce, fresh chervil, pepper and plenty of freshly grated parmesan.

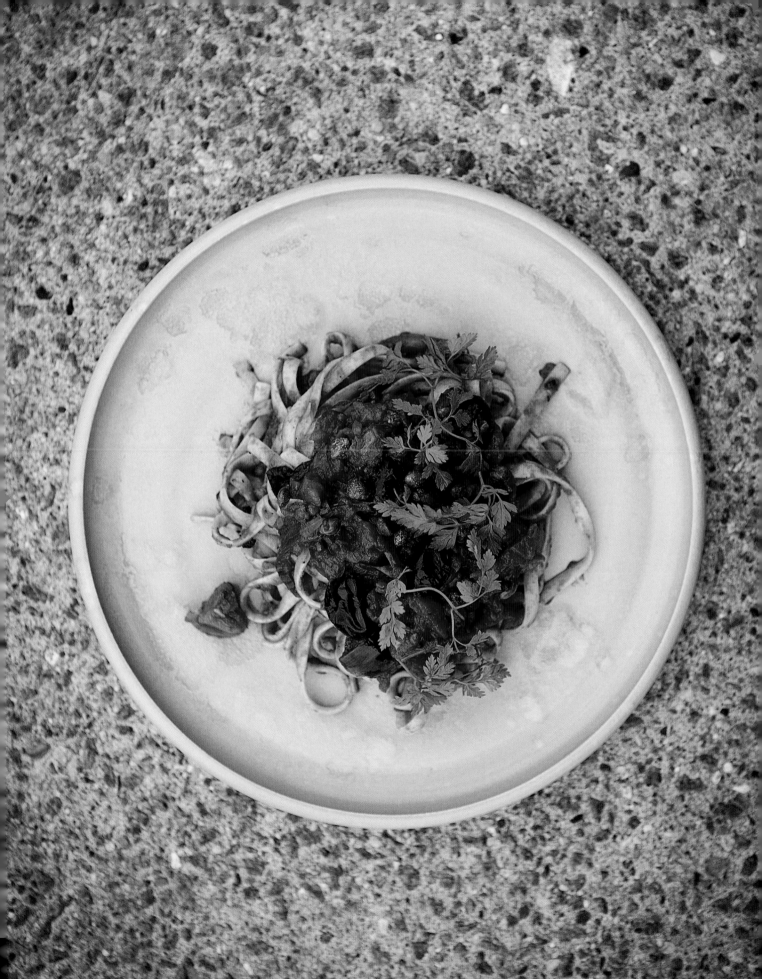

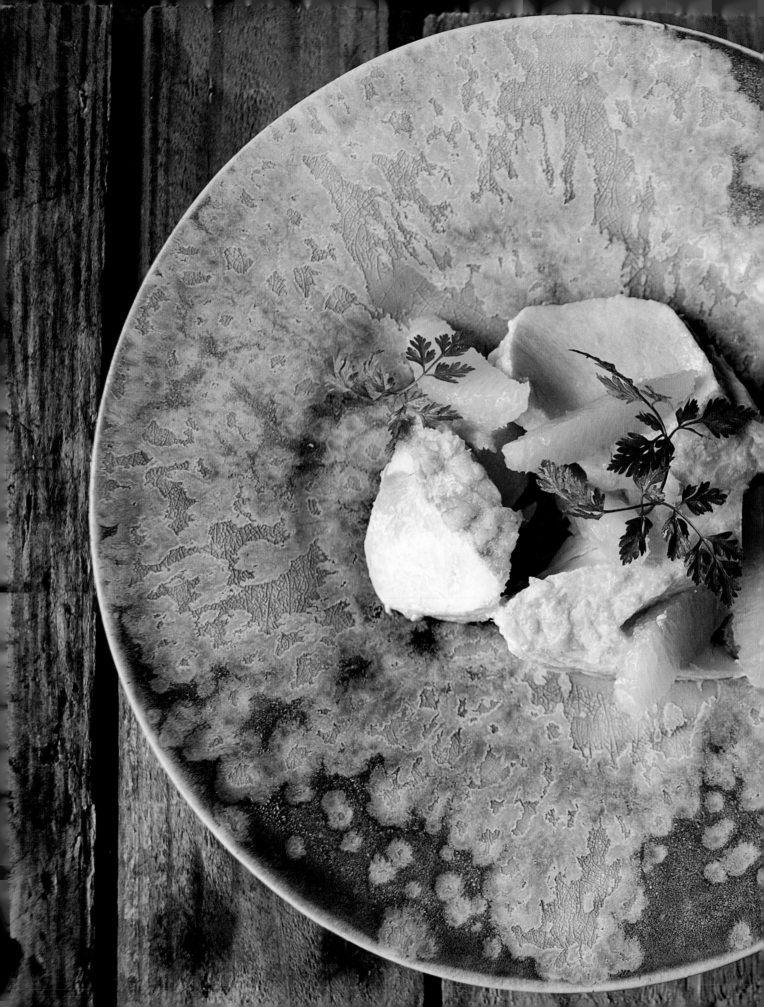

SALMON *with* ORANGE AND GINGER

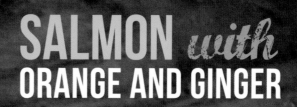

(G) (D) (N)

1 KG SALMON FILLET
1 TSP SALT
JUICE AND ZEST OF 2 ORGANIC ORANGES
100 G GINGER
1 TBSP CLEAR HONEY
½ BUNCH CHERVIL

Preheat the oven to 170°C.

Clean and trim the salmon fillet, pick out the bones and sprinkle with salt. Peel and grate the ginger. Wash and zest the oranges. Cut off the tops and bottoms and cut away the peel. Slice between the membranes so the segments fall out. Squeeze the juice out of the membranes into a bowl with the grated ginger, orange zest and honey. Mix, pour over the fish, cover and refrigerate for at least 30 minutes.

Bake the salmon for 10-12 minutes, the fish is done when a cake tester slides through the flesh without resistance. Rinse and pick the chervil. Serve the fish warm or cold with the orange segments and chervil.

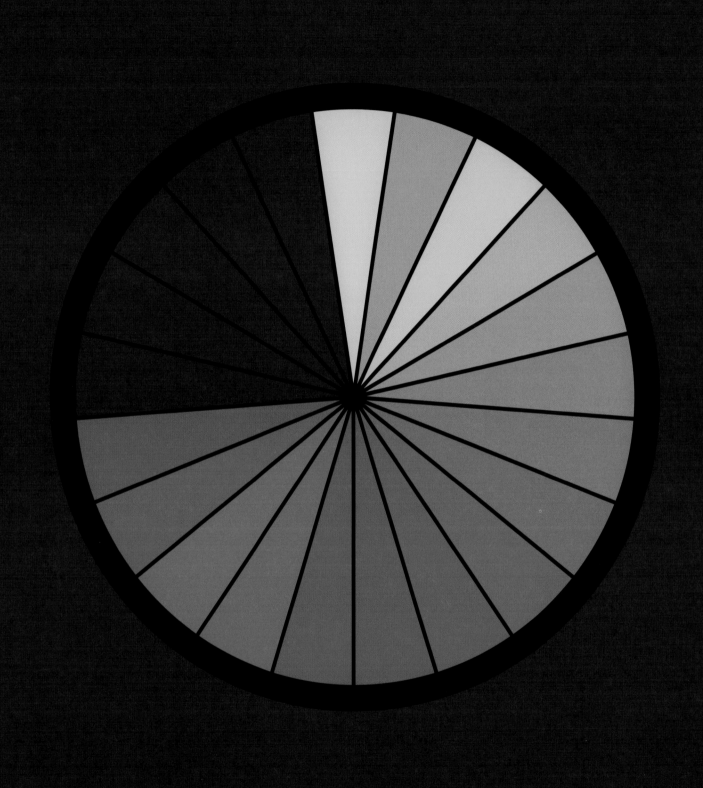

DAY 16

STAGE 15

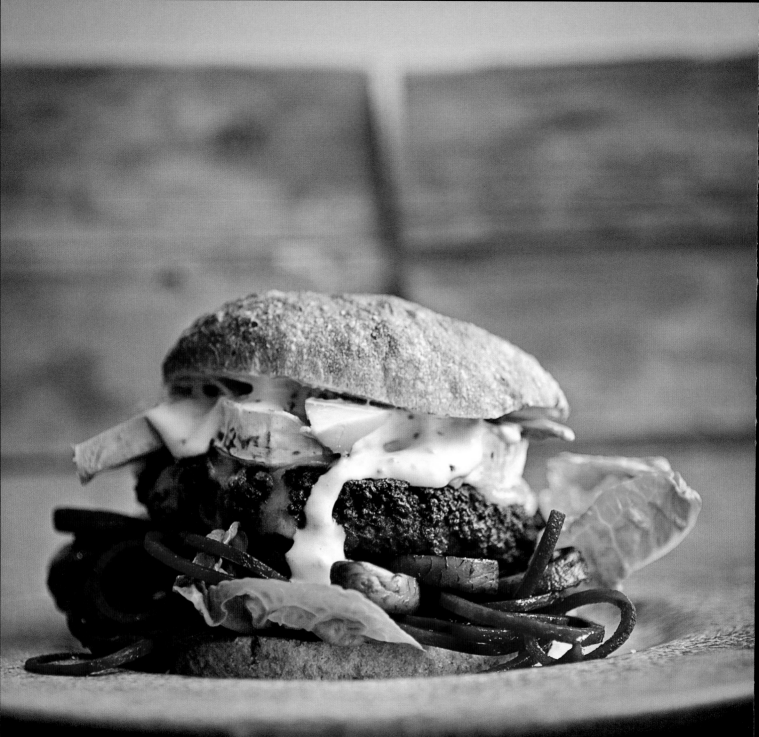

BURGER MANIA

4 BURGER BUNS (SEE PAGE 337)
1 KG MINCED BEEF
12 SLICES OF BACON
4 EGGS

A make-your-own burger is always a success and given the diversity of people on a cycling team, a great way to make sure there is something tasty to satisfy everyone. This is just one idea for a burger, but of course you can put on whatever you want: burger caprese with buffalo mozzarella, beef tomatoes, pickled red onion and basil; burger with blue cheese and roasted Portobello mushroom; the classic Danish burger with lettuce, celeriac remoulade, pickled gherkin and fried onions; or the classic Mexican with guacamole, tomatoes, onion and salsa.

WITH GOAT CHEESE, BEETROOT AND MUSHROOMS

MELTED GOAT CHEESE
BEETROOT CRUDITÉ
ROASTED PORTOBELLO MUSHROOM
ROMAINE LETTUCE
MUSTARD MAYONNAISE
AVOCADO

MELTED GOAT CHEESE
Pre-heat the oven to 200°C. Cut the goat cheese into 1.5 cm slices and place on the grilled burger. Heat in the oven at 200°C for 5 minutes until the cheese has melted.

ROASTED PORTOBELLO MUSHROOMS
Rinse the Portobello mushrooms, cut them into ½ cm slices and pan-roast them over medium/high heat in olive oil and salt.

MUSTARD MAYONNAISE
Whisk the egg yolks with salt, vinegar and the two mustards. While whisking, drizzle in the olive oil little by little until the desired thickness is reached. Season to taste with salt, pepper and vinegar.

MUSTARD MAYONNAISE
2 EGG YOLKS, PASTEURISED
1 TBSP TARRAGON VINEGAR
1 TBSP DIJON MUSTARD
1 TBSP COARSE-GRAINED
MUSTARD VINAIGRETTE
1 TSP CLEAR HONEY
250 ML COLD-PRESSED OLIVE OIL
½ TSP SALT
FRESHLY GROUND BLACK PEPPER

COLD BUTTERMILK
SOUP WITH BEETROOT

4 TBSP CREAMED HONEY
100 ML EGG YOLK, PASTEURISED
1 LITRE BUTTERMILK
500 ML JUNKET
JUICE AND ZEST OF 1 ORGANIC LEMON
3 TBSP BEETROOT CRYSTALS
OR 50 ML REDUCED BEETROOT JUICE

Beat the egg yolks and honey together until light and airy. While stirring, slowly pour in the buttermilk and junket. Wash the lemon and zest into the soup. Add the beetroot crystals and season to taste with lemon juice and honey. Cool completely before serving.

Serve the buttermilk soup ice cold with fresh berries and crispy, baked bits of leftover cake. Depending on the leftover cake used, the soup will be gluten-free.

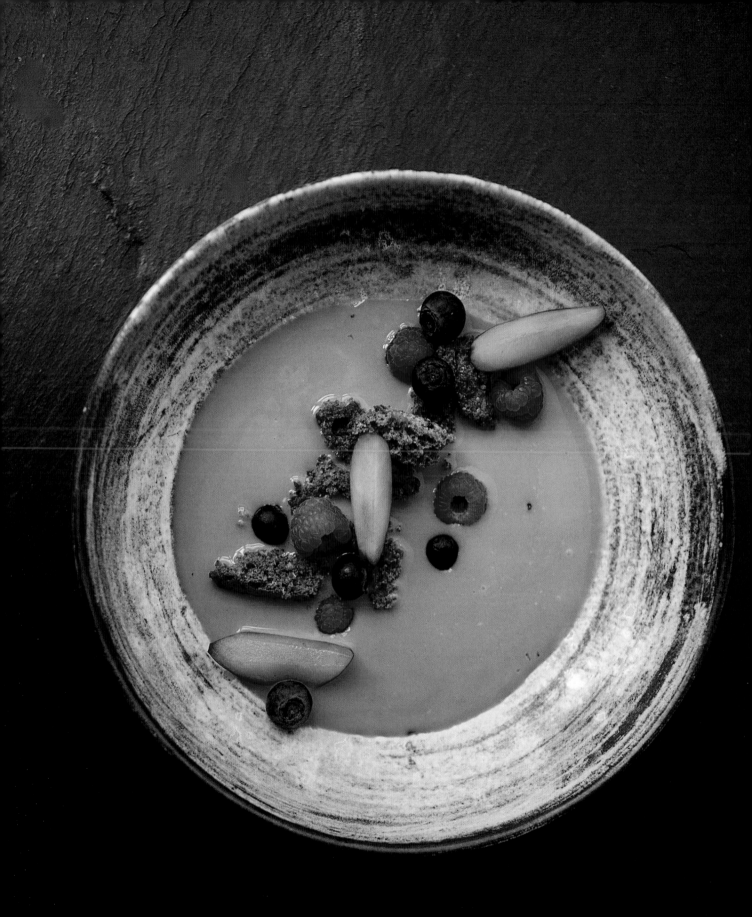

IVAN BASSO

"WHEN I KNOW THE FOOD IS THE BEST QUALITY POSSIBLE, I KNOW I CAN GIVE MY BEST."

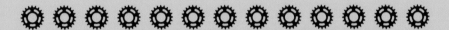

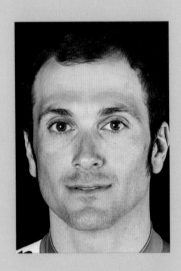

BORN: 26th November 1977
NATIONALITY: Italian
EXPERIENCE: Professional since 1998

Hannah (H): How important is the correct diet for you as a professional cyclist?
Ivan Basso (IB): For me it's very important to fuel correctly. The food that you eat provides the energy for the next day's ride, so I value good quality ingredients and the craftsmanship of a good meal. When I know the food is the best quality possible, I know I can give my best. Diet is not only eating the right things, it's also eating them at the right time, a crucial factor for optimal recovery. If you don't replenish your energy stores in the 20-minute-window after a hard day, it takes much longer for the body to get ready to ride again.

H: Can you feel the difference in your performance when you eat the right food?
IB: Yes, I have more energy and I recover faster. I also feel better in general, which is crucial for making it through a long stage or stage race. The times when I do have to eat processed, low quality food, I don't have the energy to give it my all. So for me, I can absolutely feel the difference.

H: How does eating right affect your weight? What works for you?
IB: It does! When I was younger I could eat almost anything I wanted without having to worry about gaining weight. But as I got older, my metabolism changed and I had to start thinking about what I ate and when so I would not put on weight. This resulted in me eating a lot more vegetables at all my meals and cutting down on starchy carbs at all meals except breakfast, where I eat what I want and need for a long stage.

H: What works best for you on an important race day? What do you typically eat on a day like this?
IB: In the morning I always have rice or pasta with a ham and cheese omelet and olive oil. This really keeps me going all day on the bike.

H: What is your favourite food in the race season?
IB: Good pasta with really good olive oil and parmesan cheese. I like simple, well-cooked food made from high quality products. It is important to me that the food is made with respect and care, which shows in the meal when it is served.

H: What is your advice for an amateur rider who wants to lose weight?
IB: You don't need any pasta or rice if you are riding for less than two hours. If you fill yourself with carbohydrates when they are not needed you will gain weight, so make sure to only eat carbs when they are needed. Cut down on sugar and have meals made with high quality ingredients, then you won't need as much to eat.

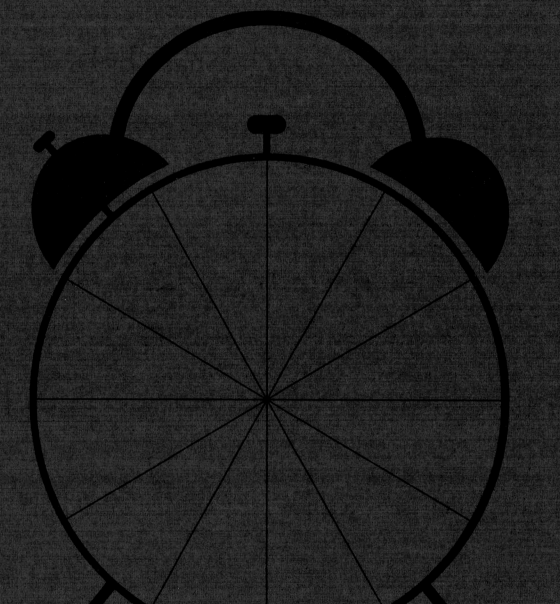

REST DAY

LUNCH

SALAD *with* EGGS, AIR-DRIED HAM AND PICKLED TOMATOES

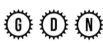

6 EGGS
12 SLICES OF AIR-DRIED HAM
200 G CHERRY TOMATOES
200 ML PICKLING LIQUID #3
(SEE PAGE 334)
2 ROMAINE LETTUCE HEARTS
100 ML COARSE-GRAINED MUSTARD
VINAIGRETTE (SEE PAGE 323)

Place the eggs in salted boiling water, boil for 8 minutes and immediately cool in cold water. Peel and halve the boiled eggs. Wash the cherry tomatoes and pluck off the stalks. Put into a saucepan with 1 tsp salt, add the pickling liquid, bring to a boil and simmer for 2 minutes. Remove the pan from the heat and let the tomatoes rest in the pickling liquid. Tear the romaine lettuce into bite-sized pieces, rinse and spin.

Arrange the egg, tomato, romaine lettuce and air-dried ham on a plate. Top with the mustard vinaigrette.

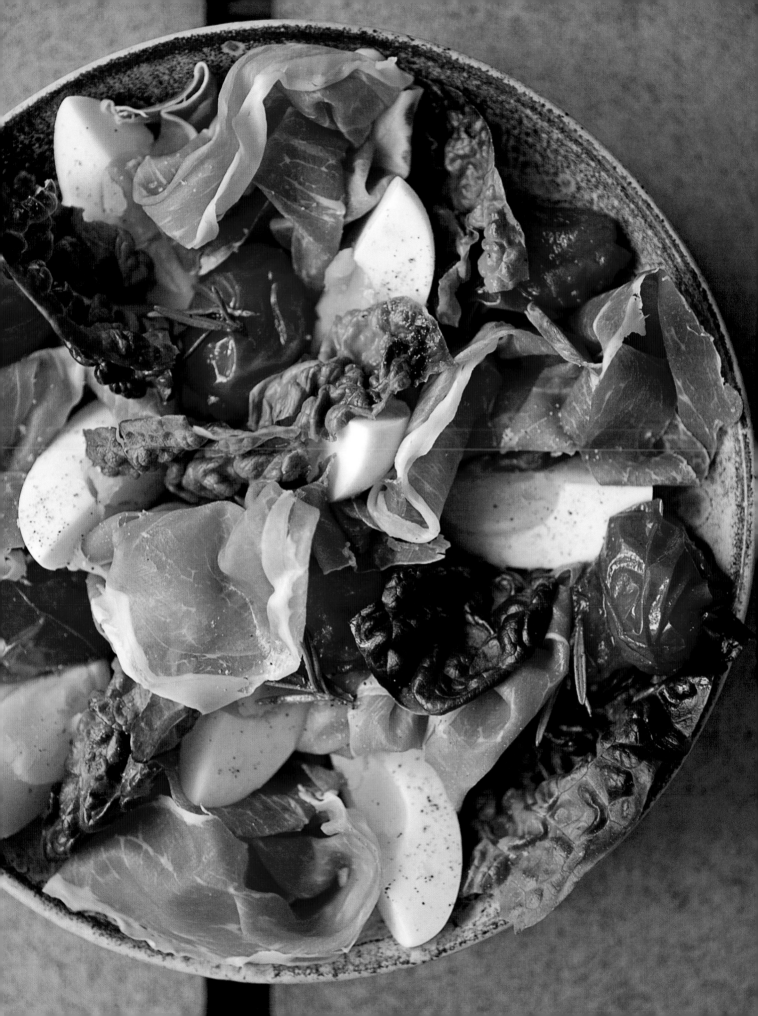

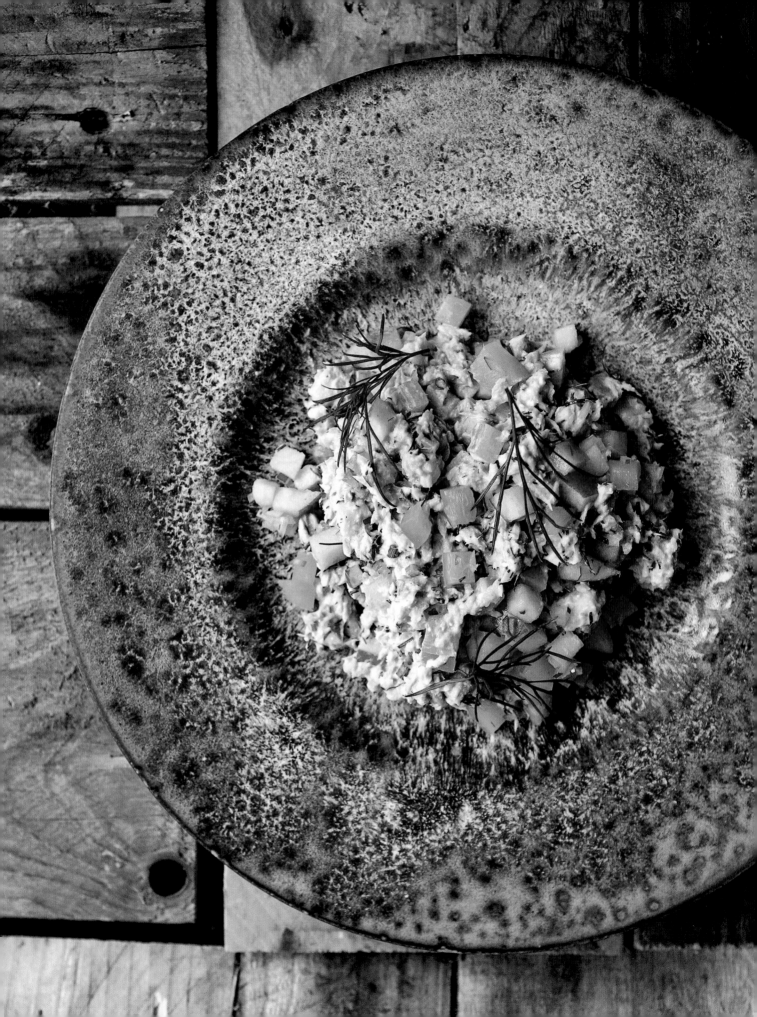

LUNCH

TUNA SALAD *with* FETA, YELLOW PEPPER AND APPLE

2 CANS OF TUNA (300 G TOTAL)
2 YELLOW PEPPERS
1 RED ONION
100 ML PICKLING LIQUID #2
(SEE PAGE 334)
½ BUNCH TARRAGON
JUICE AND ZEST OF 1 ORGANIC LIME
2 TBSP GREEK YOGHURT
100 G FETA
4 TBSP OLIVE OIL
SALT AND FRESHLY GROUND
BLACK PEPPER

Drain the tuna and transfer to a bowl. Wash the peppers, halve, scrape out the seeds and dice. Peel the onion, dice and cover with the warm pickling liquid. Cool before serving.

Tear the leaves off the tarragon and rinse, dry and chop them. Add the tarragon to the tuna, together with the pepper, lime zest and the cooled pickled onions. Mix everything with the olive oil, yoghurt and feta. Season to taste with salt, pepper and lime juice. Serve with bread.

CHICKEN, *quinoa,* MANDARIN AND SUNFLOWER SEEDS

600 G PLUCKED, COOKED CHICKEN
500 G QUINOA, BOILED
2 RED ONIONS
100 ML PICKLING LIQUID #1
(SEE PAGE 334)
4 MANDARINS
½ BUNCH PARSLEY
50 G SUNFLOWER SEEDS
100 ML HAZELNUT VINAIGRETTE
(SEE PAGE 322)
SALT
CIDER VINEGAR

Peel the onion, slice into thin rings and cover with pickling liquid. Peel the mandarins and cut into slices across the segments. Tear the parsley off the stalk, rinse and chop. Mix all the ingredients together and season with salt and cider vinegar.

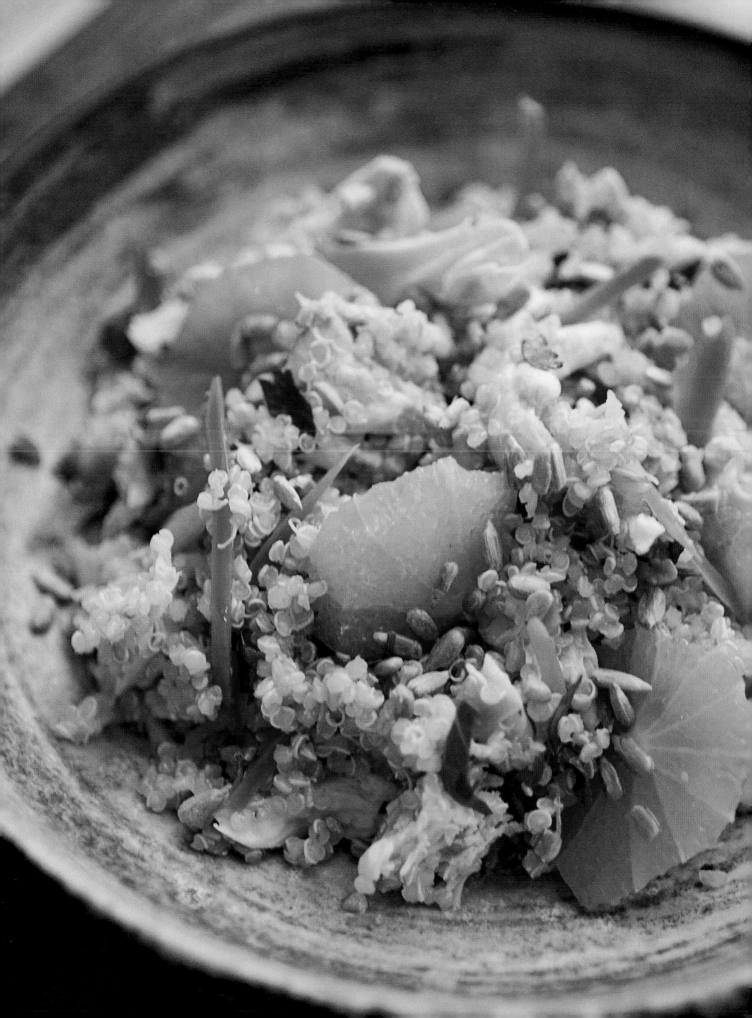

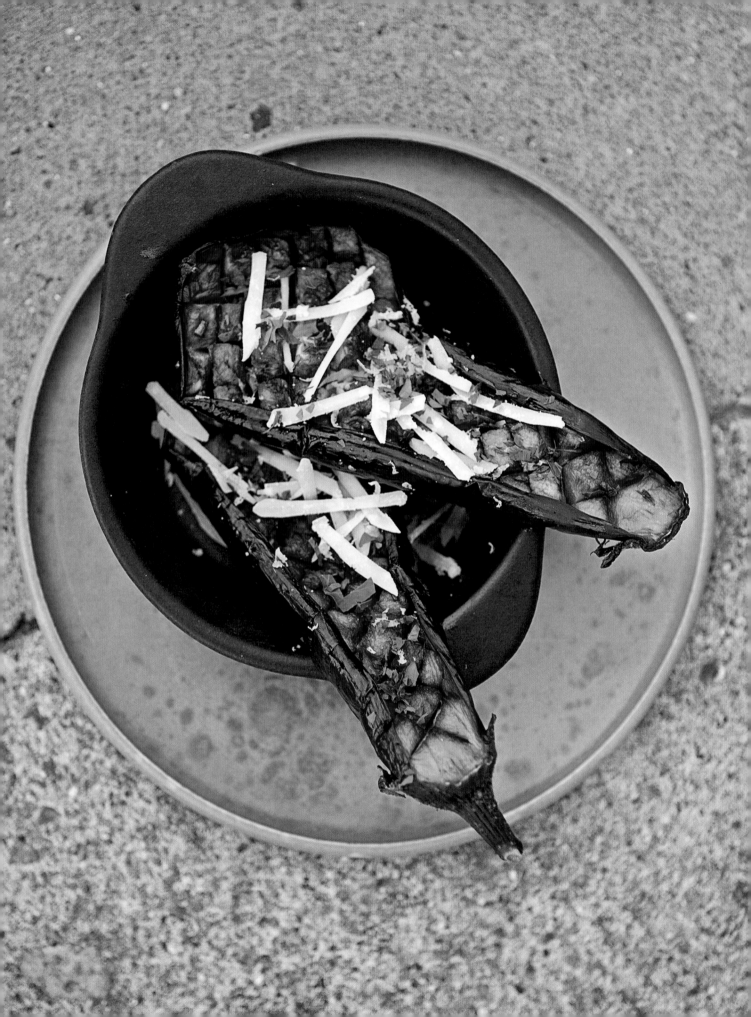

DINNER

BAKED AUBERGINE
WITH GARLIC AND PARMESAN

2 AUBERGINES
3 CLOVES GARLIC
4 TBSP OLIVE OIL
SALT AND FRESHLY GROUND
BLACK PEPPER
½ BUNCH PARSLEY
ZEST OF 1 ORGANIC LEMON
50 G SHAVED PARMESAN

Preheat the oven to 200°C.

Rinse the aubergines and halve lengthwise. Score the flesh deeply with a paring knife. Peel the garlic, chop, mix with the olive oil and rub onto the cut surfaces of the aubergines. Make sure the oil gets into the aubergine.

Season with salt and pepper and bake the aubergines in the oven until completely tender – about 30-35 minutes. At the same time, rinse the parsley and chop finely. Zest the lemon. Sprinkle the aubergines with freshly shaved parmesan, parsley and lemon zest just before serving.

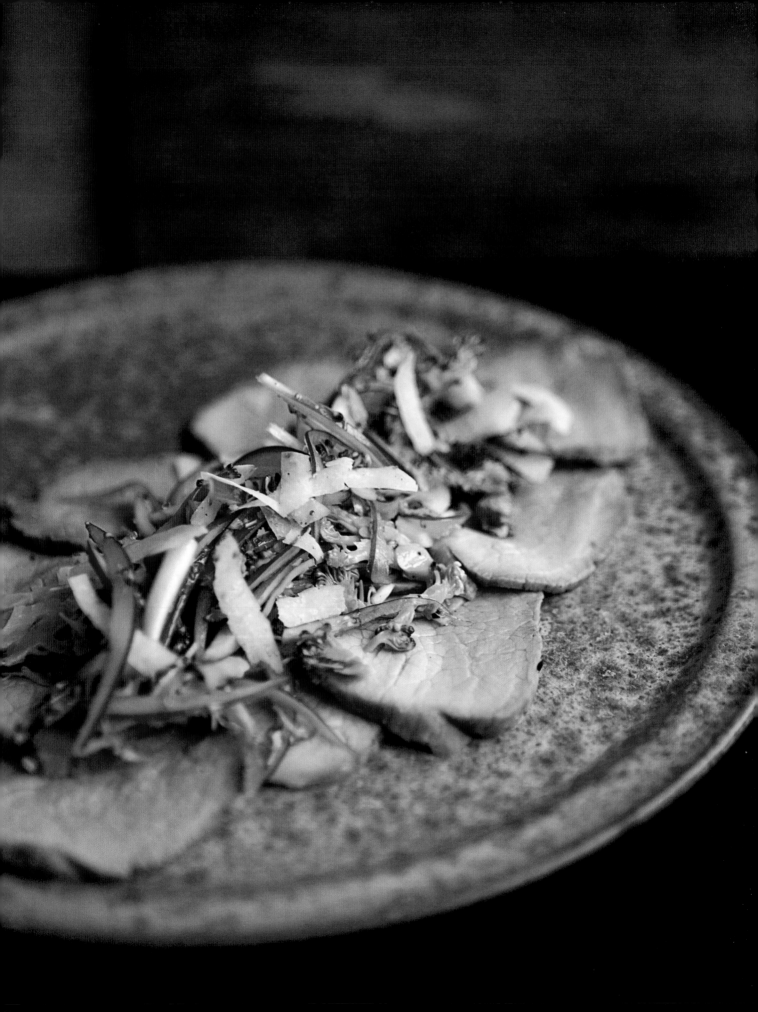

DINNER

COLD VEAL,
BROCCOLI CRUDITÉ AND
RAW PICKLED ONIONS

500 G VEAL TOP ROUND
1 RED ONION
100 ML CIDER VINEGAR
1 HEAD OF BROCCOLI
50 G PARMESAN
100 ML LEMON VINAIGRETTE
(SEE PAGE 325)
ZEST OF 1 ORGANIC LEMON
OLIVE OIL
SALT AND FRESHLY GROUND
BLACK PEPPER

Preheat the oven to 200°C.

Tie the veal with butchers twine, rub with olive oil and season with salt and pepper. Roast the veal in intervals: first for 20 minutes in the oven on a rack above a roasting pan. Then remove it from the oven and let it rest for 20 minutes before roasting for another 15 minutes. Let it rest for 15 minutes or until completely cool. The core temperature should be between 54 - 56°C.

Peel the onion, slice finely and cover with the cider vinegar. Rinse the broccoli, cut into florets and slice finely using a mandolin. Slice the veal into thin slices, drain on a paper towel and season with salt and pepper. Toss the onion and broccoli together with the dressing and arrange on top of the veal slices.

Top with lemon zest and shaved parmesan.

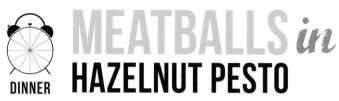

MEATBALLS *in* HAZELNUT PESTO

DINNER

500 G MINCED PORK
½ TSP SALT
2 EGGS
200 ML GLUTEN-FREE OATMEAL
200 ML RICE MILK OR MILK
2 ONIONS
2 CLOVES GARLIC
1 TBSP GROUND CORIANDER
1 PINCH GROUND CLOVES
FRESHLY GROUND BLACK PEPPER
OLIVE OIL
200 ML HAZELNUT PESTO
(SEE PAGE 329)

PICKLED CHERRY TOMATOES
500 G CHERRY TOMATOES
200 ML BALSAMIC VINEGAR
200 ML OLIVE OIL
1 TSP SALT
4 SPRIGS THYME
1 SPRIG ROSEMARY

Preheat the oven to 200°C.

Mix the meat thoroughly with salt. Mix in the eggs and oatmeal. Warm the milk to bathwater temperature and pour into the mince a little at a time until the mixture has a soft, homogeneous consistency. Peel the onions and garlic, finely chop both and add them to the mince mixture along with the ground coriander, cloves and pepper. Refrigerate for 30 minutes.

Shape the meatballs with a spoon and place them on a baking tray covered with baking paper. Drizzle with olive oil and bake until the meatballs are totally firm – about 10-12 minutes.

PICKLED CHERRY TOMATOES

Rinse the thyme and rosemary. Rinse the tomatoes, prick with a sharp knife, place them in a saucepan and add the vinegar, oil, salt, thyme and rosemary. Bring to a simmer over medium heat and cook for 2 minutes. Remove the pan from the heat and let it rest until needed.

Serve the meatballs with warm pickled tomatoes and whole grain or gluten-free pasta tossed in hazelnut pesto.

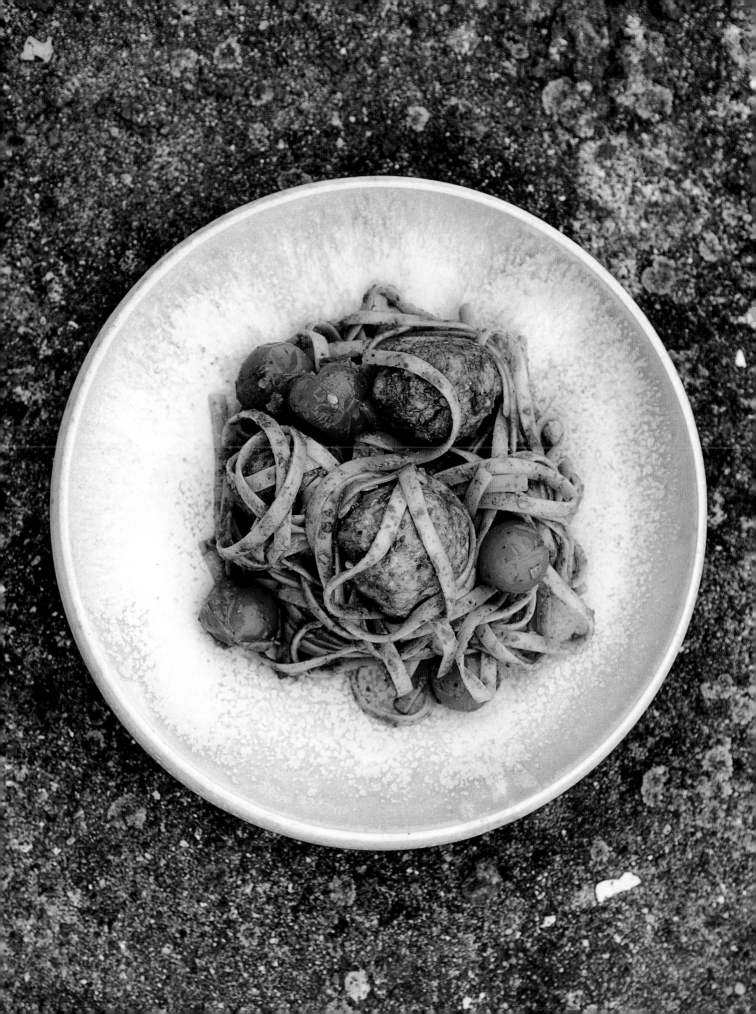

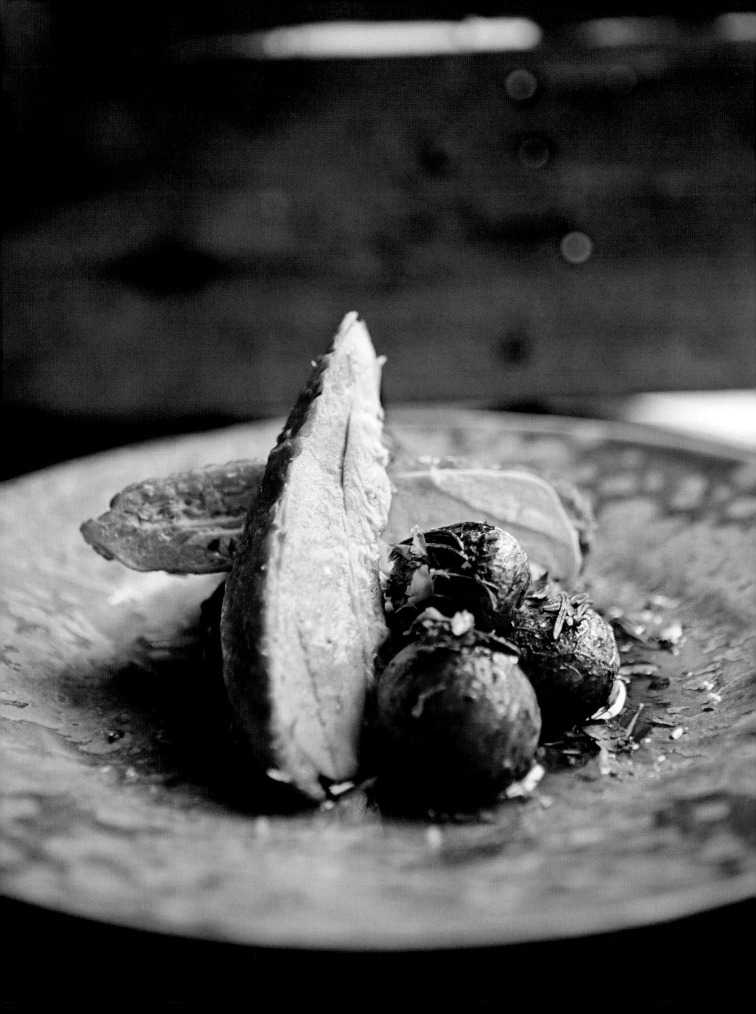

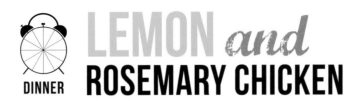

LEMON *and*
ROSEMARY CHICKEN

DINNER

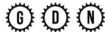

1 CHICKEN (1.2-1.4 KG)
4 TBSP HONEY
JUICE AND ZEST OF 2 ORGANIC LEMONS
EXTRA LEMON ZEST FOR SERVING
½ BUNCH FRESH ROSEMARY
50 ML OLIVE OIL
SALT
500 G NEW POTATOES
¼ BUNCH PARSLEY

Wash the rosemary, tear the leaves off the stems and chop. In a bowl, whisk together the honey, lemon juice, lemon zest, rosemary, olive oil and salt. Put the chicken in a plastic bag and pour in the marinade. Firmly rub the marinade into the meat. Close the bag and let the chicken marinate for at least 1 hour or preferably overnight.

Preheat the oven to 175°C.

Place the chicken directly on a rack over a roasting pan and roast until the juice runs clear – about 60 minutes. At the same time, scrub the potatoes and toss them in olive oil and salt. In the roasting pan under the chicken, add the potatoes so the juices from the chicken drip over them and roast for 30-35 minutes. Rinse, spin and chop the parsley. Serve the chicken with potatoes, sprinkle with chopped parsley and lemon zest.

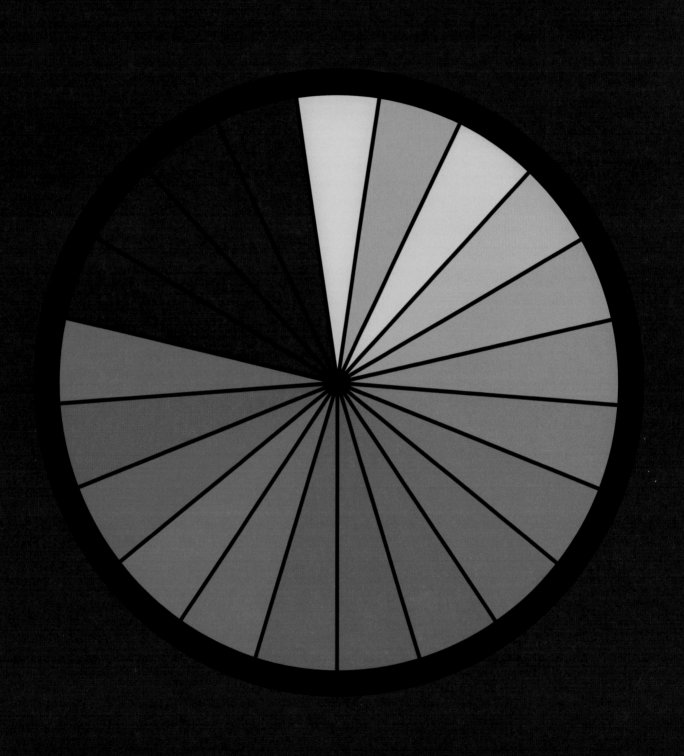

DAY

STAGE 16

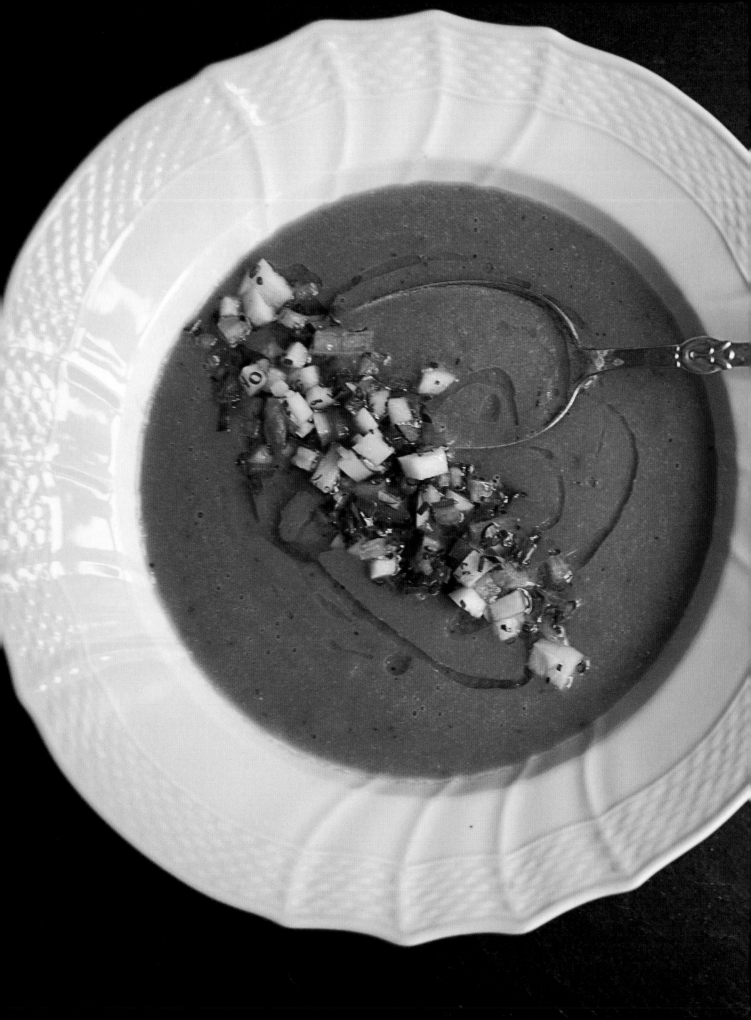

GAZPACHO *with*
APPLE AND YELLOW PEPPER

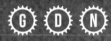

600 G RIPE TOMATOES
1 CUCUMBER
3 RED PEPPERS
½ SHALLOT
3 CLOVES GARLIC
100 ML COLD-PRESSED OLIVE OIL
3 TBSP SHERRY VINEGAR
SALT

GARNISH
2 YELLOW PEPPERS
2 APPLES
½ BUNCH PARSLEY
½ BUNCH CHIVES
COLD-PRESSED OLIVE OIL

Wash the tomatoes and cut each into 8 wedges. Peel the cucumber and cut into thick slices. Peel and chop the shallots and garlic. Scrape the seeds from the peppers and chop into chunks.

Blend the tomato, cucumber, onion, garlic and pepper to a fine purée. While still blending, slowly pour in the olive oil. Season the soup with salt and vinegar.

For the garnish, rinse the peppers, apples, parsley and chives. Scrape the seeds from the peppers. Quarter and core the apples. Dice both. Chop the parsley finely and cut the chives.

Serve the soup ice cold with the cold-pressed olive oil and garnish.

FRESH SPRINGROLLS
with ## RICE NOODLES, MINT AND PEANUT SAUCE

200 G RICE NOODLES, COOKED
4 TBSP SOY SAUCE
1 TSP SESAME OIL
1 AVOCADO
2 CARROTS
½ BUNCH MINT
16 SHEETS RICE PAPER

PEANUT SAUCE
4 TBSP UNSWEETENED
PEANUT BUTTER
50 ML OLIVE OIL
50 ML WATER
2 TBSP SOY SAUCE
1 TBSP HONEY
JUICE AND ZEST OF
2 ORGANIC LIMES

Toss the rice noodles with the soy sauce and sesame oil. Cut the avocado in half and remove the stone. Carefully scrape out the flesh in one piece with a spoon and cut into 3 mm slices. Peel the carrots and cut into thin strips. Rinse the mint and tear the leaves off the stalk.

Soak a sheet of rice paper in a bowl of cold water for 1 minute. Lay out on a dry cutting board, place two mint leaves in the middle of the rice paper, two slices of avocado on top of the mint, a bit of carrot and finish with a few rice noodles.

Fold the rice paper like an envelope around the ingredients. First fold in the sides, then the bottom, tighten the filling together and roll up to the top of the rice paper. Repeat the procedure until all the rice paper and filling has been used. It takes a little practice to get perfectly round rolls, but they taste great, even when a little uneven. Serve with peanut sauce.

PEANUT SAUCE
Mix the peanut butter with olive oil. Add the water, soy sauce, honey, lime zest and lemon juice. If necessary, season with more soy sauce and lime juice.

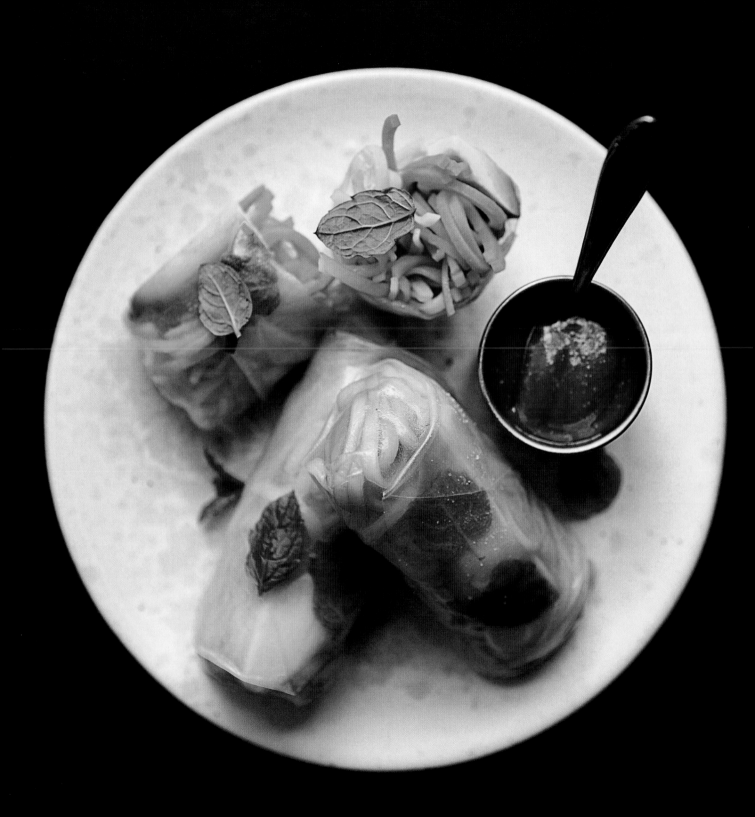

SLOW-ROASTED
SHOULDER OF PORK WITH WHITE BEAN SALAD AND GINGER SAUCE

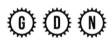

1 SHOULDER OF PORK (APPROX. 3 KG)
2 TBSP HONEY
2 TBSP SALT
500 ML WHITE WINE

WHITE BEANS WITH FRESH HERBS
250 G DRIED WHITE BEANS
1 PIECE KOMBU SEAWEED
½ BUNCH THYME
¼ BUNCH PARSLEY
2 STAR ANISE
4 BAY LEAVES
1 TSP SALT
¼ BUNCH TARRAGON
2 CLOVES GARLIC
50 ML OLIVE OIL
ZEST OF 2 ORGANIC LEMONS
SALT AND FRESHLY GROUND
BLACK PEPPER

6-8 SERVINGS

For this recipe, you should prepare the shoulder of pork a day in advance, so start by marinating two days before planning to serve.

Trim the pork shoulder and rub it with honey mixed with salt. Cover with cling film and refrigerate for at least 6 hours or preferably overnight.

Preheat the oven to 100°C.

Place the pork shoulder on a rack above a roasting pan filled with the white wine. Roast the shoulder in the oven for 12 hours. Once an hour, baste it with the wine and juices. When the meat can be pulled off the bone without resistance, it is ready.

The pork shoulder can be eaten immediately or cooled and served later.

WHITE BEANS WITH FRESH HERBS
Soak the beans in cold water overnight. Rinse and dry the thyme. Rinse the parsley and tear the leaves off the stalks. Drain the beans and add to a saucepan along with fresh water, the kombu, thyme, parsley stalks (save the leaves for later), star anise, bay leaves and salt. Bring to a boil, reduce the heat and simmer the beans until tender – about 30 minutes. Regularly skim off any impurities. Cool the beans in the cooking liquid.

Rinse and chop the tarragon and parsley leaves. Grate the garlic with a Microplane. Drain the beans and add the olive oil, tarragon, parsley, garlic and lemon zest. Season with salt and pepper.

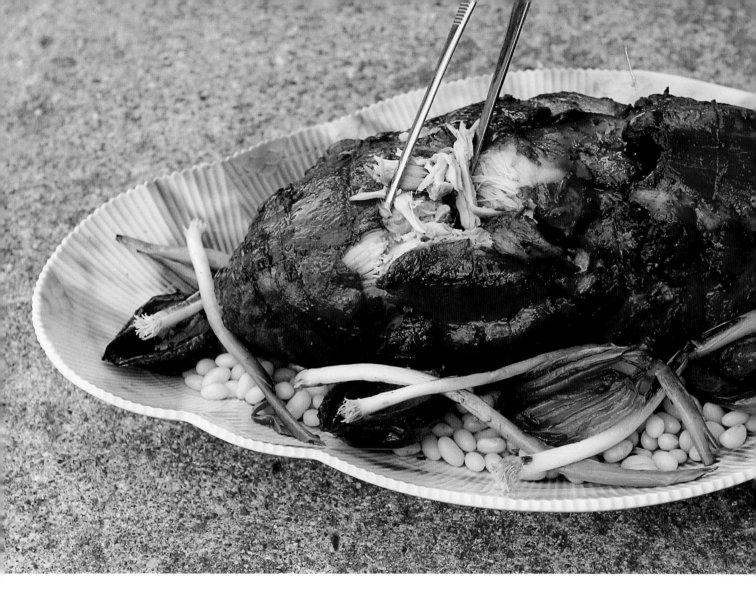

SWEET ONIONS

2 BUNCHES SPRING ONIONS
3 RED ONIONS
3 ONIONS
3 TBSP OLIVE OIL
SALT

SWEET ONIONS

Clean the spring onions and cut the roots and tops off. Peel and halve the onions. Place cut-side down in a frying pan with olive oil and salt. Cover the pan with aluminium foil and set over a low heat. Let the onions caramelise and steam slowly until ready – about 30 minutes. Set a saucepan on top of the spring onions and roast the spring onions in a dry frying pan over high heat until they are completely dark on one side and steamed through.

GINGER SAUCE

100 G FRESH GINGER
200 ML OLIVE OIL
4 TBSP SOY SAUCE
2 TBSP CLEAR HONEY
2 TBSP CIDER VINEGAR

GINGER SAUCE

Peel the ginger and cut into small pieces. Blend with the olive oil. Stir in soy sauce, honey and vinegar to taste.

An hour before serving, heat the pork shoulder in a 150°C oven. Serve with the white beans, fresh herbs, sweet onions and ginger sauce.

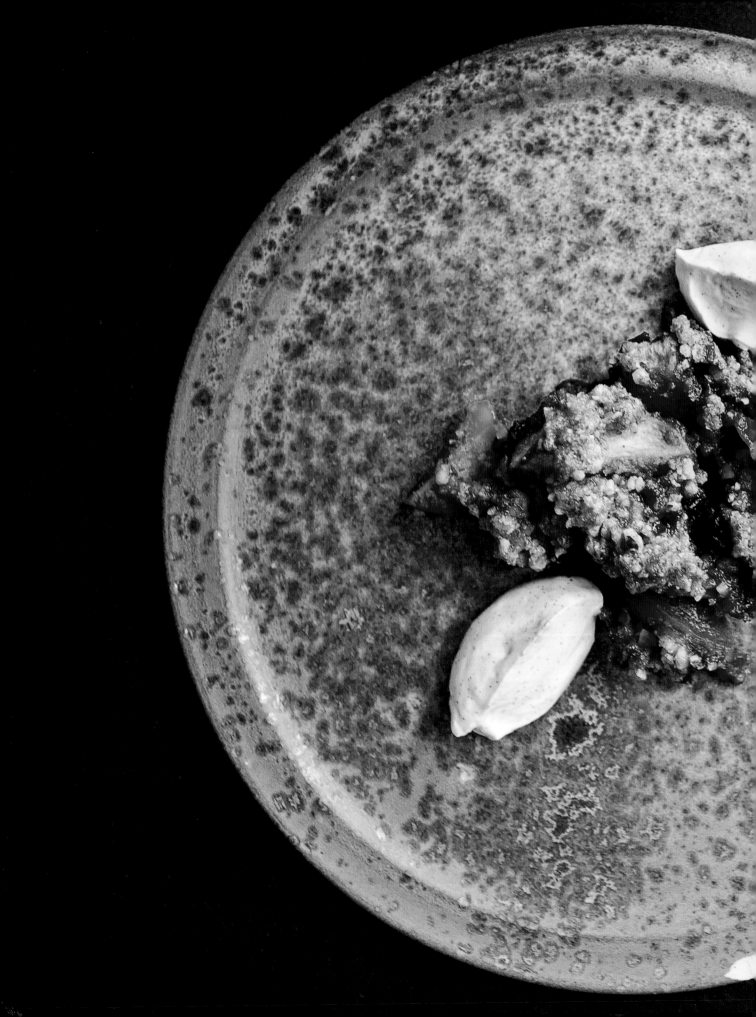

APPLE
AND BLUEBERRY CRUMBLE

(G)

50 G ALMOND FLOUR
50 G ROLLED OATS
50 G BUTTER
50 G CANE SUGAR
4 APPLES
300 G FRESH OR FROZEN BLUEBERRIES
3 TBSP CLEAR HONEY

Preheat the oven to 170°C.

With your hands, rub the almond flour, oats, butter and sugar into a crumbly dough. Peel the apples, quarter, remove the cores and cut the wedges into large chunks. Place the apples in an ovenproof dish with a little butter and spread the blueberries on top. Spread the dough across the baking dish, covering the apples and blueberries and bake until the top is nice and golden and the apples and berries are cooked – about 15-20 minutes.

Serve warm with Greek yoghurt/skyr and drizzled honey.

PETER SAGAN

"DIET IS ONE OF THE BASICS OF PERFORMANCE"

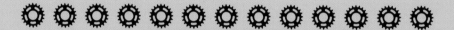

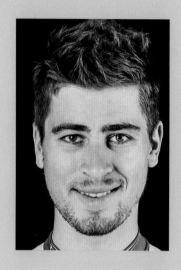

BORN: 26th January 1990
NATIONALITY: Slovakian
EXPERIENCE: Professional
since 2009

Hannah (H): How important is the right diet for you as a professional cyclist?

Peter Sagan (PS): Like any other professional sportsman, it's part of our commitment. I have to feed my body properly when training or racing, otherwise it will strike, which means that we cannot win races.

H: How do you think diet changes an athlete's performance?

PS: Diet is one of the basics of performance, even just for getting sufficient amount of energy into the system. Depending on the length of a stage or a training session, you need to adjust portions' sizes so you can make it through the day. For example, if I don't eat enough, my energy levels drop and my mind is focused on food all the time, which makes it hard for me to perform at my best.

H: Can you feel the difference in your performance when you eat the right food?

PS: Yes, definitely. Riders need to eat a proper diet on a daily basis and, of course, a well-balanced, good, nutritious meal before a hard training session or a long stage race. Also, eating the right food at the right time is crucial for the optimal recovery, so riders can be ready for the next day.

H: How did eating right affect your weight?

PS: Well, I'm not the type of rider that has to be extremely careful about their weight, but I feel better when I eat good, high quality food. I prefer to eat organic food if I have the option.

H: What works best for you on an important race day? What do you typically eat on a day like this?

PS: Everything that's on the table! As I said, I have to eat a lot to get through a day on the bike. Normally I like something sweet, muesli, good quality bread with jam, chocolate spread, sometimes pasta and definitely a nice coffee.

H: Has changing your diet affected you physically or mentally?

PS: I ride well if I eat a good, varied diet. I know that I get nervous when I'm hungry, so I always make sure to eat well.

H: When not racing, what do you eat before, during and after a typical day of training?

PS: When I'm at home, I start my day with freshly-squeezed juice and a cappuccino – that's my ritual. As for breakfast, something salty, like poached eggs with whole grain or muesli bread, but there always has to be something sweet, too. My favourite is pancakes or waffles with organic Jerusalem artichoke syrup and organic Jerusalem artichoke and blueberry jam. During my training I always grab a cappuccino and croissant. After training, I make sure to load up on pasta, rice or soup.

H: Is the taste and appearance of food important to you on a long stage race where you tend to lose your appetite?

PS: For me, the most important thing is that the food is of good quality. As long as I can get the fuel I need before and after a long day on the bike, I am happy.

H: What is your favourite food in the race season?

PS: When I'm in the season I like to eat everything, and a lot of it!

H: What is your favourite food out of season?

PS: I don't have any favourite foods, no cravings for anything specific. I like everything.

H: Can good food help make the difference between whether you win or not?

PS: Hard to say, I would say a proper diet is one of many factors that can influence my performance to a great extent.

H: How has your opinion on food for athletes changed in the last couple of years?

PS: When I was a non-professional rider, I ate very non-professionally, not thinking about recovery and the days to come. I learned a lot since I became a pro-rider, it's important to fuel correctly.

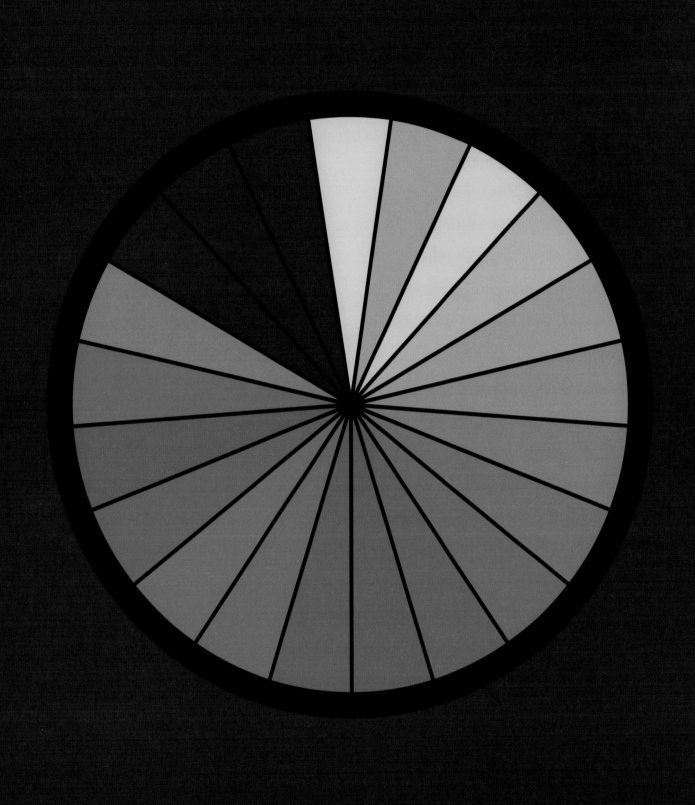

DAY 13

STAGE 17

MOZZARELLA,
BLACKBERRIES, MARJORAM AND APPLE

(G) (N)

2 X BUFFALO MOZZARELLA
3 APPLES
JUICE OF 1 LIME
½ BUNCH MARJORAM
100 G FRESH BLACKBERRIES
4 TBSP OLIVE OIL
SALT AND FRESHLY GROUND BLACK PEPPER

Drain the mozzarella and tear it into small pieces. Wash the apples, quarter, remove the cores, cut the quarters into thin slices and marinate in the lime juice. Rinse and tear the leaves off the marjoram. Rinse blackberries and halve half of them. Serve the mozzarella, blackberries and apple with olive oil, pepper and salt.

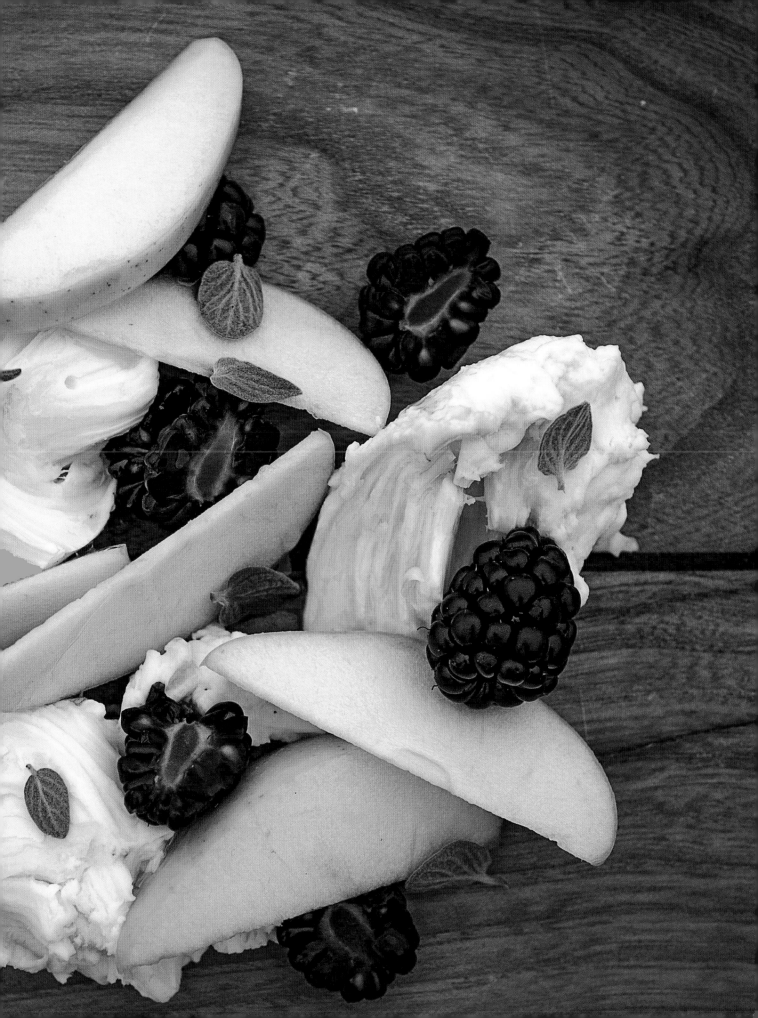

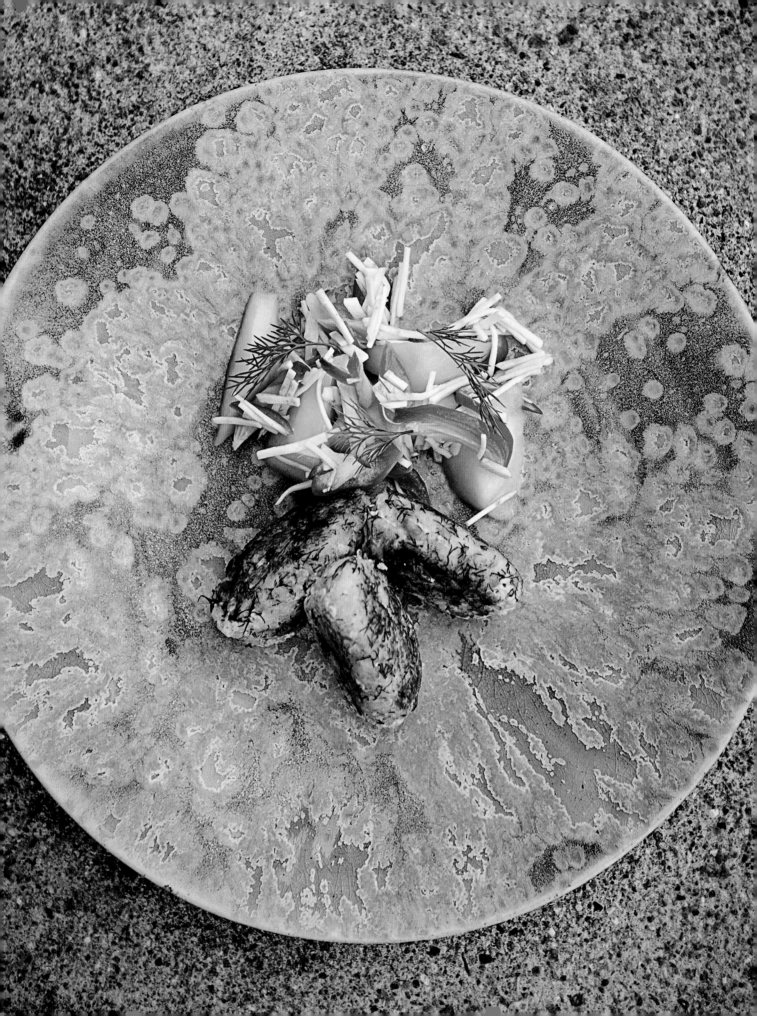

FISH CAKES *with* MANGO SALAD

600 G FILLET OF COD OR POLLACK
½ TSP SALT
3 EGGS
2 TBSP GLUTEN-FREE FINE ROLLED OATS
100 ML MILK (ROOM TEMPERATURE)
2 SHALLOTS
1 CLOVE GARLIC
50 G FRESH GINGER
½ BUNCH DILL
4 TBSP OLIVE OIL
FRESHLY GROUND BLACK PEPPER

MANGO SALAD

2 MANGOS
1 RED ONION
1 HEAD OF CELERIAC
100 ML PICKLING LIQUID #1
(SEE PAGE 334)
4 TBSP OLIVE OIL
JUICE OF 1 LIME
SALT AND FRESHLY GROUND
BLACK PEPPER

Preheat the oven to 175°C.

Cut half of the fish into 1x1 cubes. Blend the rest with salt to a fine consistency in a food processor. Add the eggs one at a time, blending until the mixture is homogenous. Continuing to blend, add the oats and slowly pour in the milk.

Peel and mince the shallots and garlic. Peel and grate the ginger. Rinse the dill, tear off the leaves and chop finely. Transfer the blended fish mixture to a bowl. Mix in the cubed fish, onion, garlic, half of the dill, ginger and pepper. Fry a teaspoon of the mixture in a frying pan to check the seasoning.

Shape the fish cakes with a tablespoon, brown on both sides in a non-stick frying pan in 1 tbsp olive oil. Transfer the fish cakes to an oven-proof dish and bake in the oven for 6-7 minutes until firm and done.

MANGO SALAD

Peel the red onion, halve and slice lengthwise. Put the slices in a bowl, pour the pickling liquid over them and refrigerate. Halve the mango, remove the stone, peel and dice. Peel the celeriac and grate using a grater or a food processor. Toss the celeriac, mango and onion with olive oil and season with lime juice, salt and pepper.

Serve the fish cakes with mango salad and topped with dill.

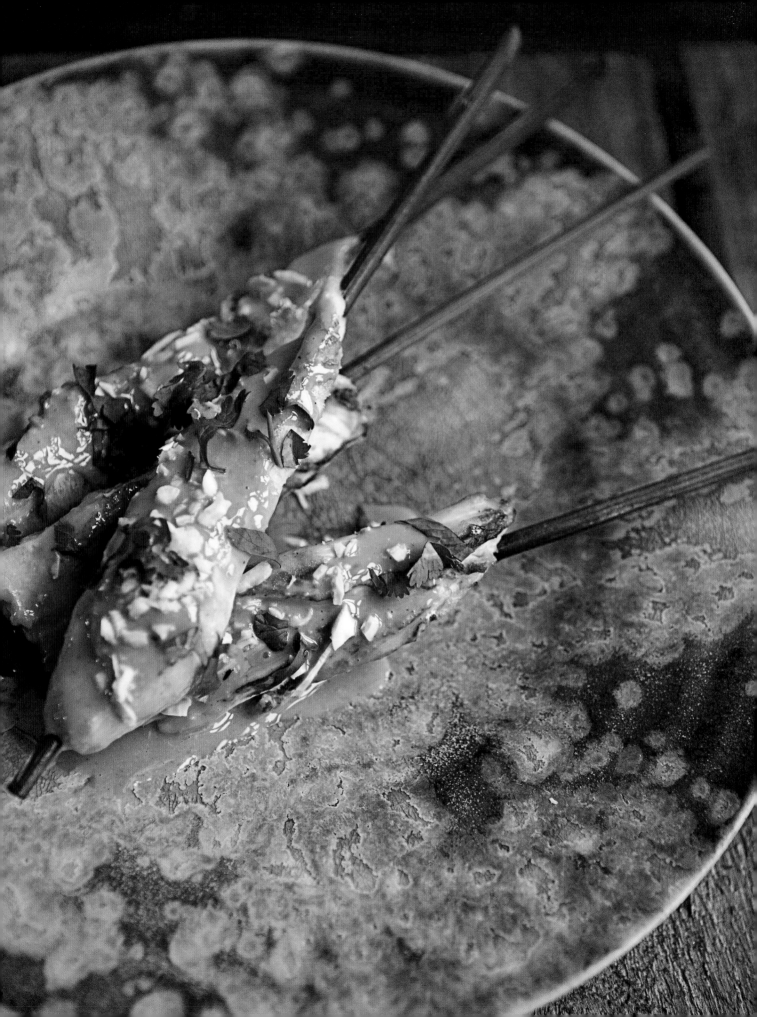

PEANUT CHICKEN
KEBABS

4-6 CHICKEN BREASTS (800 G TOTAL)
12 WOODEN SKEWERS
4 TBSP UNSWEETENED PEANUT BUTTER
4 TBSP SOY SAUCE
1 TBSP HONEY
1 CLOVE GARLIC
JUICE AND ZEST OF 2 ORGANIC LIMES
2 TBSP CHOPPED CASHEWS
1 BUNCH CORIANDER

Soak the wooden skewers in water for 5 minutes to prevent from burning in the oven. Preheat the oven to 175°C.

Mix the peanut butter with the soy sauce, honey, grated garlic, lime zest and lime juice. Cut each chicken breast lengthwise into thirds, salt and thread the pieces onto the wooden skewers. Roast the kebabs until the chicken is cooked through and firm – about 7-8 minutes. Meanwhile, rinse and chop the coriander.

Pour the sauce over the chicken kebabs and top with the chopped cashews and coriander.

POACHED *pears,* YOGHURT AND CHOCOLATE

4 PEARS
500 ML WHITE WINE
500 ML WATER
250 G CANE SUGAR
1 CINNAMON STICK
2 STAR ANISE
1 VANILLA POD
200 ML GREEK YOGHURT
1 TBSP HONEY
JUICE AND ZEST OF 1 ORGANIC LEMON
100 G 70% DARK CHOCOLATE

Bring water, wine, sugar and spices to a boil. Peel the pears and place them in the sugar syrup. Cover with a sheet of baking paper and a small plate to keep the pears in the syrup. Bring the syrup back to a boil, reduce the heat and simmer until the pears are tender – about 15 minutes. Let the pears cool in the syrup. Using a teaspoon, dig the core from the bottom of each pear.

Mix the yoghurt with honey and lemon zest. Flavour the yoghurt cream with lemon juice. Serve the pears with the yoghurt cream and chopped dark chocolate.

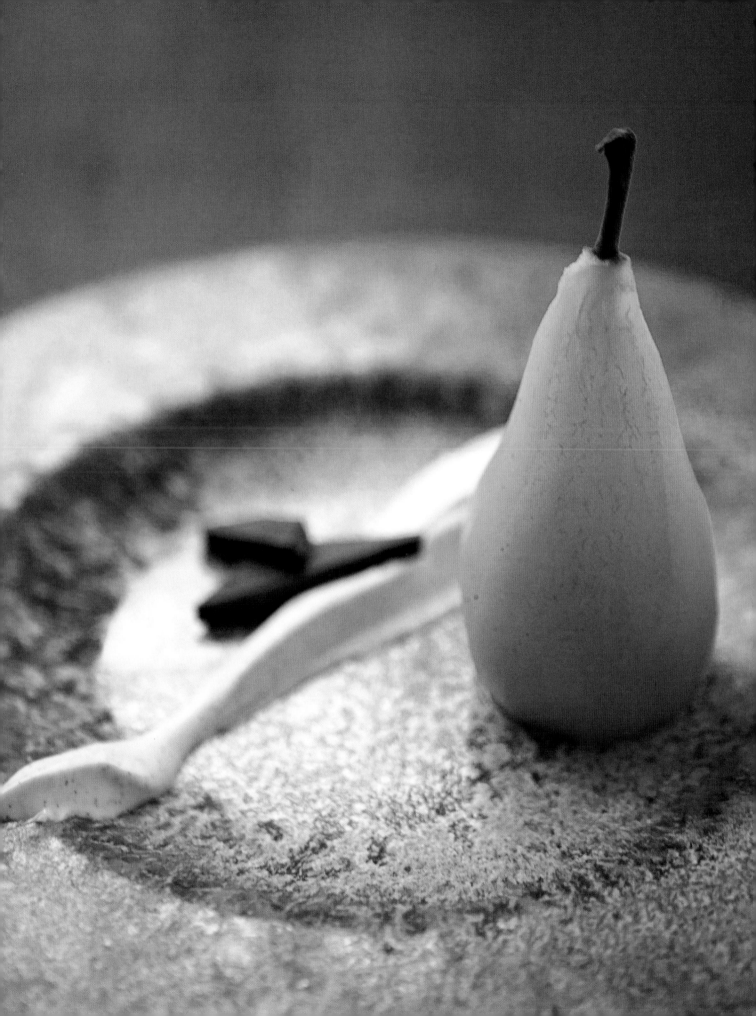

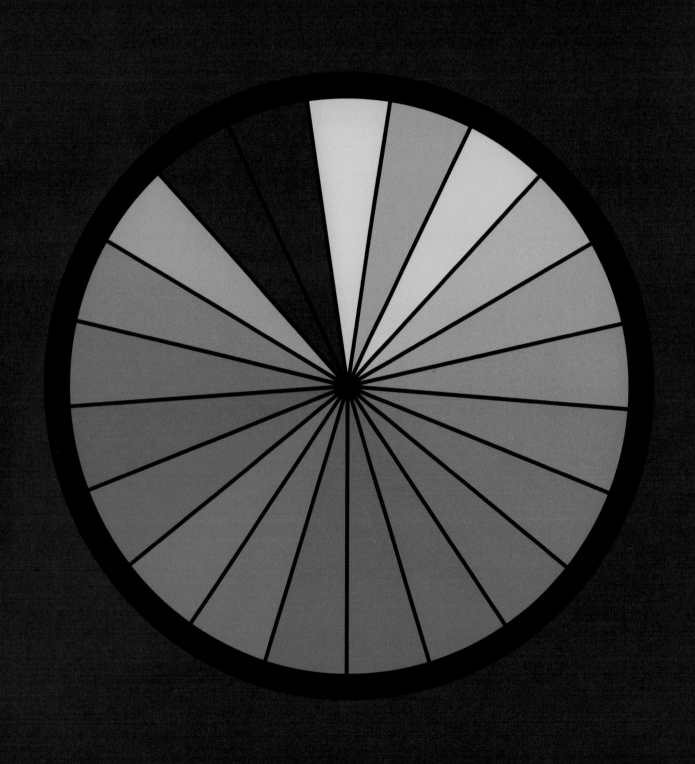

DAY 18

STAGE 18

RATATOUILLE

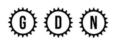

2 COURGETTES
1 AUBERGINE
2 RED PEPPERS
1 YELLOW PEPPER
4 RED ONIONS
4 SPRIGS ROSEMARY
4 SPRIGS THYME
¼ BUNCH PARSLEY
2 STAR ANISE
3 BAY LEAVES
1 CAN PEELED TOMATOES
1 CAN CONCENTRATED
TOMATO PURÉE (70 G)
2 TBSP HONEY
100 ML BALSAMIC VINEGAR
SALT AND PEPPER
OLIVE OIL FOR FRYING

Rinse the courgettes, aubergine and peppers and chop into to bite-sized pieces. Peel the onions and cut into ½ cm thick rings. Rinse and tear the leaves off the rosemary, thyme and parsley. Roughly chop the parsley and rosemary and put in separate bowls.

Pan-roast all vegetables separately on high heat with olive oil and salt until nicely caramelised. Transfer all the vegetables to a pot along with the thyme, rosemary, star anise, bay leaves, peeled tomatoes and tomato purée. Bring to a boil over a low heat.

At the same time, in a small saucepan, warm the honey over medium heat until it begins to bubble. Pour in the balsamic vinegar and reduce by half. Once the vegetables and puree have come to a boil, pour in the honey mixture and simmer for 10 minutes. Season the ratatouille with salt, pepper and balsamic vinegar. Remove the pot from the heat and mix in the parsley just before serving.

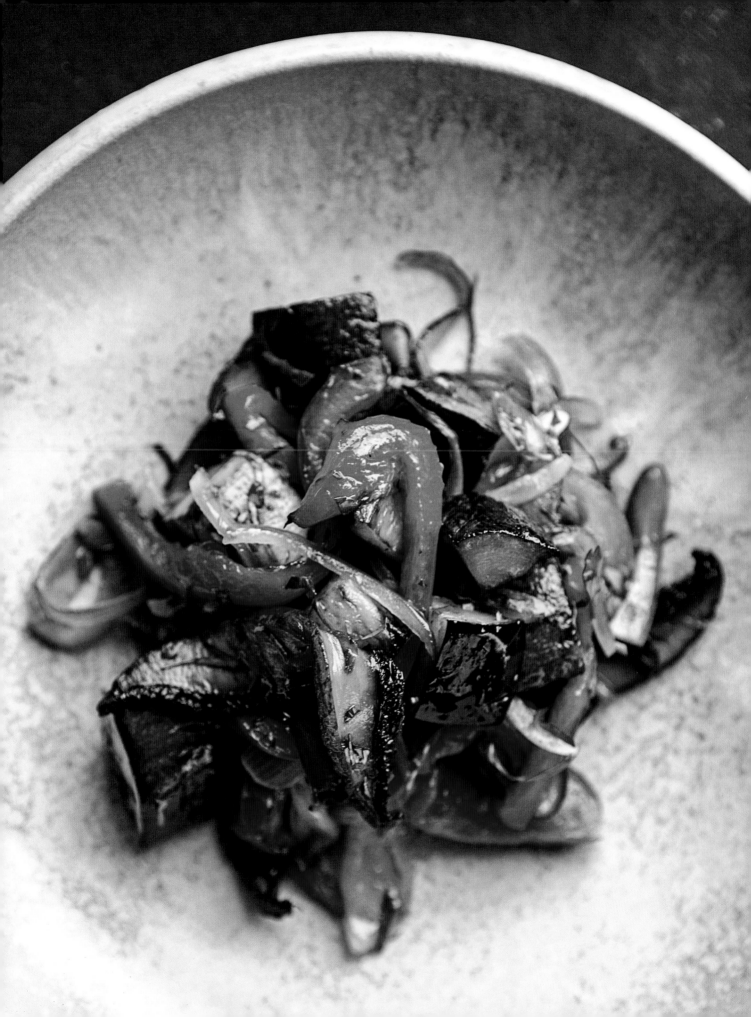

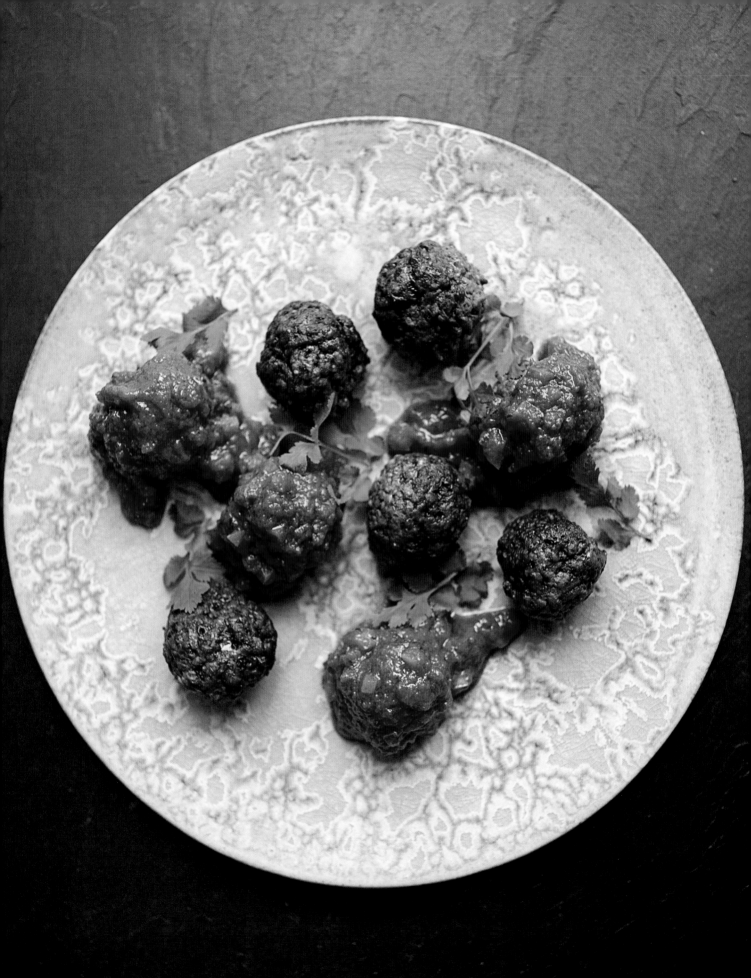

MEATBALLS *with*
CORIANDER AND
SPICY TOMATO SAUCE

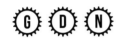

500 G MINCED BEEF
2 EGGS
200 ML GLUTEN-FREE OATMEAL
200 ML RICE MILK OR MILK
2 ONIONS
2 CLOVES GARLIC
50 G GINGER
1 TBSP GROUND CORIANDER
½ TSP SALT
FRESHLY GROUND BLACK PEPPER

1 LITRE TOMATO SAUCE OF YOUR
OWN CHOICE (SEE PAGE 330-331)
½ TSP CINNAMON
½ TSP CUMIN
3 TBSP HONEY
3 CLOVES GARLIC
2 TBSP CIDER VINEGAR
1 BUNCH CORIANDER

Mix the mince thoroughly with salt, eggs and oatmeal. Warm the milk and pour it in a little at a time until the mince mixture has a soft, homogeneous consistency. Peel the onions and garlic and chop finely. Peel the ginger and grate finely. Add the onion, garlic, ginger, ground coriander and freshly ground black pepper to the mince mixture. Let the mince stand in the refrigerator for 30 minutes.

Preheat the oven to 200°C.

Fry a mini meatball in olive oil to check the seasoning. Shape the meatballs with a tablespoon and place on a baking tray covered with baking paper brushed with olive oil. Roast until the meatballs are cooked through and firm – about 8-10 minutes.

Bring the tomato sauce to a boil. Peel the garlic, chop finely and sauté it in 1 tbsp olive oil. Season the sauce with cinnamon, cumin, honey, vinegar and garlic.

Serve the meatballs with the sauce and freshly chopped coriander.

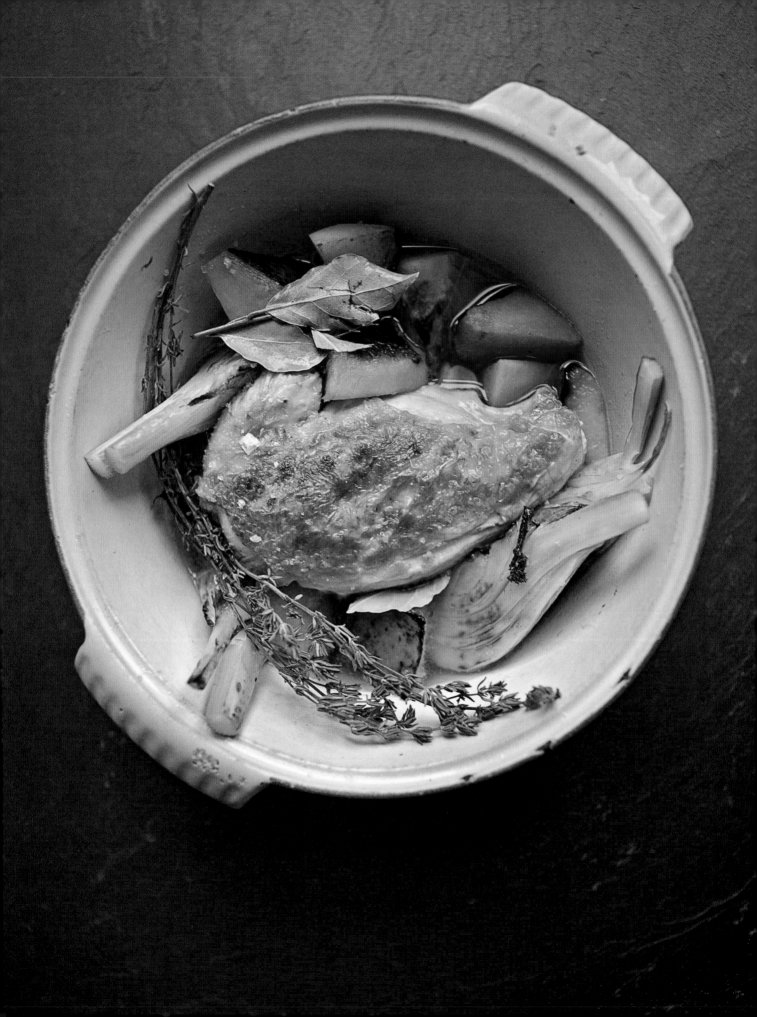

CHICKEN CASSEROLE
with BUTTERNUT SQUASH AND FENNEL

1 CHICKEN (1.4-1.6 KG)
1 BUTTERNUT SQUASH (500 G)
3 FENNEL BULBS
½ BUNCH THYME
2 BAY LEAVES
200 ML WHITE WINE
200 ML CHICKEN STOCK (SEE PAGE 332)
3 TBSP CIDER VINEGAR
2 TBSP HONEY
4 TBSP OLIVE OIL
SALT AND FRESHLY GROUND
BLACK PEPPER

Clean the chicken and cut off the tail and wings. Divide the chicken into 2 legs and 2 breasts on the bone. Brown the skin in a little olive oil and salt. Peel the butternut squash and chop into large chunks, then brown in olive oil and salt. Clean the fennel and cut each into 6 wedges. Brown the pieces on each side in olive oil and salt.

Transfer the chicken to a cast iron casserole with the butternut squash, fennel, thyme and bay leaves. Pour the wine and stock over the chicken, stir in the honey, cover and simmer until the juices run clear – about 30-35 minutes. Strain the liquid and season with salt and cider vinegar.

Serve with brown rice or crushed potatoes with fresh herbs.

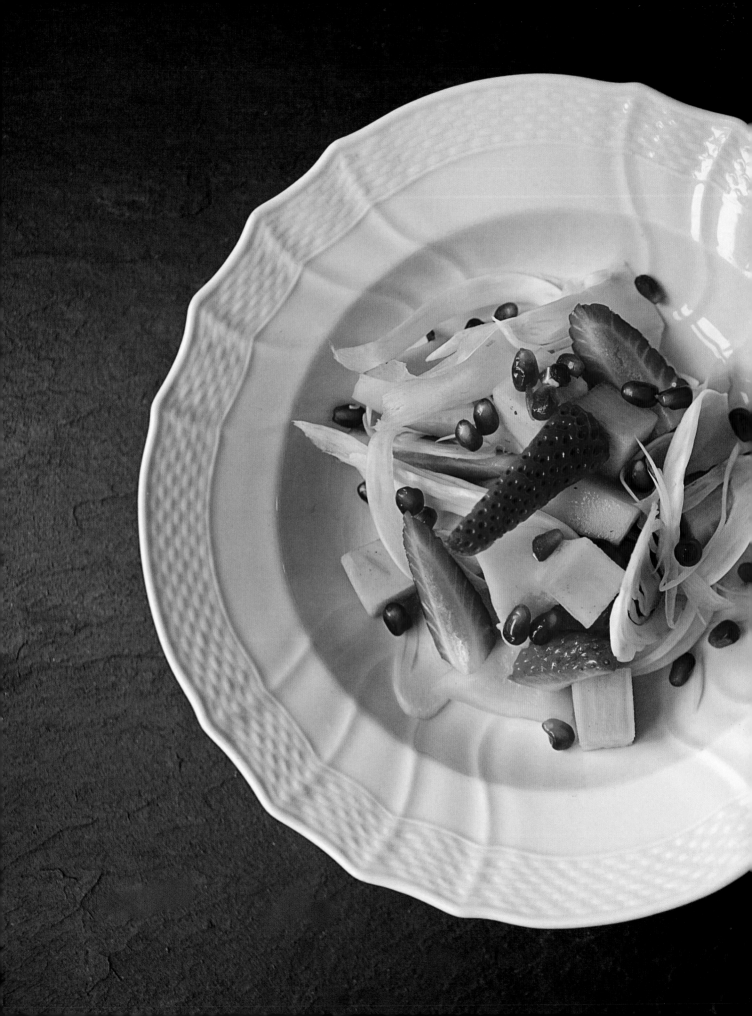

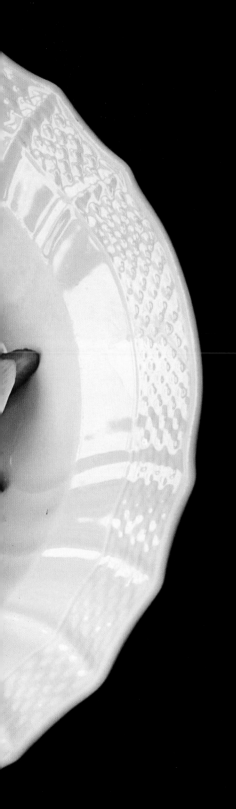

FRUIT SALAD *with* FENNEL

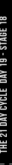

(G) (D) (N)

2 MANGOES
200 G STRAWBERRIES
2 FENNEL BULBS
1 PERSIMMON
1 POMEGRANATE
LIQUID HONEY
LEMON JUICE

Halve the mangoes, remove the stone, peel and dice. Rinse the strawberries and cut them into quarters. Rinse the fennel bulbs, slice them diagonally into thin strips using a mandolin and submerge them in cold water with lemon juice. Peel the persimmon and dice it.

Using a wooden spoon, bang the seeds out of the two pomegranate halves onto a paper towel. Remove any white membranes. Mix all the fruit with the fennel and flavour with honey and lemon juice. Sprinkle over the pomegranate seeds before serving.

MICHAEL VALGREN

"A BODY GETTING THE CORRECT NUTRITION FROM REAL, HEALTHY FOOD CAN GIVE 110% EVERYDAY"

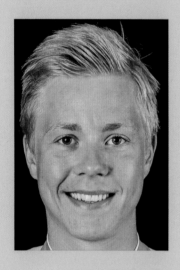

BORN: 7th February 1992
NATIONALITY: Danish
EXPERIENCE: Professional since 2014

Hannah (H): How important is the right diet for you as a professional cyclist?
Michael Valgren (MV): In the times that we live in now, diet is the alpha and omega. The correct diet and right nutrition means everything when it comes to recovery, performance and physical condition. So, yes! The diet, the correct diet, is very, very important!

H: Do you think that food can change an athlete's performance?
MV: Yes, absolutely, food can indeed change a lot in an athlete's performance. For example, compared to a diet consisting of factory-made, fake foods with lots of additives and unknown ingredients, a body getting the correct nutrition from real, healthy food can give 110% everyday. It's important to say that what you fuel your body with will show in your training and your racing performance. If you eat poorly, your performance will be too. On the other hand, if you eat nutritious, natural food, you will perform much better and you might even get that win.

H: Can you feel the difference in your performance when you eat well?
MV: I personally feel a big difference. If I eat too much junk, I bonk really fast and if I do not eat well enough before and during some tough workouts, I simply can't finish. When I have been eating healthy food, it not only makes my body feel great, but it also makes my mind happy, making me confident so I can perform at my best.

H: Does it affect your weight when you eat right?
MV: After I turned professional with Tinkoff-Saxo, I reduced my body fat substantially and added a good deal of muscle mass, which I consider a good sign. I ate right and I lost weight, which is important if you want to be the fastest. For me, what works really well is avoiding lots of carbohydrates after breakfast. Breakfast is the most important meal, the source of energy for the day's training or race, so I always eat a good portion of oatmeal with extra oats, nuts and seeds on top. In the evening I focus on eating mostly vegetables and fish or meat, I watch my carbohydrate intake when I don't need it.

H: What works best for you on an important race day and what do you typically eat?

MV: Well, for me, a quiet morning is important, it's nice to be able to sit and enjoy your morning coffee and hot oatmeal. I would rather sleep 15 minutes less and have time at the table to fill my energy stores before an important race. As I said, I normally eat a good portion of rolled oats or porridge for breakfast with mixed nuts and seeds on top and whole milk yoghurt on the side. I might also eat an omelette and one of your super delicious breakfast rolls with a little chocolate spread for my sweet tooth! I usually always eat oats, I have always done this before races and I know it works.

H: How has altering your diet affected you physically and mentally?

MV: At some point I changed my mentality and started thinking like a professional rider. I eat more vegetables, less sugar and I don't snack as much as I used to do. For example, when it comes to losing weight, there is a huge difference between eating correctly and starving yourself. The times I've tried to lose weight in the past, I've done it wrong. I learned the hard way that when I eat too little, I become grumpy and agitated, I end up snacking way too much on the wrong stuff and I feel even worse. Now, thanks to the team and your food, I know what I should eat and what I can eat as much of as I want to without jeopardizing my physical condition. Most importantly of all, I have lots more energy for riding day after day.

H: When not racing, what do you eat before, during and after a typical day of training?

MV: On a typical training day, I stick to the same breakfast I have been having for years, porridge or oatmeal with corn flakes and yoghurt. During my training session, depending on how long it is, I eat a homemade energy bar and maybe a few bananas. After training, I make an omelette. I love omelettes and usually just put all the vegetables I have in the fridge into them, add a little ham, sit down and enjoy.

H: Is the taste and appearance of food important to you on a long stage race, where you tend to lose your appetite?

MV: On a grand tour you easily lose your appetite, so it's very important that your food looks delicious and appealing. When food looks great, you have to dig in and taste it. It's really good that we can have beautiful, well-tasting food during a three-week stage race, since we need the energy to get through.

H: What is your favourite food in and out of the race season?

MV: In season, always salmon, anything with salmon. Out of the race season, it's a steak with béarnaise, fries and a nice glass of red wine.

H: What's your best advice for a young rider/amateur who wants to eat correctly, have more energy and lose weight?

MV: First of all, they should not stress over losing weight. That actually makes it harder to shed those kilos. But basically, eat a good breakfast, cut down portions the rest of the day and try and avoid eating after 8 o'clock at night. Eat a lot of vegetables and colourful, healthy food that makes you happy.

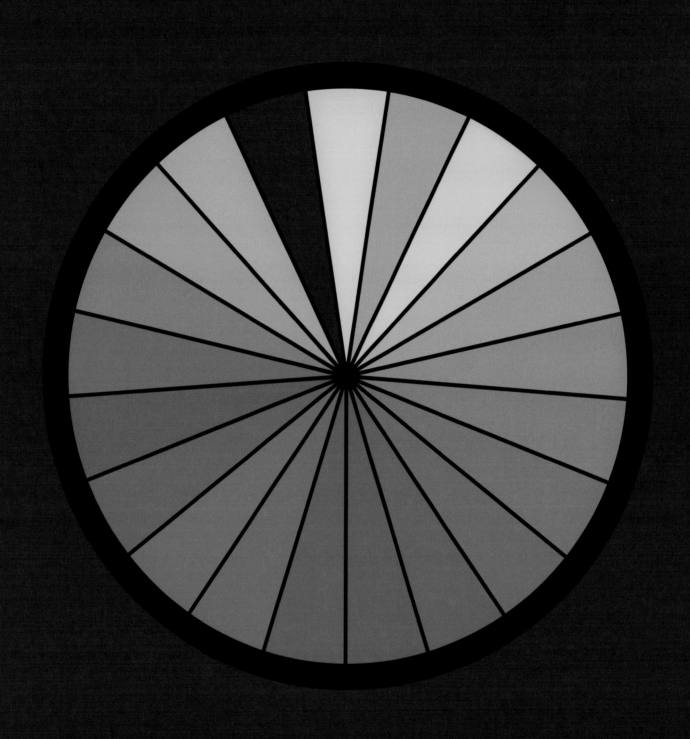

DAY

STAGE 19

BEETROOT, *green* BEANS AND TAHINI DRESSING

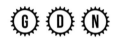

500 G BEETROOT
250 G GREEN BEANS
2 TBSP TAHINI
1 TBSP HONEY
1 CLOVE GARLIC
JUICE AND ZEST OF 1 ORGANIC LEMON
3 TBSP WATER
100 ML OLIVE OIL
¼ TSP SALT

Boil the beetroot in salted water until tender. Rinse the beans, trim the ends and blanch for 20 seconds in boiling salted water. Immediately cool in cold water. Mix the tahini, honey, grated garlic, lemon zest, lemon juice and salt. Slowly whisk in the olive oil. Adjust the dressing to a suitable consistency with water. Season with salt, honey and lemon juice.

Squeeze the skin off the beetroot and cut them into bite-sized pieces. Plate the beans with the beetroot and drizzle with tahini dressing.

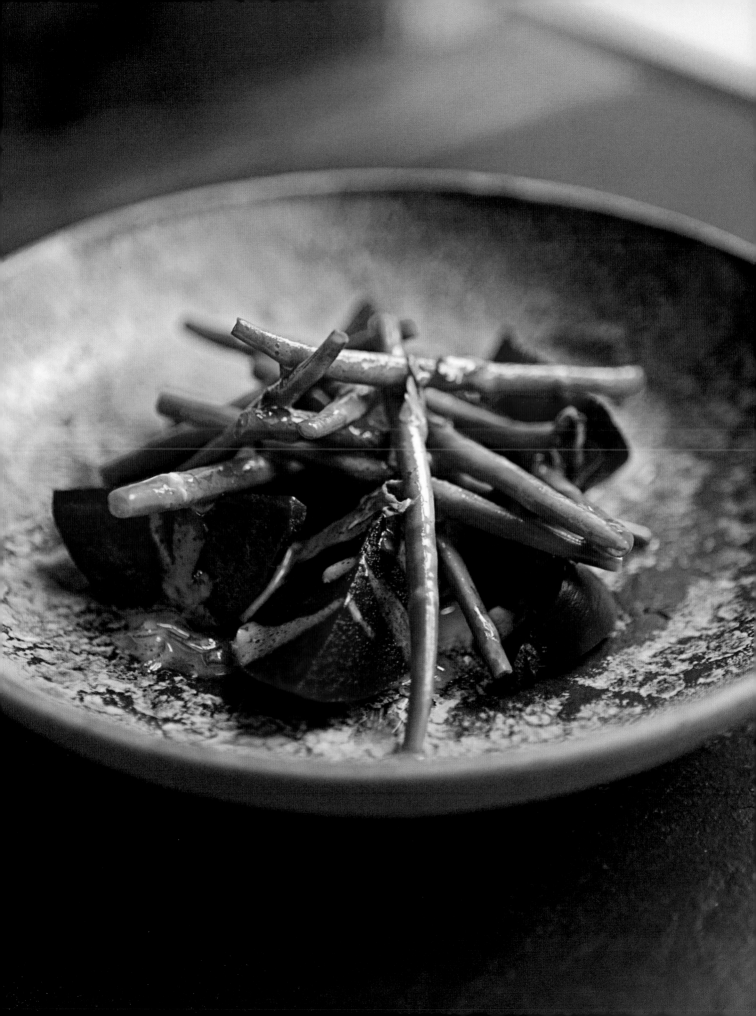

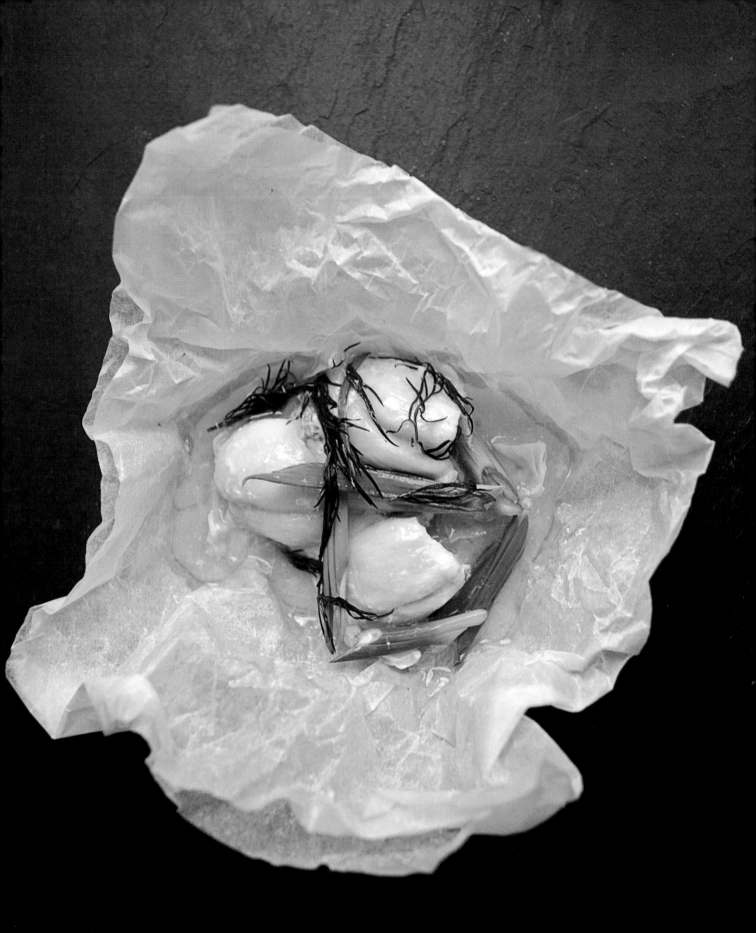

BAKED MONKFISH
CHEEKS, SPRING ONIONS *and* POINTED CABBAGE

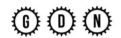

800 G MONKFISH CHEEKS, CLEANED
12 SPRING ONIONS
1 POINTED CABBAGE
1 BUNCH DILL
200 ML WHITE WINE
4 TBSP OLIVE OIL
SALT

Preheat the oven to 175°C.

Clean the spring onions and cut into 4 pieces. Cut the pointed cabbage into 1 cm slices. Rinse and tear the dill off the stalk. Lay two layers of foil on the counter with baking paper on top (the two pieces of foil placed so they overlap, then a piece of baking paper on top). Fold the foil to form a bowl. Divide the monk fish cheeks, spring onions, cabbage, white wine and olive oil between the four foil bowls and season with salt. Fold the packages together and steam in the oven until a cake tester can pierce the fish with no force – about 20-25 minutes. Serve the fish in the packages with potatoes or quinoa salad.

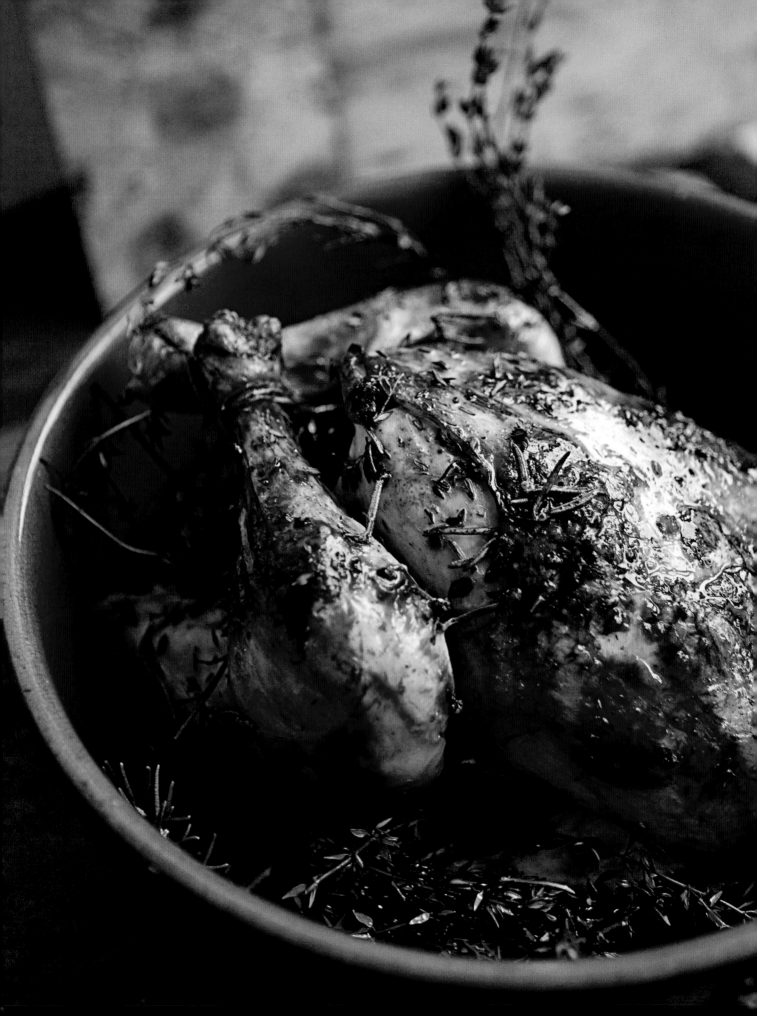

WHOLE ROAST
CHICKEN WITH HERBS

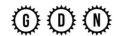

1 CHICKEN (1.2-1.4 KG)
3 CLOVES GARLIC
1 BUNCH THYME
1 BUNCH ROSEMARY
4 TBSP OLIVE OIL
SALT AND FRESHLY GROUND
BLACK PEPPER

Preheat the oven to 175°C.

Peel the garlic cloves and chop finely. Rinse the thyme and rosemary. Remove the leaves and chop, mix with the garlic and rub the mixture under the chicken skin. Rub the skin with salt and drizzle with olive oil. Roast the chicken until the skin is crisp and the juices run clear – about 45 minutes. Let the chicken rest for 15 minutes before carving.

Serve with several finely chopped herbs of your choice and roast or crushed potatoes.

BROWNIE

375 G BUTTER
375 G 70% DARK CHOCOLATE
6 LARGE EGGS
375 G CANE SUGAR
225 G GROUND ALMONDS
1 TSP FINE SALT
150 G CHOPPED NUTS

Preheat the oven to 175°C.

Melt the butter and chocolate in a double boiler covered with cling film. Beat the eggs with the sugar – preferably in a food mixer. Stir the melted chocolate into the eggs and then stir in the ground almonds, salt and chopped nuts. Transfer the dough to a greased cake tin (A4 size) and bake for 20-25 minutes.

Cool before cutting or eat warm with a spoon.

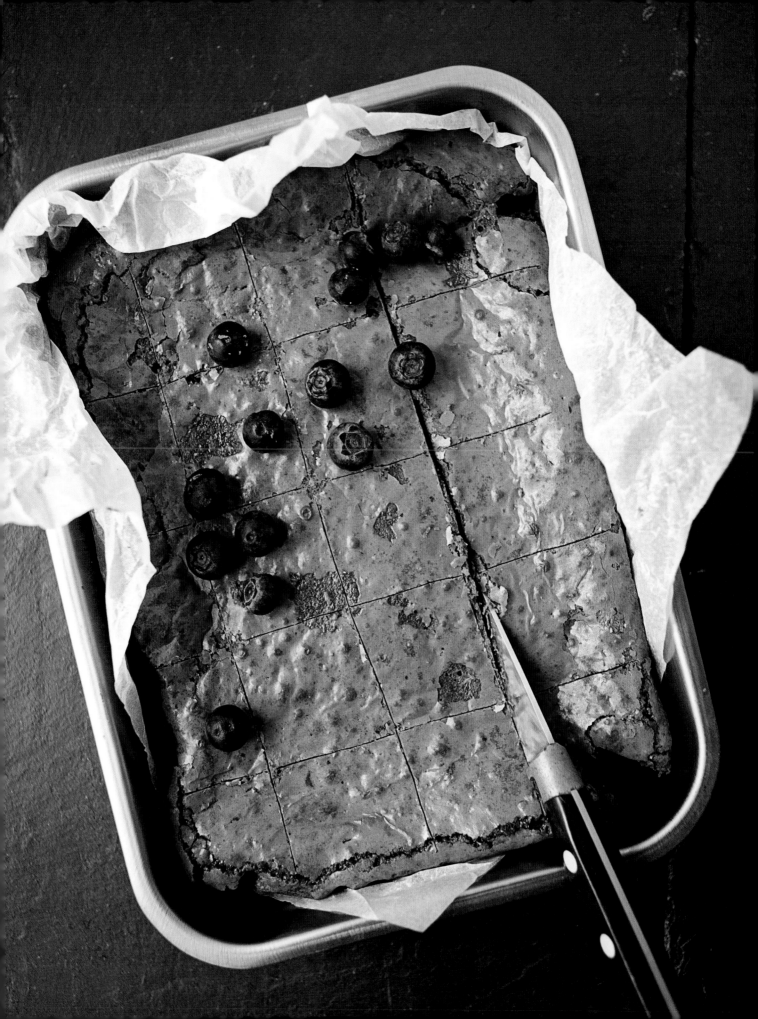

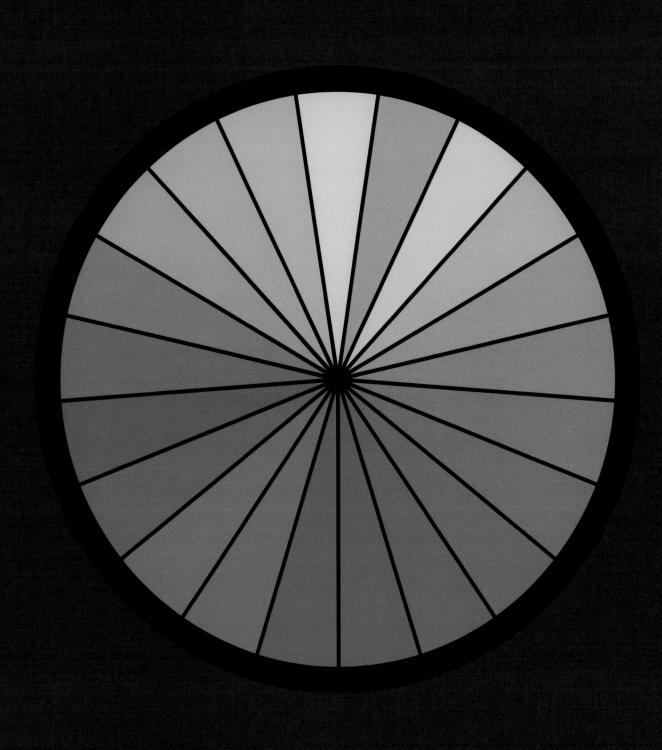

DAY

STAGE 20

PIZZA and BUBBLY

6-8 PIZZAS

500 ML COLD WATER
40 G FRESH YEAST
2 TSP HONEY
300 G FLOUR
300 G FINE DURUM FLOUR
250 G SEMOLINA FLOUR
2 TSP FINE SALT
2 TBSP OLIVE OIL
1 LITRE TOMATO SAUCE OF YOUR
OWN CHOICE (SEE PAGES 330-331)
2 X BUFFALO MOZZARELLA
PIZZA TOPPING OF YOUR CHOICE

After the last stage, the tradition is that the staff and riders celebrate with pizza and champagne in front of the team bus with family and friends.

Start the day before. Stir the water, yeast and honey together. Mix the three types of flour together, add the first 2/3 to the yeast mixture and knead to a consistent dough. Add salt and oil and knead again. Knead in the remaining flour a little at a time until the dough is smooth and shiny – about 10-12 minutes. This is easy to do with a mixer and a dough hook. Depending on the type of flour, you can adjust the dough with more or less flour and/or water until the dough is smooth and soft. Refrigerate overnight or until it has at least doubled in size.

Knead the dough thoroughly and divide into 6-8 balls, cover and leave to rise at room temperature until doubled in size.

Preheat the oven to 250°C well ahead of time, so it is good and hot when you need to bake the pizzas. Roll out the dough balls on baking paper and spread the tomato sauce in a very thin layer over the entire pizza.
Scatter the mozzarella over the pizza, drag onto a hot baking sheet or pizza stone and bake until the bottom is a crisp with a lovely golden colour.

Remove the pizza and top with roasted mushrooms, air-dried ham, pesto, rocket or whatever else you crave after a long, hard race.

Serve with champagne!

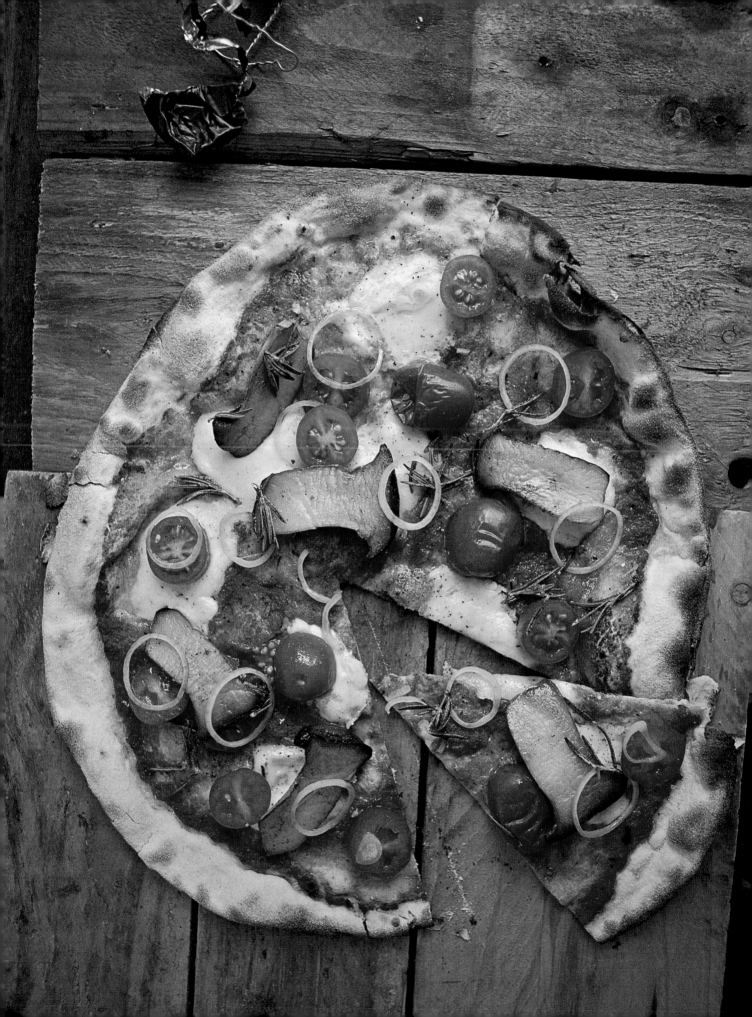

CHRISTOPHER JUUL JENSEN

"PROPER FOOD MAKES A MASSIVE DIFFERENCE IN TERMS OF PERFORMANCE"

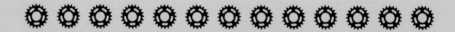

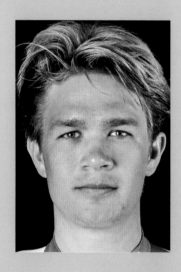

BORN: 6th July 1989
NATIONALITY: Danish
EXPERIENCE: Professional since 2012

Hannah (H): How important is the right diet for you as a professional cyclist?
Christopher Juul (CJ): I find that diet is one of the most important aspects of being a bike rider. In order for the body to be able to perform and recover properly, it's obvious that it needs the right diet. A car wouldn't go particularly far if you only filled it with 2 litres of petrol.

H: How do you think the right food changes an athlete's performance?
CJ: Personally, I've noticed that some riders tend to have a slightly dated approach to food and diet. The old school opinion is typically "the less you eat the better." As a bike rider, weight is an important factor. However, people often forget that they need to lose weight and perform at the same time, which involves eating as little as possible and trying to burn as much as possible. Eating the right food in the right amount is essential when the body needs to be able to do both. If it's fed with enough of the right fuel, the body will automatically start to work properly. Proper food makes a massive difference in terms of performance. The body will benefit from being fed with what it needs during both performance and recovery. Wow, I sound like a real food nerd! Maybe I should go on a morning TV show, like you?

H: Can you feel the difference in your performance when you eat the right food?
CJ: Yes! It's obvious during very long and hard races. I don't get hunger flats if I make sure to load before the race with all the correct nutrients. If I were to fill myself with toast and croissants before a race, I wouldn't even make it to the end of the neutral start.

H: How does eating correctly affect your weight? What works for you?
CJ: Whenever I want to lose weight I usually eat a lot, which sounds odd. But I find that if my body is properly fed, it doesn't become stressed during hard training periods or racing. When I was younger, I thought that the best way to lose weight was to try and starve my body: eat a small breakfast, burn a lot during training and eat as little as possible afterwards. It sounds stupid, I know! I completely wasted my legs after a couple days of training without losing any weight. At one point I was even convinced my scales were in need of new batteries every morning! I eventually realised that this method didn't make any sense. I was stressing my body, working hard and getting no results

on or off the bike. Now I eat enough before and after riding to make sure that I've ticked off the essential boxes. Gradually, my body starts to get rid of the extra weight it doesn't need and, at the same time, I don't feel exhausted during training. To be honest though, I don't weigh myself constantly. When I feel that everything is running smoothly, I'm pretty relaxed about my weight. Like Oprah once said, "it's about looking in a mirror and feeling good about yourself." Not that I watch Oprah. I don't! Honestly. It was my mum who told me... it was!

H: What do you typically eat on an important race day?
CJ: Before a big race, stage or training ride I typically eat a massive breakfast consisting of nuts, seeds and carbohydrates. At home, the prospect of having to clean my blender often leads me to skip making a smoothie, but luckily at races you usually have them made for us before we have even woken up! Oh, I can't forget two very important aspects of my breakfast: chocolate spread and coffee. Not together though.

H: How has altering your diet affected you physically and mentally?
CJ: I admit to being one of those gluten- and lactose-free kinds of people. I'm not obsessed with avoiding them, but whenever the option is there, I chose to leave them out. I prefer gluten-free because, without going into too much detail, I can clearly feel the benefit it has on my stomach. Everything functions a lot more smoothly.

H: When not racing, what do you eat before, during and after a typical day of training?
CJ: Breakfast and lunch are more or less the same. During training periods I don't eat too many carbohydrates for dinner, mainly greens and meat or fish. When I'm training I especially like to stop for a coffee, as I always end up eating whatever I have in my pockets already within the first hour of riding. Whoops!

H: Is the taste and appearance of food important for you on a long stage race?
CJ: During a long stage race it's always nice that the food looks and tastes good and for meals to have a variety of flavours. Otherwise things can get a little boring, especially as the mind starts to slow down and everything becomes routine. Having something to look forward to for dinner is always nice. Although sometimes, I catch myself feeling a little sad when I'm eating one of your meals. They taste so good, but I get to a point where I know it's almost finished. Luckily though, I remind myself that breakfast is just around the corner and the routine goes on and on and on!

H: What is your best advice for an amateur who wants to eat properly, maintain good energy levels and lose weight?
CJ: Stick to the basics and make sure no habit becomes too extreme. Find the personal modifications to any diet that work for you. As long as the body is fed with the essentials before, during and after riding, I can't imagine that things could go particularly wrong. Starving yourself doesn't work and neither does binging. Finding the healthy balance is what will make everything work nice and smoothly. Also, remember to allow yourself the satisfaction of all the bad stuff once in a while!

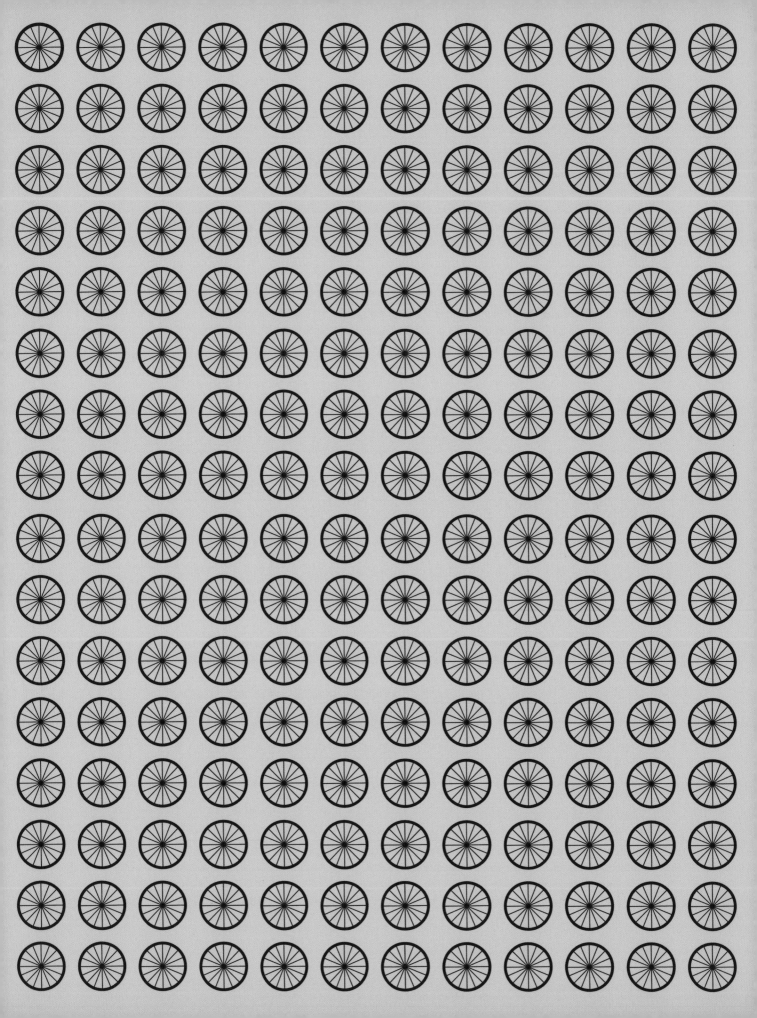

Race & snacks RECOVERY FOODS

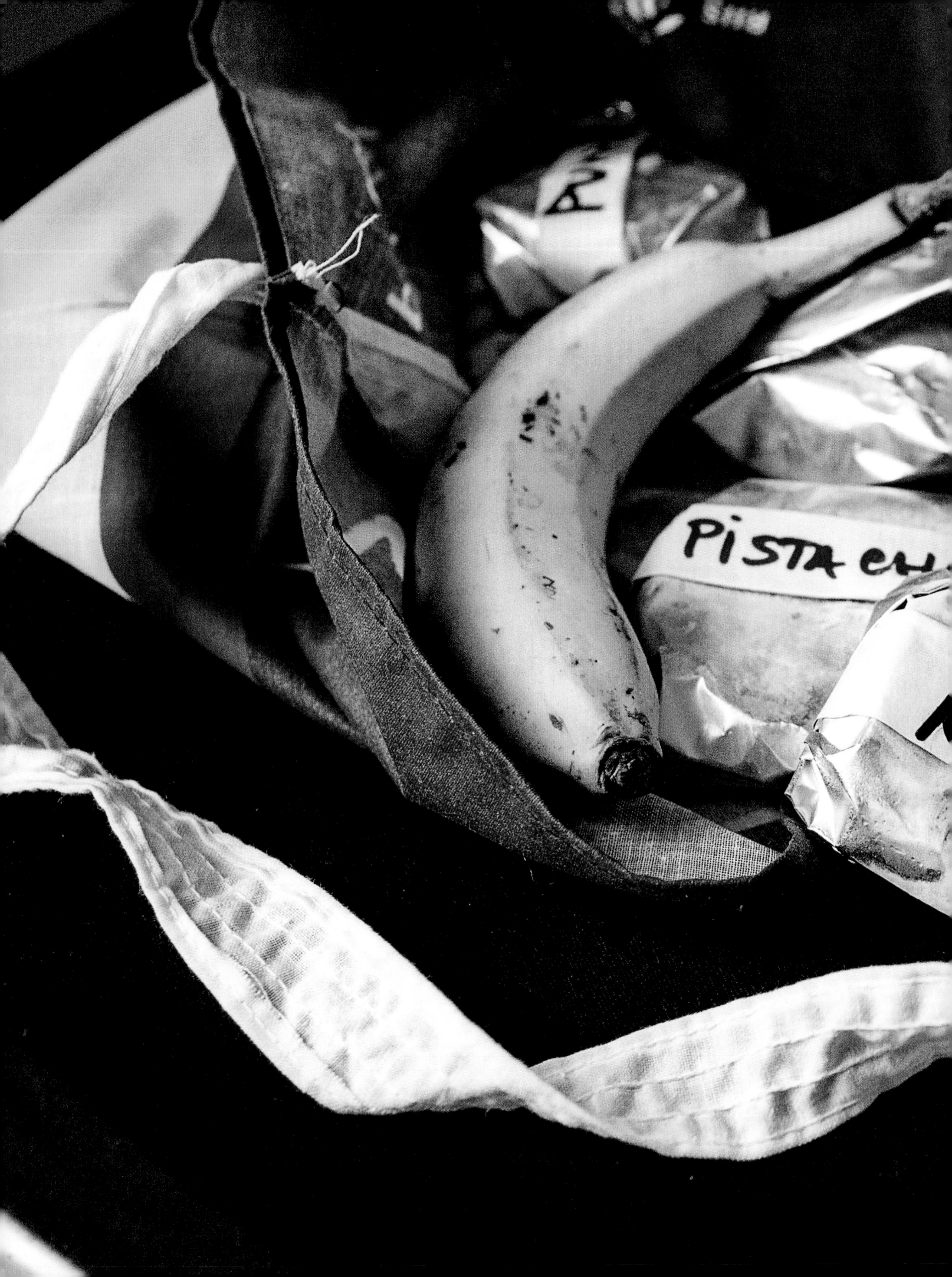

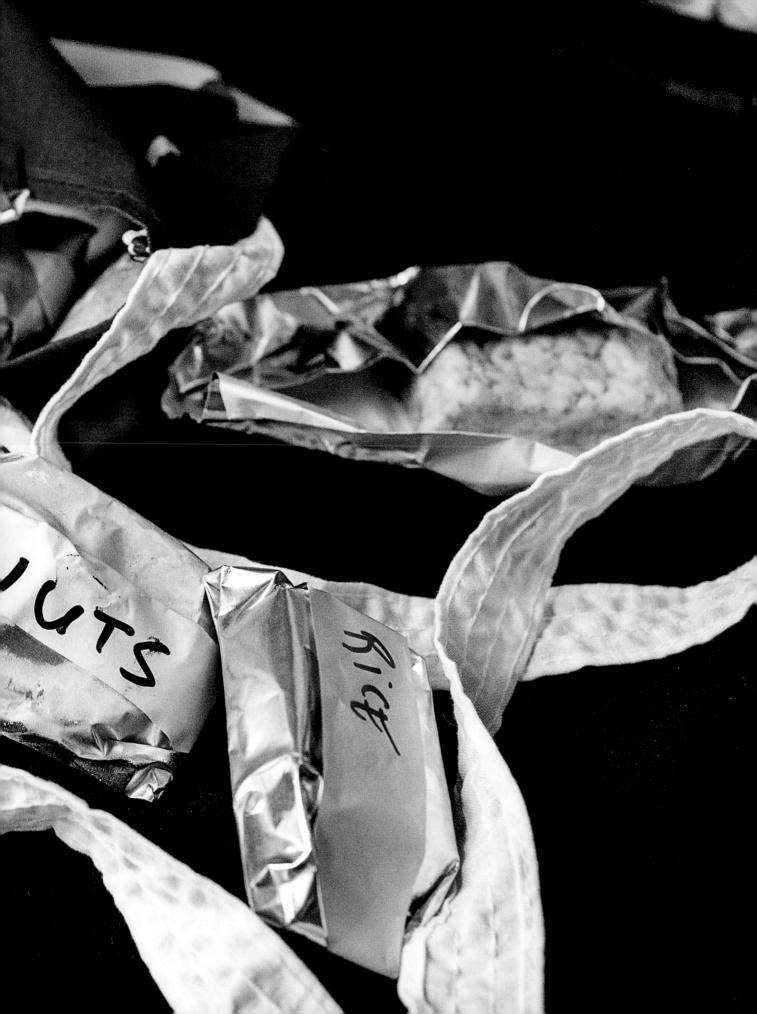

RACE
SNACKS

During a long race it is important to grab a quick bite to maintain the energy needed to complete the day's work. Race snacks are prepared before the race and handed out in feed bags (musettes) in the feed zone of the stage.

WHAT DOES A FEED BAG CONTAIN?
3-4 small sandwiches, wraps or cakes, a banana, energy bars and energy gels. The contents vary depending on the length and gradient of the stage and the diet and tastes of the individual cyclist.

SOFT SANDWICHES ON BURGER BUNS WITH FILLING OF:
Banana and fig
Chicken and guacamole
Ham and mozzarella
Toasted almond spread
and apple wraps
Cocoa, date and mango
Apple compote and pulled pork

DANISH STYLE TORTILLAS
Potato and spinach
Bacon and quinoa

CAKES & BARS
Brownie (page 290)
Date brownie (page 103)
Carrot cake
Fig bar with lime
Soft rice cakes

SOFT RICE CAKES
Boil 500 g of pudding rice in 700 ml of water and 1 can of coconut milk. Turn down the heat, cover and let simmer. Stir regularly. When the rice is soft and the liquid has boiled away, stir in 3 tbsp brown sugar, 1 tsp cinnamon and a little salt. Transfer the pudding to a resealable plastic container lined with cling film, seal and refrigerate overnight.

The following day, cut the rice cakes into convenient sizes and pack them and put them in the feed bags.

Instead of cinnamon, you can add 1 diced apple and 3 tbsp peanut butter or 50 g of chocolate chips and 1 banana. Play around with the ingredients to your taste.

RECOVERY
FOODS

Right after the finish of a race, it is important to have protein and then carbohydrates to replenish the muscle glycogen stores and add building blocks to quickly repair the broken down muscle fibres. This is often done in the form of a protein drink followed by a generous portion of high-carb food, which is packed in the morning and refrigerated until just after the race.

The combinations are straightforward, simple in taste and consist mostly of leftovers from dinner combined in various ways and packed in small individual plastic containers. That makes it easy and practical, because it saves using extra time in the kitchen preparing a substantial supply of recovery foods. It also means that less food gets wasted.

Pasta and tomato sauce
Pasta with pesto
Pasta or noodles and chicken with soy and sesame oil
Rice with cinnamon, honey and blueberries
Rice with coleslaw
Rice, egg and ham
Rice noodles with nori seaweed, pickled ginger and lime
Quinoa with chicken and roasted vegetables
Quinoa, pineapple and mint
Potatoes with pesto
Potatoes in mustard vinaigrette
Couscous with apple, cucumber and fresh parsley
Couscous with lamb, tomatoes and almonds
Bulgur wheat with orange, honey and hazelnuts
Meatballs
Danish-style tortilla with spinach and feta
Fruit salad

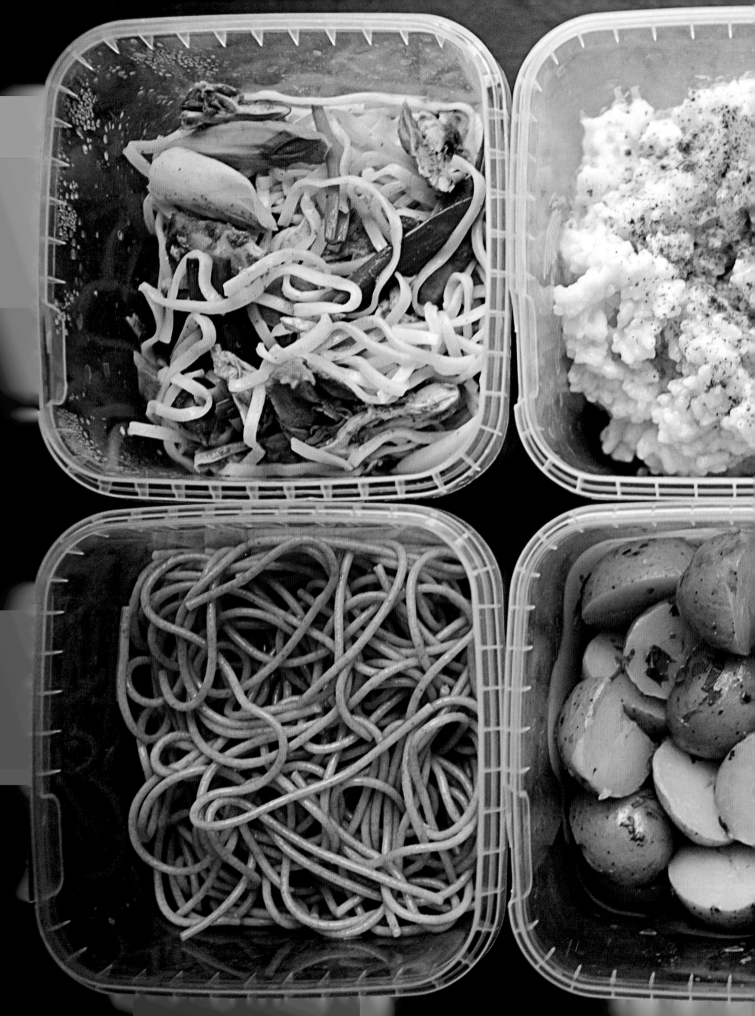

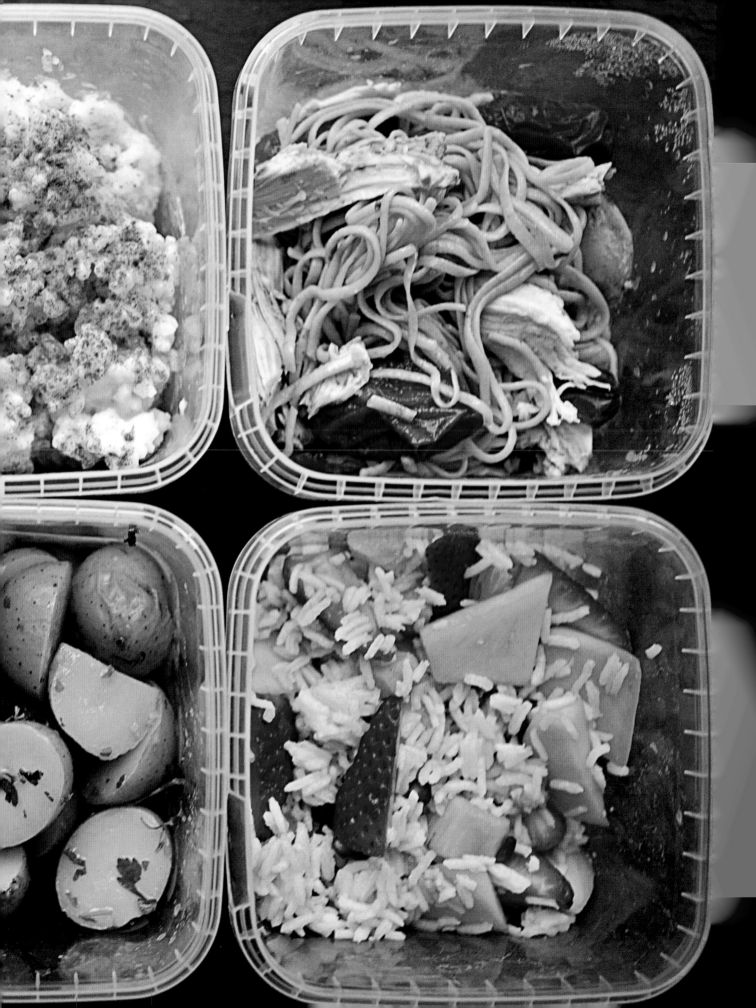

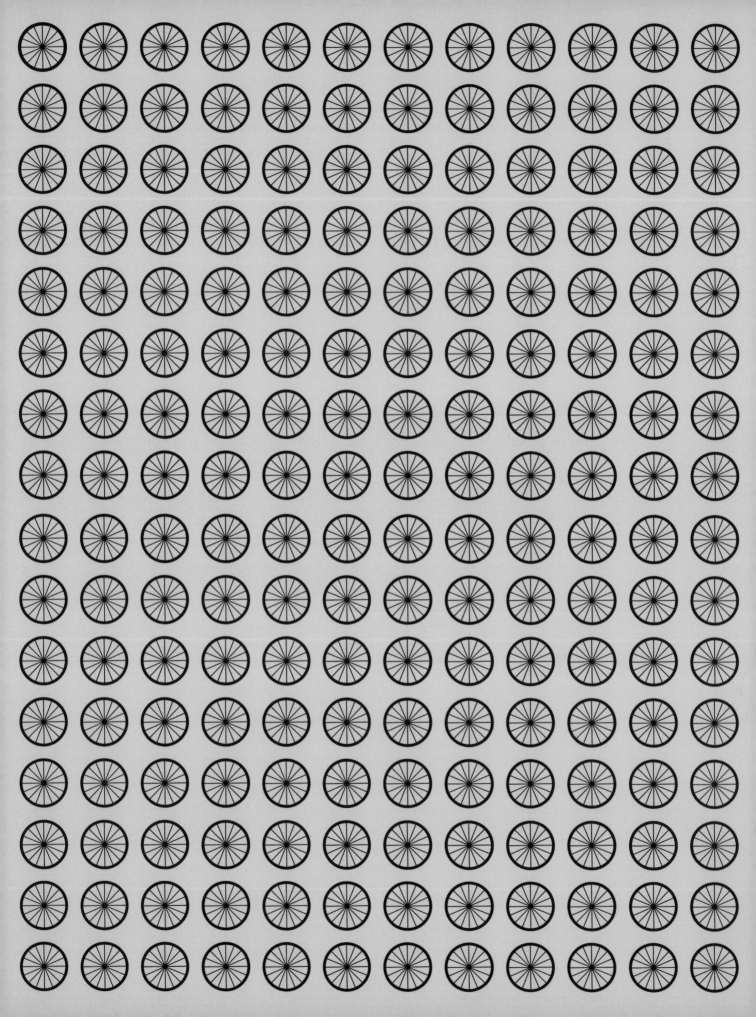

BREAK*fast*

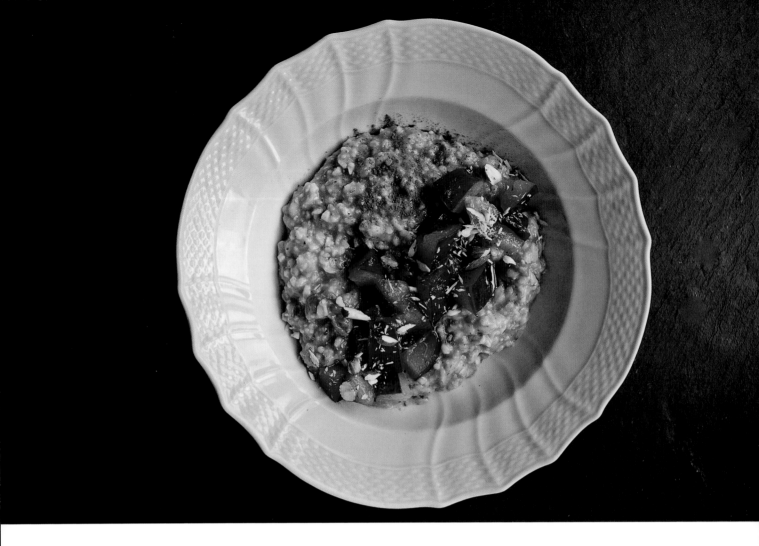

PORRIDGE *with* PLUMS AND ALMONDS

200 G GLUTEN-FREE OATMEAL
600 ML WATER
50 G DRIED GOJI BERRIES
1 TSP GROUND CINNAMON
½ TSP ALLSPICE
50 G CHOPPED ALMONDS
¼ TSP SALT
4 PLUMS
HONEY

Bring the water to a boil with the goji berries, allspice and half of the almonds. Add the oatmeal and cook the porridge, stirring constantly. Turn down the heat and let the porridge simmer until it has the desired consistency. Add more water if desired. Season the porridge with salt. Rinse the plums and cut into wedges. Serve the porridge with plums, the rest of the chopped almonds and topped with honey.

If the day's training is going to be particularly tough, you can add 1 tsp organic, unsweetened protein powder.

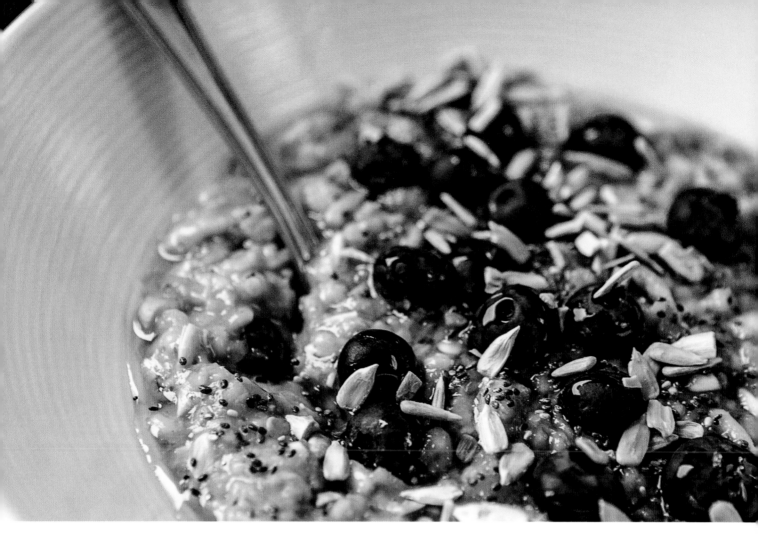

PORRIDGE *with*
BLUEBERRIES AND CHIA SEEDS

200 G GLUTEN-FREE OATMEAL
700 ML WATER
½ TSP GROUND CINNAMON
¼ TSP DRIED GINGER
¼ TSP GROUND NUTMEG
50 G SUNFLOWER SEEDS
3 TBSP CHIA SEEDS
¼ TSP SALT
100 G FRESH BLUEBERRIES
HONEY

Bring the water to a boil with the spices, sunflower seeds and chia seeds. Add the oatmeal and cook the porridge, stirring constantly. Turn down the heat and let the porridge simmer until it has the desired consistency. Add more water if desired. Season the porridge with salt and serve with the rinsed blueberries and honey.

If that day's training is going to be particularly tough, you can add 1 tsp organic, unsweetened protein powder.

The result is best when you use a mixture of fine-rolled oats and coarse oatmeal.

BREAKFAST

RASPBERRY
AND GINGER SMOOTHIE

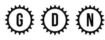

500 G FROZEN RASPBERRIES
4 BANANAS
400 ML RICE MILK OR ALMOND MILK
100 G FRESH GINGER,
PEELED AND SLICED
4 TBSP BEETROOT CRYSTALS
OR 100 ML REDUCED BEETROOT JUICE
JUICE AND ZEST OF 2 ORGANIC LIMES
4 TBSP COLD-PRESSED FLAXSEED OIL
HONEY

Blend the berries with the bananas and milk. Add the ginger, beetroot crystals, lime zest and lime juice. Slowly pour in the flaxseed oil while blending. Season with honey and lime.

AVOCADO
AND APPLE SMOOTHIE

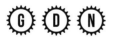

2 RIPE AVOCADOS
2 APPLES
600 ML COLD-PRESSED APPLE JUICE
100 G FRESH GINGER
50 G PARSLEY
JUICE AND ZEST OF 2 ORGANIC LIMES
4 TBSP COLD-PRESSED FLAXSEED OIL
HONEY

Blend the avocado and apples with the apple juice. Peel and cut the ginger into thin slices. Add the ginger, rinsed parsley and lime juice and zest. Slowly pour in the flaxseed oil while blending. Season with honey and lime.

STRAWBERRY
AND COCONUT SMOOTHIE

500 G STRAWBERRIES
4 BANANAS
2 PASSION FRUIT
200 ML COCONUT MILK
200 ML ALMOND MILK
4 TBSP COLD-PRESSED FLAXSEED OIL
JUICE AND ZEST OF 2 ORGANIC LIMES
HONEY

Blend the strawberries, bananas and passion fruit with the coconut and almond milk. Slowly pour in the flaxseed oil while blending and season with the lime juice, lime zest and honey.

GINGER
SHOTS

1 KG FRESH GINGER
1 L WATER

Ginger shots can be made in large quantities and stored in the refrigerator for quite some time. To prevent inflammation, you should consume 20 g ginger per day. If you have inflammation, you should consume 100 g per day.

Peel the ginger and cut it into thin slices across the fibres. Blend the ginger and cold water into a fine purée in a food processor or powerful blender. Press it through a sieve using a ladle and store it in a resealable container in the refrigerator. Drink it as a shot, mix it into smoothies or tea. You can save the ginger pulp to use in stews, breads and cakes.

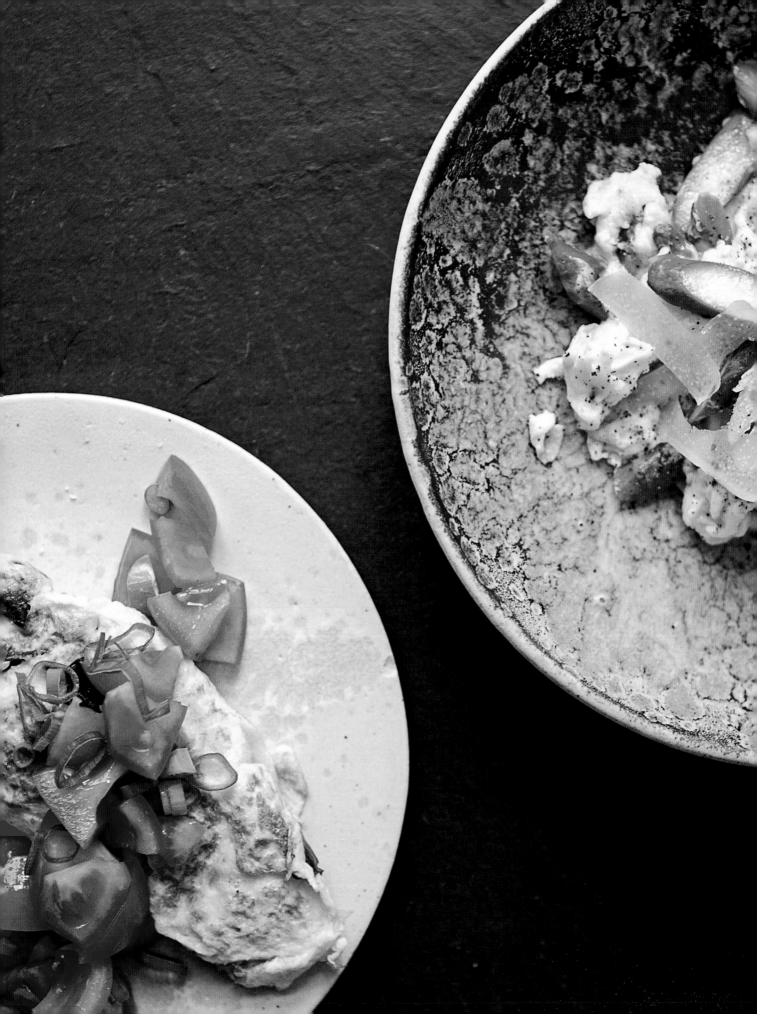

OMELETTE *with* TOMATO AND SPRING VEGETABLES

1 TOMATO
1 SPRING ONION
1 TBSP BALSAMIC VINEGAR
3 EGGS
2 TBSP OLIVE OIL
1 TBSP GRATED PARMESAN
SALT AND FRESHLY GROUND
BLACK PEPPER

Rinse and dice the tomato. Rinse the spring onion and slice finely. Mix both with the balsamic vinegar and salt and leave in the refrigerator until needed.

Beat the eggs with salt and pepper. Pour into a very hot, but not smoking, frying pan coated with olive oil. Sprinkle with Parmesan. When the egg has slightly set at the bottom, fold it over to one side with a palette knife or a spatula. Repeat this process until the omelette is set softly and nicely layered. Tip the omelette onto a plate and serve with the tomato salad.

SCRAMBLED EGGS *with* ASPARAGUS AND PARMESAN

3 EGGS
3 TBSP RICE MILK OR MILK
NUTMEG
SALT AND FRESHLY GROUND
BLACK PEPPER
3 GREEN ASPARAGUS SPEARS
2 TBSP COCONUT OIL
PARMESAN

Beat the eggs and milk together with a fork. Add salt, pepper and grated nutmeg to taste.

Rinse the asparagus, break off the woody parts and slice them into small pieces. Sauté in the coconut oil in a non-stick frying pan. Pour in the egg and stir with a spatula until the eggs have a nice, soft consistency. Serve with freshly shaved Parmesan.

You can replace the asparagus with any kind of vegetable according to season and taste.

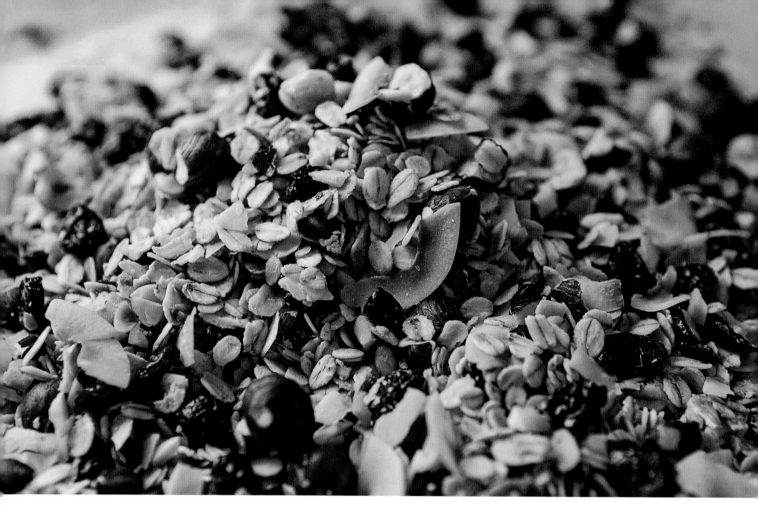

TOASTED CINNAMON
MUESLI WITH SEEDS

250 G GLUTEN-FREE ROLLED OATS
25 G COCONUT FLAKES
25 G SUNFLOWER SEEDS
25 G PUMPKIN SEEDS
25 G CHOPPED HAZELNUTS
½ TSP GROUND CINNAMON
1 PINCH SALT
3 TBSP CLEAR HONEY
2 TBSP OLIVE OIL
25 G DRIED BLUEBERRIES

Preheat the oven to 170°C.

Mix the dry ingredients together. Add the honey and oil and thoroughly stir together. Spread the muesli on a baking tray covered with baking paper and bake for 10-12 minutes until the mixture is golden and completely dry. Occasionally during baking, mix the muesli so it bakes evenly. Let the mixture cool completely before mixing in the blueberries. Store in an airtight container.

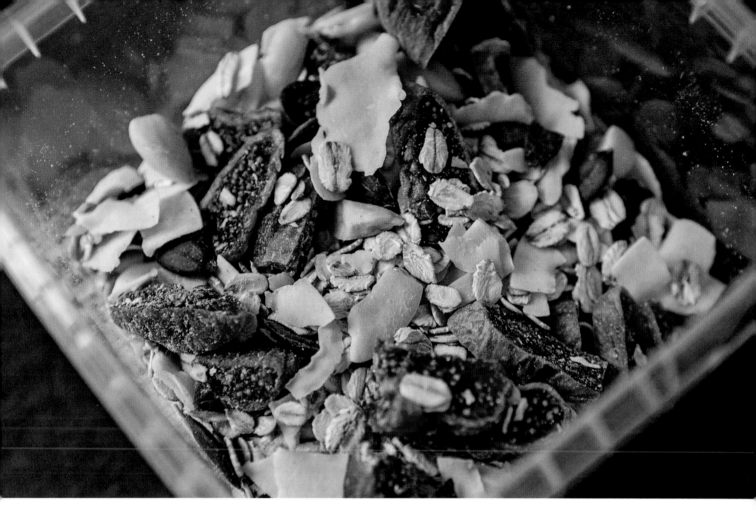

RAW MUESLI
WITH SEEDS

250 G GLUTEN-FREE ROLLED OATS
50 G DRIED FIGS, FINELY CHOPPED
25 G COCONUT FLAKES
50 G CHOPPED ALMONDS
50 G ROASTED HAZELNUTS

Mix all the ingredients together.

Store in an airtight container.

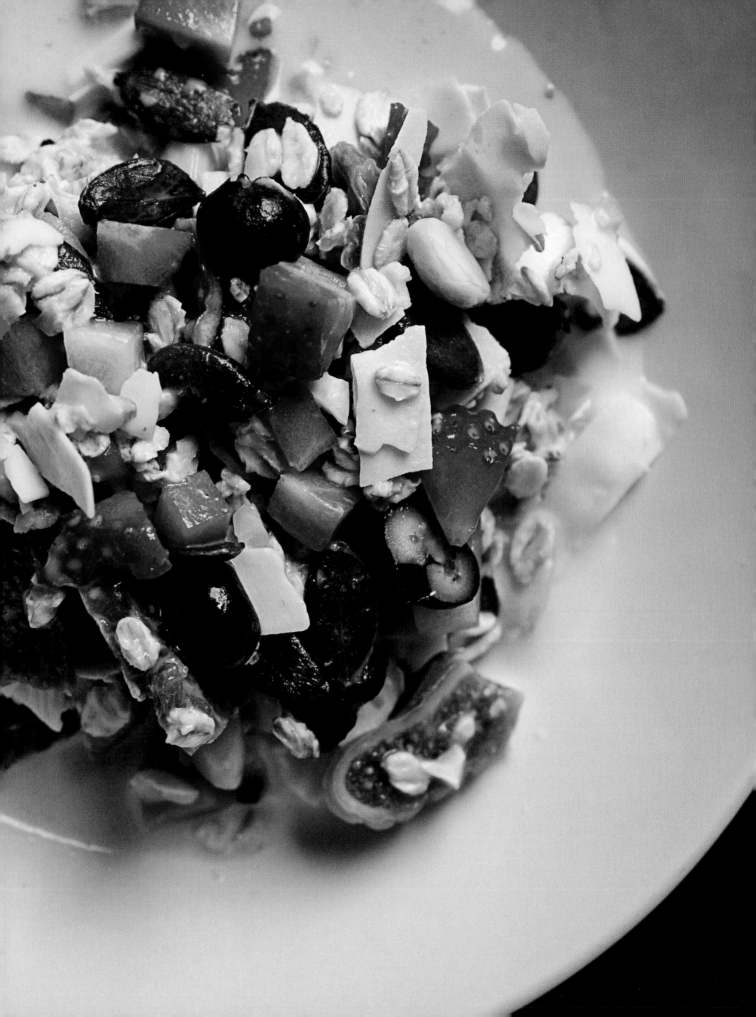

RICE MILK-SOAKED
MUESLI WITH FRESH BERRIES

250 G RAW MUESLI (SEE PAGE 313)
50 G STRAWBERRIES
50 G BLUEBERRIES
500 ML RICE MILK
2 TBSP CLEAR HONEY

Rinse the berries and quarter the strawberries. Mix the muesli, berries and rice milk. Sweeten with honey.

Mix it up ready for the next morning.

TOASTED ALMOND
SPREAD WITH CINNAMON

500 G ALMONDS
½ TBSP COCONUT OIL
1 TSP CINNAMON
1 TBSP CREAMED HONEY
½ TSP SALT FLAKES

Preheat the oven to 170°C.

Toast the almonds in the oven until golden, about 8-10 minutes. Blend in a food processor while they are still warm. Initially the almonds will turn to flour, then to liquid. Add the coconut oil, cinnamon, honey and salt and blend thoroughly into a completely homogeneous mixture. Transfer the almond spread to a jar with a lid or resealable container. The spread is excellent on bread, especially gluten-free bread.

HAZELNUT SPREAD
with 70% CHOCOLATE

500 G SHELLED HAZELNUTS
100 G 70% CHOCOLATE
3 TBSP DARK COCOA POWDER,
UNSWEETENED
¼ TSK SALT FLAKES
1 TBSP HONEY

Preheat the oven to 170°C.

Toast the hazelnuts in the oven until golden – about 8-10 minutes. Blend in a food processor while they are still warm. Initially they will turn to flour, then to liquid. Melt the chocolate in a double boiler and add to the hazelnut mixture with the cocoa powder and salt. Blend into a completely homogeneous mixture. Flavour with honey and transfer the nut spread to a jar with a lid or resealable container and refrigerate.

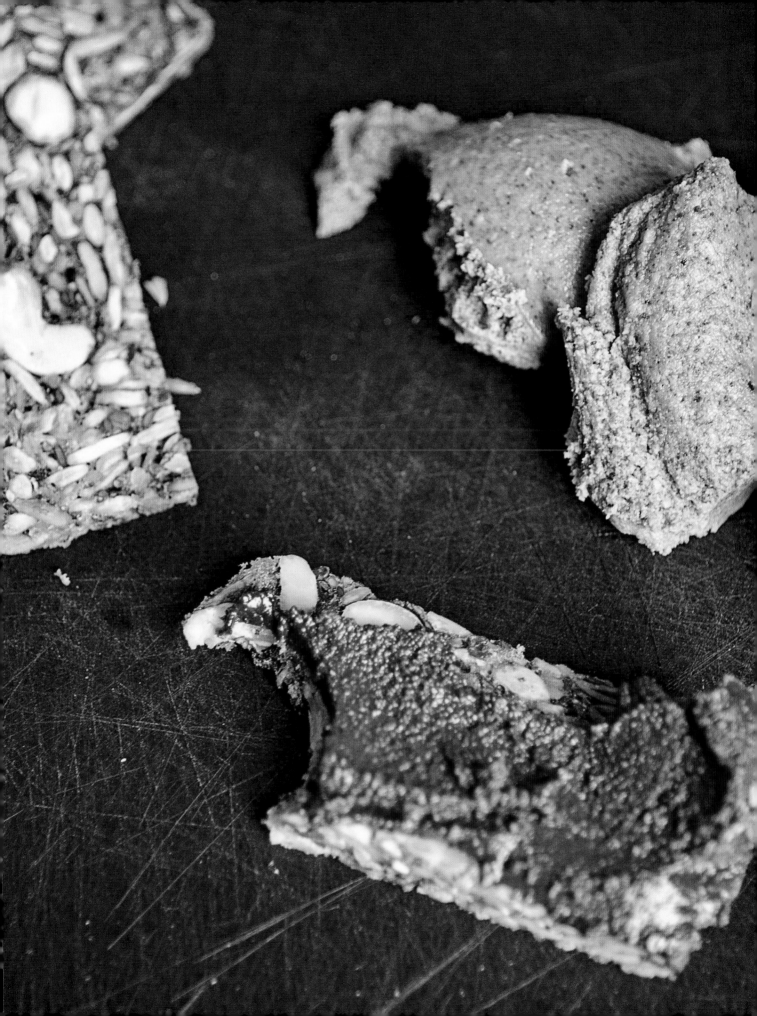

KRISTOFFER GLAVIND KJÆR
"GOOD FOOD SUPPORTS THE BODY"

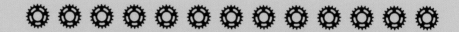

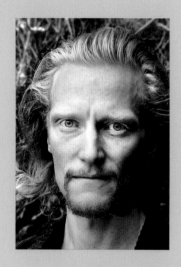

JOB: Body therapist, with
Tinkoff-Saxo since 2011
BACKGROUND:
Social psychologist, author
and partner in Manuvision

Hannah (H): How do you think a good, varied diet affects a rider or an athlete in comparison with a standard hotel diet of refined foods?

Kristoffer Glavind Kjær (KGK): In terms of elite athletes, diet is very important. They often push their limits both mentally and physically and, just like a Ferrari, they must also have the very best fuel. Poor food provides less energy and problems can also arise when the body needs to clean out later. Just try to imagine cycling a Cobblestone Classic with a bloated stomach and heartburn. The liver is perhaps the most important human organ. During the major stage races, it absolutely has to be able to clean our system and help it recover. The liver has a lot of vital functions (it cleans our blood and forms enzymes to help digestion so we can absorb energy), but if it is overloaded by poor food, it can't do its best.

H: Do you think you can optimise recovery with the help of a varied diet?

KGK: In my experience, good nutrition has an impact not only on the body's general recovery, but also on wound healing, oxygen absorption and hormonal balance. Think of how ordinary recreational athletes are affected by hypoglycaemia. It certainly doesn't get any easier when you have to climb the Alpe d'Huez. It's as if the body needs variety in its diet all the time in order to wake up the digestive process.

H: Do you notice a difference in the healing process with cyclists on an improved diet?

KGK: Yes. They accumulate significantly less lactic acid in their muscles and the joints and connective tissue becomes more flexible. Good food supports the body and I can tell physically from their organs that they are soft and ready. Poor diet makes the body stiff and heavy and waste substances accumulate in the connective tissue and joints, where they do most harm. You can see the difference in the cyclists during the races when the kitchen truck is present. Both their endurance and their recovery are noticeably better.

H: Does their diet affect how tired or muscle-tired a rider gets?

KGK: Yes. There's no doubt about it. Professional cyclists work incredibly hard and it is vital for them to get the right nutrients in the right doses. They need to eat a varied diet, good ingredients (not processed) and not in excess. The issue of over-eating is particularly important for cyclists. I believe it is said that 1 kilo too heavy corresponds to 10 seconds lost at the top. So they pay a lot of attention to eating as small portions as possible. That makes perfect sense when we know how much energy the body uses to burn all the excess food we eat. But it is also true that the less you eat, the more important it is to eat the right food. There's a world of difference between the traditional mountains of pasta and your delicious quinoa salads.

H: How does diet affect an athlete's psyche?
KGK: Partly, there's the issue of hypoglycaemia – "bonking" or "hitting the wall". You can't underestimate the knowledge of having enough energy available when you have to go out and perform in the extremes. In fact, it is often a prerequisite when the riders go into a breakaway that they feel they have something extra to give off. The meal is also one of the only bright spots in an otherwise ascetic and incredibly tough working day. This is when they can enjoy a bit of a rest. That's why many riders are great food connoisseurs and they have travelled a great deal. The food is not just nutrition on the physical level. The knowledge and care that go into preparing it also feeds your happiness. You get stimulated on several levels when you sit in front of a meal like the ones you, Hannah, serve the riders. Bjarne's choice to invest in a chef and a state-of-the-art mobile kitchen was an excellent initiative. Not only do I notice the physical effect on the riders when your superfood starts to work, but I can also see their excitement when they see what's on the evening menu. For example, they have developed a points system for the desserts and they discuss the subject until the end of the world, just like when they discuss cycling.

H: Do you think that other types of athletes (runners, triathletes, swimmers, skiers etc.) could also benefit from a changed and varied diet in relation to their training?
KGK: Definitely. And fortunately, they have also started to look at the issue. For example, Indians used to run extremely long distances on a bit of water and chia seeds. I've been fasting every spring since I was 14 and I've noticed how my body's joints, muscles and circulation can change drastically when you remove food that is hard on the system. Even though your muscle mass decreases when you fast, it's amazing to notice how you can suddenly run without any resistance and acid in your musculoskeletal system.

H: What is your favourite food?
KGK: Out of your recipes, probably the lamb shank. Otherwise I'm crazy about pesto. Any salads with that on are just the best.

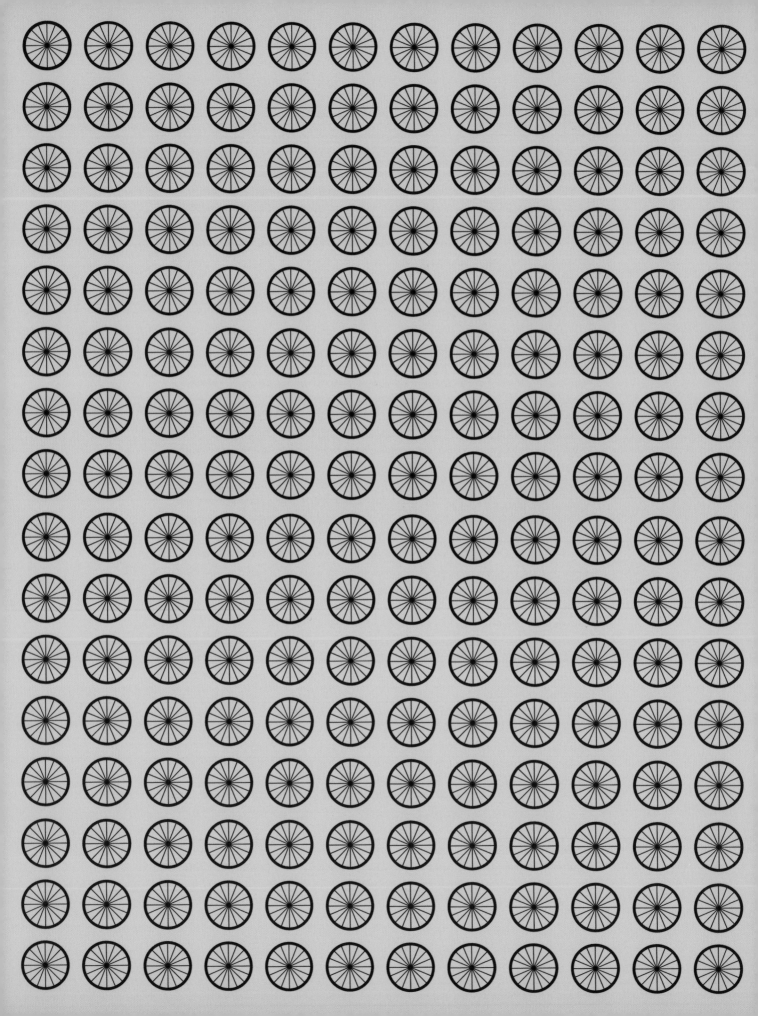

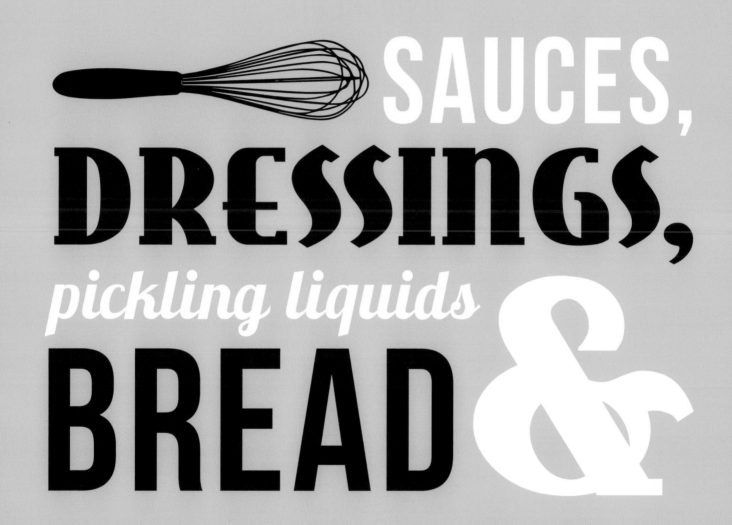

SAUCES,
DRESSINGS,
pickling liquids
BREAD &

HAZELNUT
VINAIGRETTE

50 ML CIDER VINEGAR
1 TBSP DIJON MUSTARD
1 TBSP THICK HONEY
½ TSP SALT
200 ML COLD-PRESSED OLIVE OIL
4 TBSP HAZELNUT OIL

In a bowl, whisk the vinegar, mustard, honey and salt together until the salt and honey are dissolved. While whisking, slowly add the olive oil and hazelnut oil. Whisk until it's nice and emulsified. Season with salt and vinegar.

MUSTARD
VINAIGRETTE

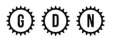

50 ML CIDER VINEGAR
3 TBSP DIJON MUSTARD
1 TBSP ACACIA HONEY
½ TSP SALT
200 ML COLD-PRESSED OLIVE OIL
FRESHLY GROUND BLACK PEPPER

In a bowl, whisk the vinegar, mustard, honey and salt until the salt and honey are dissolved. While whisking, slowly add the olive oil. Whisk until it's nice and emulsified. Season with salt, pepper and vinegar.

COARSE-GRAINED
MUSTARD VINAIGRETTE

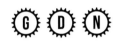

50 ML CIDER VINEGAR
3 TBSP COARSE-GRAINED MUSTARD
1 TBSP THICK HONEY
½ TSP SALT
200 ML COLD-PRESSED OLIVE OIL
2 CLOVES GARLIC
FRESHLY GROUND BLACK PEPPER

Whisk the vinegar, mustard, honey and salt together in a bowl until the salt and honey are dissolved. While whisking, slowly pour in the olive oil. Whisk until the consistency is sufficiently viscous. Mince the garlic and fold it in. Season with salt, pepper and vinegar.

CIDER VINEGAR
VINAIGRETTE

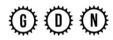

50 ML CIDER VINEGAR
1 TBSP DIJON MUSTARD
1 TBSP THICK HONEY
½ TSP SALT
200 ML COLD-PRESSED OLIVE OIL

In a bowl, whisk the vinegar, mustard, honey and salt until the salt and honey are dissolved. While whisking, slowly add the olive oil. Whisk until it's nice and emulsified. Season with salt and vinegar.

ELDERFLOWER VINAIGRETTE
Replace the cider vinegar with elderflower vinegar.

RASPBERRY VINAIGRETTE
Replace the cider vinegar with raspberry vinegar.

BALSAMIC
VINAIGRETTE

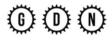

50 ML BALSAMIC VINEGAR
3 TBSP DIJON MUSTARD
3 TBSP THICK HONEY
½ TSP SALT
200 ML COLD-PRESSED OLIVE OIL
FRESHLY GROUND BLACK PEPPER

In a bowl, whisk the balsamic vinegar with mustard, honey and salt until the salt and honey are dissolved. While whisking, slowly add the olive oil. Whisk until it's nice and emulsified. Season with salt and pepper.

HONEY
VINAIGRETTE

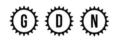

50 ML LEMON JUICE
ZEST OF 2 ORGANIC LEMONS
3 TBSP THICK HONEY
3 TBSP DIJON MUSTARD
½ TSP SALT
200 ML COLD-PRESSED OLIVE OIL
FRESHLY GROUND BLACK PEPPER

In a bowl, whisk the lemon juice and zest, honey, mustard and salt until the salt and honey are dissolved. While whisking, slowly add the olive oil. Whisk until it's nice and emulsified. Season with salt, pepper and lemon juice.

LIME
VINAIGRETTE

50 ML LIME JUICE
ZEST OF 2 ORGANIC LIMES
3 TBSP HONEY
1 TSP WASABI
½ TSP JAPANESE
GLUTEN-FREE SOY SAUCE
200 ML COLD-PRESSED OLIVE OIL

In a bowl, whisk the lime juice, lime zest, honey, wasabi and soy sauce together until the honey is dissolved. While whisking, slowly add the olive oil. Whisk until it's nice and emulsified. Season with soy sauce and lime juice.

ORANGE
VINAIGRETTE

50 ML ORANGE JUICE
ZEST OF 2 ORGANIC LEMONS
3 TBSP DIJON MUSTARD
2 TBSP CIDER VINEGAR
1 TBSP THICK HONEY
½ TSP SALT
200 ML COLD-PRESSED OLIVE OIL
FRESHLY GROUND BLACK PEPPER

In a bowl, whisk the orange juice with lemon zest, mustard, vinegar, honey and salt until the salt and honey are dissolved. While whisking, slowly add the olive oil. Whisk until it's nice and emulsified. Season with salt, pepper and vinegar.

LEMON VINAIGRETTE
Replace the orange juice with lemon juice.

MAYONNAISE

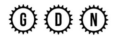

2 EGG YOLKS, PASTEURISED
½ TSP SALT
1 TBSP TARRAGON VINEGAR
1 TSP CLEAR HONEY
1 TBSP DIJON MUSTARD
1 TBSP COARSE-GRAINED MUSTARD
250 ML COLD-PRESSED OLIVE OIL
FRESHLY GROUND BLACK PEPPER

Whisk the egg yolks with salt, vinegar and the two types of mustard. Whisk the olive oil in slowly. Start with a few drops while whisking thoroughly and then continue with the rest of the oil in a thin stream. Season with salt and pepper and, if you wish, a little vinegar.

SOY SAUCE
AND SESAME DRESSING

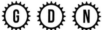

JUICE AND ZEST OF 1 ORGANIC LIME
1 TBSP HONEY
6 TBSP SOY SAUCE
4 TBSP SESAME OIL
100 ML OLIVE OIL

Mix the lime zest, lime juice, honey, sesame oil and olive oil. Season with additional soy sauce.

YOGHURT DRESSING
WITH SMOKED SALT

300 ML WHOLE MILK YOGHURT
½ TSP SMOKED FLAKY SALT
(E.G. MALDON)
JUICE AND ZEST OF 1 ORGANIC LEMON
1 CLOVE GARLIC
1 TBSP DIJON MUSTARD
FRESHLY GROUND BLACK PEPPER

Stir the yoghurt with the smoked salt, lemon zest, grated garlic, mustard and pepper. Season to taste with salt and lemon juice.

YOGHURT DRESSING
WITH DILL AND LEMON

200 ML DRAINED GREEK YOGHURT
3 TBSP DIJON MUSTARD
JUICE AND ZEST OF 1 ORGANIC LEMON
¼ BUNCH DILL, CHOPPED
SALT AND FRESHLY GROUND
BLACK PEPPER
1 TBSP HONEY

Stir the yoghurt with the mustard, lemon zest, dill, salt and pepper. Season to taste with lemon juice, salt and honey.

ROCKET
SAUCE

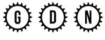

250 G ROCKET
3 TBSP WATER
3 TBSP DIJON MUSTARD
3 TBSP CIDER VINEGAR
400 ML OLIVE OIL
SALT

Rinse the rocket and blend with water, mustard and vinegar. Blend in the oil a little at a time until the consistency is sufficiently thick and creamy. Season with salt and cider vinegar.

PARSLEY
AND LEMON OIL

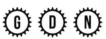

1 BUNCH FRESH PARSLEY
JUICE AND ZEST OF 1 ORGANIC LEMON
300 ML OLIVE OIL
1 CLOVE GARLIC
SALT

Rinse and tear the parsley off the stalk. Wash, zest and juice the lemon. Blend the parsley leaves with the olive oil, peeled garlic and lemon zest. Season to taste with lemon juice and salt.

If you want a smooth oil, strain through a coffee filter.

HAZELNUT
PESTO

(G)

1 BUNCH BASIL
½ BUNCH PARSLEY
3 CLOVES GARLIC
300 ML OLIVE OIL
100 G HAZELNUTS
100 G GRATED PARMESAN
JUICE AND ZEST OF 3 ORGANIC LEMONS
SALT

Rinse and tear the leaves off the basil and parsley. Peel the garlic and chop finely. Blend the herbs with the garlic and olive oil to a homogeneous consistency. Add the hazelnuts, a few at a time, and blend to a coarse purée. Add the parmesan and lemon zest. Season with lemon juice and salt.

TOMATO SAUCE #1
THE QUICK ONE

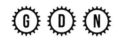

2 CLOVES GARLIC, CHOPPED
1 TBSP DRIED OREGANO
50 G CONCENTRATED TOMATO PURÉE
5 TBSP BALSAMIC VINEGAR
2 CANS CHOPPED TOMATOES
4 TBSP OLIVE OIL
SALT AND FRESHLY GROUND
BLACK PEPPER

Pour the oil into a thick-bottomed saucepan. Add the garlic and oregano and sauté. Stir in the concentrated tomato purée and sauté for a couple of minutes. Be careful not to burn the sauce. Pour in the balsamic vinegar, reduce by half and then add the chopped tomatoes. Let the sauce simmer for 10-12 minutes over low heat. Season with salt and pepper.

TOMATO SAUCE #2
THE SLOW ONE

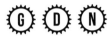

2 SHALLOTS, FINELY CHOPPED
5 CLOVES GARLIC, CHOPPED
1 TBSP DRIED OREGANO
½ BUNCH FRESH THYME, RINSED
3 SPRIGS FRESH ROSEMARY, RINSED
1 TBSP HONEY
100 ML BALSAMIC VINEGAR
140 G CONCENTRATED TOMATO PURÉE
3 CANS CHOPPED TOMATOES
3 BAY LEAVES
2 STAR ANISE
4 TBSP OLIVE OIL
SALT AND PEPPER

Heat the olive oil in a thick-bottomed saucepan over medium heat. Sauté the onion, garlic, oregano, thyme and rosemary, constantly stirring, until the onion is tender – about 2 minutes. Do not let it colour. Add honey, melt and heat until it starts to bubble. Add the vinegar and reduce by half. Add the concentrated tomato purée and let it sauté for a couple of minutes. Add the chopped tomatoes, bay leaves and star anise. Bring everything to a boil, then reduce to a low heat, cover and simmer for 30 minutes. Remove the thyme, rosemary, star anise and bay leaves. Season the sauce with salt, pepper and balsamic vinegar.

The batch makes 1.5 litres, which can either be refrigerated or frozen.

Variation # 1
SMOOTH TOMATO SAUCE
Blend the sauce to a homogeneous consistency and cream with 100 ml cold-pressed olive oil.

Variation # 2
TOMATO SAUCE COOKED IN WINE
Replace the 100 ml balsamic vinegar with 200 ml wine and reduce by 3/4. Season with balsamic vinegar.

CHICKEN STOCK

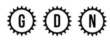

2 CHICKEN CARCASSES, BONES AND WINGS
3-4 LITRES WATER
2 CARROTS
2 ONIONS
1 LEEK
½ BUNCH THYME
2 STAR ANISE
2 BAY LEAVES
1 TBSP CORIANDER SEEDS

Preheat the oven to 250°C.

Clean the chicken carcasses thoroughly, rinse well and dry. Brown in a roasting tin in the oven until well roasted but not burnt – about 10 minutes – turning occasionally.

Peel the carrots and onions. Slice the leek lengthwise and rinse thoroughly. Chop everything into 3-4 cm chunks. Rinse the thyme.

Place the chicken carcasses in a large stock pot and cover with the cold water. While bringing to a boil, skim off impurities with a slotted spoon. Once boiling, turn down the heat and remove all the impurities and fat from the surface with a ladle. Add the herbs and spices. Let the stock simmer for 1 hour, skimming regularly.

Remove the pot from the heat, skim the stock one last time and strain through a cloth into a clean saucepan. Reduce by half and divide in small resealable containers so the stock can be easily portioned later. Cool before sealing. Freeze or refrigerate for up to two weeks.

VEAL STOCK

3 KG VEAL BONES
6 LITRES WATER
2 CARROTS
1 HEAD CELERIAC
3 ONIONS
1 HEAD GARLIC
½ BUNCH THYME
OLIVE OIL
2 STAR ANISE
2 BAY LEAVES
1 TBSP CORIANDER SEEDS
1 TSP BLACK PEPPERCORNS

Preheat the oven to 250°C.

Rinse the veal bones and dry them. Brown them in the oven for approximately 25 minutes until they are well roasted but not burnt, turning them occasionally.

Peel the carrots, celeriac and onions and split the garlic. Chop everything except the garlic into 3-4 cm chunks. Rinse the thyme thoroughly. Pan-roast the vegetables in olive oil until they have a lovely dark colour.

Place the veal bones in a large stock pot and cover with cold water. Bring to the boil over a medium heat and skim off any impurities along the way with a slotted spoon. When it boils, turn down the heat and remove all the impurities and fat from the surface with a ladle. Let the stock simmer for 4 hours, regularly skimming off impurities and fat. If necessary, add a little extra water in the process so the bones are always covered.

After 4 hours, add the herbs and spices and simmer the stock for 1 more hour. Remove the pot from the heat and skim the stock one last time before straining it through a cloth into a clean saucepan. Reduce by a half and divide it in small plastic boxes so you have small portion whenever you need them later. Allow to cool before putting lids on. Keeps for about two weeks in the refrigerator and longer in the freezer.

PICKLING LIQUID #1

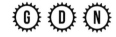

SIMPLE PICKLING LIQUID

200 ML CIDER VINEGAR
50 ML WATER
100 G HONEY

Bring the vinegar, water and honey to a boil and simmer for 1 minute. Cool and pour into a resealable container.

PICKLING LIQUID #2

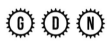

SPICY PICKLING LIQUID

200 ML CIDER VINEGAR
50 ML WATER
100 G HONEY
2 STAR ANISE
1 CINNAMON STICK
3 ALLSPICE BERRIES
1 TSP CORIANDER SEEDS
6 BLACK PEPPERCORNS

Bring the vinegar, water, honey and spices to a boil and simmer for 2 minutes. Cool and strain into a resealable container.

You can vary the spices according to taste. Try using fennel seeds, cloves, thyme etc.

PICKLING LIQUID #3

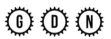

BALSAMIC PICKLING LIQUID

200 ML BALSAMIC VINEGAR
50 ML WATER
100 G HONEY
2 SPRIGS ROSEMARY

Bring the vinegar, water, honey and rosemary to a boil and simmer for 1 minute. Cool and pour it into a resealable container.

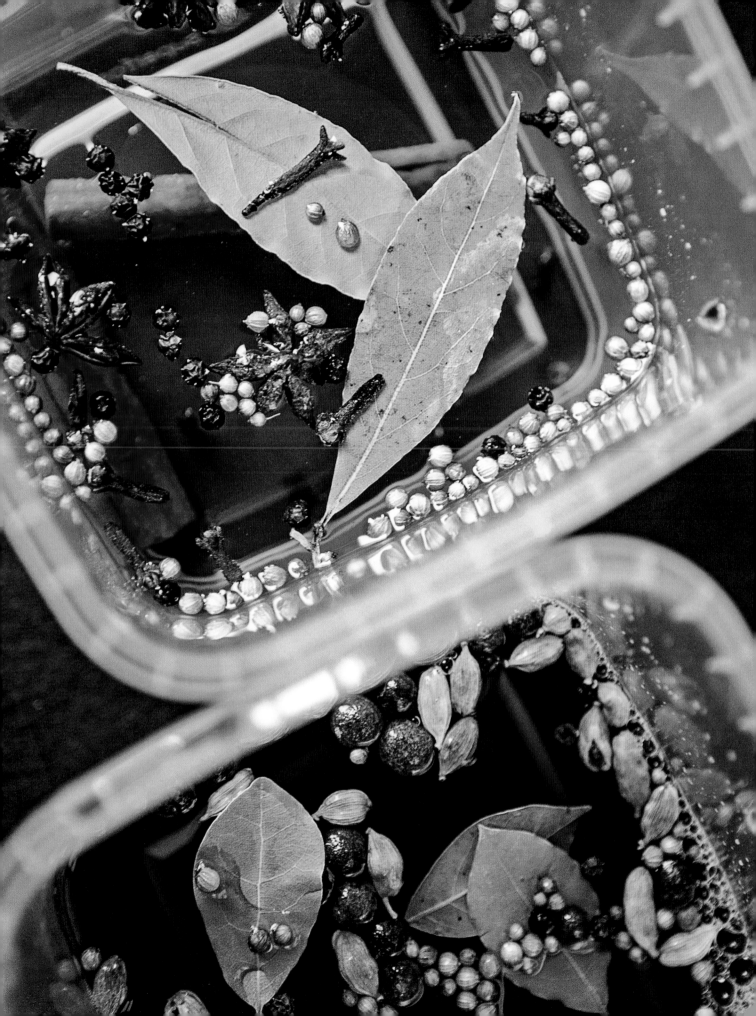

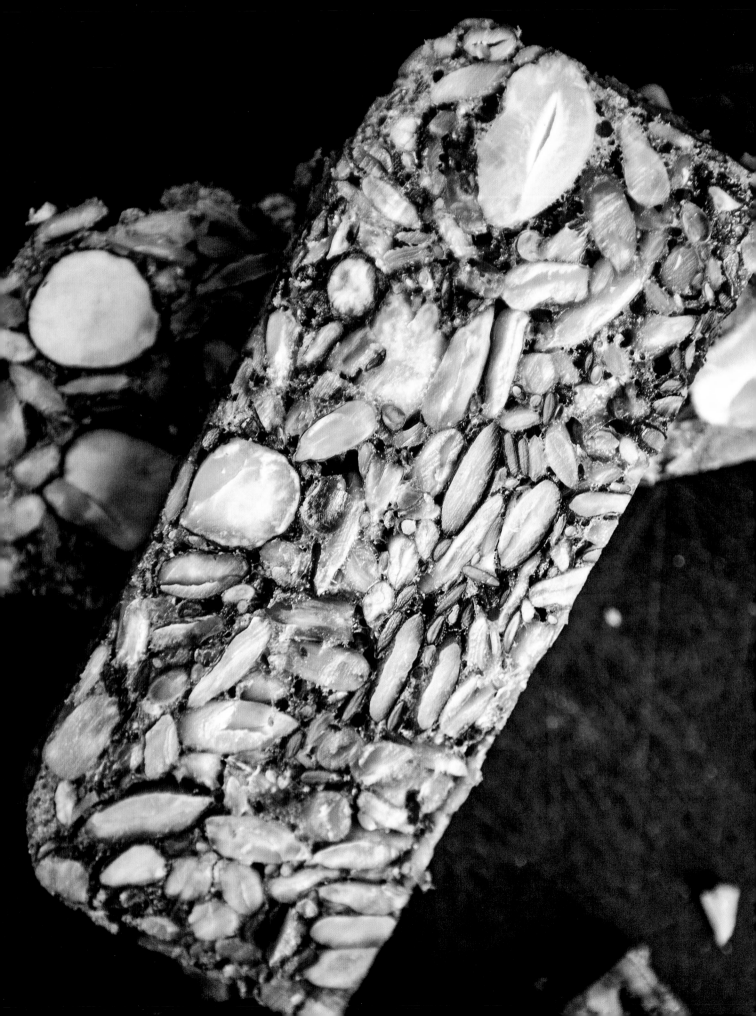

BASIC SPELT BREAD

4 LOAVES

25 G FRESH YEAST
50 G SOURDOUGH
500 ML WATER
25 G SALT
250 G DURUM FLOUR
250 G WHOLE WHEAT FLOUR
250 G SPELT FLOUR
A LITTLE OLIVE OIL FOR THE BREAD TINS

In a large bowl, dissolve the yeast and the sourdough in water and knead in all the flour and salt. Cover the dough with cling film and leave to rise at room temperature until doubled in size, then knead it again, preferably using a mixer with dough hook. Knead until the dough is smooth and supple. Remove the sourdough for reuse. Divide the dough into four greased loaf tins, cover in cling film and let the loaves rise until doubled in size or refrigerate overnight. The next day, take the dough out of the refridgerator and bring to room temperature before baking.

Preheat the oven to 220°C. Drizzle the loaves with olive oil and bake for 20-25 minutes before flipping them upside-down and baking for another 5 minutes. Remove them from the tins and leave to cool on a wire rack. Can be frozen. Wrap the bread in cling film in the evening if you have not eaten it. It can be re-baked the next day by spraying it with water and baking it for 7 min at 220°C.

BURGER BUNS

8-10 BUNS

20 G FRESH YEAST
500 ML WATER
20 G FINE SALT
250 G FLOUR
250 G WHOLE WHEAT FLOUR
300 G DURUM FLOUR
A LITTLE OLIVE OIL

Dissolve the yeast in water, add the salt and then the flour and knead the dough for 5 minutes. Alternatively, use a mixer with a dough hook. Allow the dough to rise for 1 hour at room temperature or overnight in the refrigerator.

Preheat the oven to 200°C. Shape the burger buns and place them on baking tray sprinkled with flour or in round baking tins sprinkled with flour. Drizzle the dough with olive oil and cover loosely with cling film. Let the dough rise until doubled in size. Bake the buns until the surface is nice and golden and the buns sound hollow when you tap them – about 20-25 minutes. Leave the buns to cool before serving.

MUESLI BREAD

(D)

4 LOAVES

12.5 G FRESH YEAST OR 5 G DRY YEAST
100 G SOURDOUGH
600 ML LUKEWARM WATER
250 G FINE DURUM FLOUR
250 G SPELT FLOUR
250 G WHOLE WHEAT FLOUR
12.5 G FINE SALT
100 G RAW, UNSWEETENED MUESLI +
A LITTLE EXTRA FOR THE BREAD TINS
(SEE PAGE 313)
½ TSP GROUND CINNAMON
2 TBSP COLD-PRESSED OLIVE OIL +
A LITTLE EXTRA FOR THE TINS

Dissolve the yeast and sourdough in the lukewarm water and then add all the flour and mix thoroughly. Add the salt and knead until firm. Knead in the muesli, cinnamon and oil. The dough may stick to your fingers the first time you knead it. Depending on the muesli used, adjust the dough with more or less flour, until it is firm, but still moist.

Cover the bowl with cling film and leave the dough to rise for 30 minutes at room temperature. Knead the dough again and let it sit in the refridgerator over night. Divide into 4 bread tins and cover with cling film, prove until doubled in size.

Bake the loaves in an oven preheated to 220°C until they are golden and crisp – about 20-25 minutes. Flip them out of the tins and bake for another 5 minutes. Tap the bread on the bottom. If it sounds hollow, the loaves are ready. Cool on a wire rack before slicing.

FOCCACIA

(D) (N)

20 G FRESH YEAST
500 ML LUKEWARM WATER
2 TBSP HONEY
20 G FINE SALT
250 G ORGANIC FLOUR
250 G WHOLE WHEAT FLOUR
300 G DURUM FLOUR
4 TBSP OLIVE OIL
1 TSP SALT FLAKES
½ BUNCH ROSEMARY
50 G OLIVES, PITTED

Dissolve the yeast in the lukewarm water and add the honey. Mix in the flour and knead the dough for 5 minutes or use a mixer with a dough hook. Allow the dough to rise for 1 hour at room temperature or overnight in a refrigerator.

Preheat the oven to 200°C. Transfer the dough to a large baking tray lined with greased baking paper. Rinse the rosemary and remove the leaves. Sprinkle the dough with the rosemary and olives and press 20-25 holes into it using your fingers. Cover the dough with cling film and leave it to rise until doubled in size. Sprinkle with salt flakes and bake for 25 minutes until the surface is nice and golden, flip the bread out and bake for another 5 minutes until the bread sounds hollow when you tap on the bottom. Cool on a wire rack before slicing.

GLUTEN-FREE
NUT AND SEED BREAD

#1: LIGHT GLUTEN-FREE GRAIN BREAD WITH NUTS

6 EGGS

50 ML OLIVE OIL

½ TSP FINE SALT

300 G SUNFLOWER SEEDS

200 G PUMPKIN SEEDS

100 G ALMONDS OR HAZELNUTS

FLAX SEEDS FOR THE TIN

#2: DARK GLUTEN-FREE GRAIN BREAD WITH NUTS

6 EGGS

50 ML OLIVE OIL

½ TSP FINE SALT

300 G FLAX SEEDS

100 G BRAZIL NUTS

200 G ALMONDS OR HAZELNUTS

FLAX SEEDS FOR THE TIN

Preheat the oven to 160°C. Whisk the eggs, olive oil and salt together. Mix all the seeds and nuts and add to the egg mixture. Grease 1 large bread tin (25x10 cm) or 2 small tins with olive oil and sprinkle with flaxseed or almond flour. Pour the egg mixture into the tins and bake until the bread is firm and golden – about 40-45 minutes. Cool on a wire rack before serving. To store, cling film and keep in the refrigerator.

The bread can be frozen and easily made in larger portions.

GLUTEN-FREE
SODABREAD

GLUTEN-FREE FLOUR MIX
2 KG BROWN RICE FLOUR
500 G FINE CORNMEAL (NOT CORNFLOUR)
500 G GLUTEN-FREE OAT FLOUR
1 KG POTATO FLOUR

THE BREAD
500 ML GLUTEN-FREE FLOUR MIXTURE
1 TSP FINE SALT
1 TSP BAKING POWDER
1 TSP BICARBONATE OF SODA
½ TSP XANTANA
1 EGG
250 ML MILK
2 TBSP SHERRY VINEGAR
2 TBSP CLEAR HONEY
50 G GINGER PULP (OPTIONAL)
(SEE PAGE 309)

2 LOAVES

Preheat the oven to 175°C. Mix the ingredients for the gluten-free flour mix and set 500 ml aside.

Mix 500 ml gluten-free flour mix, salt, baking powder, baking soda and xantana in a bowl. Whisk the egg, milk, vinegar, honey and ginger pulp together in another bowl. Stir the two mixtures together with a wooden spoon until homogeneous. Remove the dough from the bowl and knead thoroughly on a surface sprinkled with the gluten-free flour mixture. Divide the dough into two parts and shape into two small round loaves before making three slits across the top of each one.

Bake the loaves on baking paper for about 35-40 minutes. Test by sticking a toothpick or wooden skewer into the baked bread. If the toothpick comes out clean, the bread is done. Let the bread cool completely before serving. Store at room temperature in an airtight container.

If you cannot find gluten-free oat flour, you can use gluten-free porridge oats blended into flour.

RECIPE INDEX

All the recipes are for 4 people,
unless otherwise noted.

STAGE OVERVIEW

PROLOGUE
Tomato, avocado, pine nuts and feta ... 33
Quinoa, broccoli, apple and pomegranate ... 34
Salad with duck, pickled shallots, ... 37
red currants and walnuts ... 38
Chicken with pickled and roasted
mushrooms and sautéed leek ... 40

STAGE 1
Red cabbage, fennel and grapes ... 43
Roasted broccoli, blackberries and walnuts ... 45
Poached chicken, leeks and fried apple ... 46
Leg of lamb with parsley, lemon ... 48
and crushed potatoes ... 51
Polkadot mountain jersey dessert ... 52

STAGE 2
Pickled white asparagus, soft-boiled
eggs and caper vinaigrette ... 57
Meatballs and sautéed cabbage ... 59
with fennel and blueberries ... 61
Coconut chicken with ginger and lime ... 62
Old-fashioned apple cake ... 65

STAGE 3
Goat cheese, figs and raspberries ... 67
Bulgur wheat salad with nectarine ... 69
and yellow pepper ... 70
Moroccan-style chicken with black olives ... 73
Baked cod with radish crudité, dill and samphire ... 74
Carrot cake with vanilla yoghurt and apricots ... 77

STAGE 4
Cauliflower soup with dill and ... 81
roasted cauliflower ... 82
Roasted celeriac, apple, spinach and raspberries ... 85
Bolognese sauce ... 86
Balsamic and honey marinated chicken ... 89

STAGE 5
Cod brandade, chervil and cranberries ... 91
Watermelon, feta and black cumin ... 93
Chicken with peach, capers and tarragon ... 94
Ossobuco ... 97

Date brownie ... 101

STAGE 6 ... 105
Chicken and noodles in lime and
ginger broth ... 106
Beetroot, orange and toasted hazelnuts ... 109
Chicken, cashew and sage with
lemon-steamed cabbage ... 110
Lasagne ... 113

STAGE 7 ... 115
Warm potato salad with broccoli and cranberries ... 117
Celeriac, savoy cabbage, apricot ... 118
and sunflower seeds
Whole roast chicken with apple ... 121
and hazelnut stuffing ... 122
Flounder with steamed cauliflower ... 127
and new potatoes ... 129

STAGE 8 ... 130
White bean dip with baby vegetables ... 133
Chickpeas, fennel, pineapple and mint ... 134
Chicken meatballs with rocket sauce ... 137
Sea bream with sweetcorn and tarragon ... 139

STAGE 9 – THE DAY BEFORE THE FIRST REST DAY
Cured salmon, dill, apple and sheep's yoghurt ... 140
Roast veal, sweet potato compote ... 142
and cooked onion ... 147
Chocolate mousse 70% ... 148

REST DAY 1 ... 151
LUNCH ... 152
Eggs, tomato and baked salmon
Salad with chicken, fresh plums, ... 155
cranberries and hazelnuts ... 157
Charcuterie, fennel, pickled ... 158
red onion and caperberries ... 161

DINNER ... 167
Sugar snap pea and cabbage salad ... 169
Miso soup, carrot noodles and wakame seaweed ... 170
Sashimi ... 173
Chicken teriyaki skewers ... 174

STAGE 10
Caramelised cauliflower and almond salad
Pearl barley, roasted fennel, mango and mint
Danish Style whole roast chicken,
pear compote and new potatoes
Pork cheeks, salt-baked celeriac,
beetroot and savoy cabbage

Baked fruit with vanilla skyr ... 177

STAGE 11 ... 179
Couscous with melon and orange ... 180
Kale, red cabbage, apple and pistachios ... 182
Chicken in turmeric and lemon ... 185
Braised lamb shank ... 186

STAGE 12 ... 191
Ruby grapefruit, avocado and pine nuts ... 192
Caramelised onion soup ... 194
Chicken, red pepper salsa and pearl barley risotto ... 196
Duck breast, pan-roasted carrots,
orange and radicchio ... 198

STAGE 13 ... 201
Red quinoa tabbouleh ... 203
Brown rice, celeriac and figs ... 204
Soy-sesame chicken with buckwheat noodles ... 207
Mango, junket panna cotta and pomegranate ... 208

STAGE 14 ... 213
Cauliflower and celeriac soup ... 215
Baked butternut squash, feta and mint ... 217
Pasta puttanesca ... 218
Salmon with orange and ginger ... 221

**STAGE 15 – THE DAY BEFORE
THE SECOND REST DAY** ... 223
Burger mania: burger with
goat cheese and beetroot ... 225
Cold buttermilk soup with beetroot ... 226

REST DAY 2 ... 231
LUNCH
Salad with eggs, air-dried ham
and pickled tomatoes ... 232
Tuna salad with feta, yellow pepper and apple ... 235
Chicken, quinoa, mandarin and sunflower seeds ... 236

DINNER
Baked aubergine with garlic and parmesan ... 239
Cold veal, broccoli crudité and raw pickled onions ... 241
Meatballs in hazelnut pesto ... 242
Lemon and rosemary chicken ... 245

STAGE 16 ... 247
Gazpacho with apple and yellow pepper ... 249
Fresh spring rolls with rice noodles,
mint and peanut sauce ... 250
Slow-roasted shoulder of pork with
white bean salad and ginger sauce ... 252

Apple and blueberry crumble 255

STAGE 17 259
Mozzarella, blackberries, marjoram and apple 260
Fish cakes with mango salad 263
Peanut chicken kebabs 265
Poached pears, yoghurt and chocolate 266

STAGE 18 269
Ratatouille 270
Meatballs with coriander and spicy tomato sauce 273
Chicken casserole with butternut squash and fennel 275
Fruit salad with fennel 277

STAGE 19 281
Beetroot, green beans and tahini dressing 282
Baked monkfish cheeks, spring
onions and pointed cabbage 285
Whole roast chicken with herbs 287
Brownie 288

STAGE 20 291
Pizza and bubbly 292

RACE SNACKS 300
Soft rice cakes 300

RECOVERY FOODS 301

BREAKFAST 305
Porridge with plums and almonds 306
Porridge with blueberries and chia seeds 307
Raspberry and ginger smoothie 308
Avocado and apple smoothie 308
Strawberry and coconut smoothie 309
Ginger shots 309
Omelette with tomato and spring vegetables 311
Scrambled eggs with asparagus and parmesan 311
Toasted cinnamon muesli with seeds 312
Raw muesli with seeds 313
Rice milk-soaked muesli with fresh berries 315
Toasted almond spread with cinnamon 316
Hazelnut spread with 70% chocolate 316

**SAUCES, DRESSINGS,
PICKLING LIQUIDS & BREAD** 321
Hazelnut vinaigrette 322
Mustard vinaigrette 322
Coarse-grained mustard vinaigrette 323
Cider vinegar vinaigrette 323
Elderflower vinaigrette 323
Raspberry vinaigrette 323

Balsamic vinaigrette 324
Honey vinaigrette 324
Lime vinaigrette 325
Orange vinaigrette 325
Lemon vinaigrette 325
Mayonnaise 326
Soy sauce and sesame dressing 326
Yoghurt dressing with smoked salt 327
Yoghurt dressing with dill and lemon 327
Rocket sauce 328
Parsley and lemon oil 328
Hazelnut pesto 329
Tomato sauce # 1: The quick one 330
Tomato sauce # 2: The slow one 331
Chicken stock 332
Veal stock 333
Pickling liquid #1 – Simple pickling liquid 334
Pickling liquid #2 – Spicy pickling liquid 334
Pickling liquid #3 – Balsamic pickling liquid 334
Basic spelt bread 337
Burger buns 337
Muesli bread 338
Foccacia 339
Gluten-free nut and seed bread: 340
    Light gluten-free grain bread with nuts 340
    Dark gluten-free grain bread with nuts 340
Gluten-free soda bread 341

RECIPE INDEX —
IN ALPHABETICAL ORDER
AND ACCORDING TO CATEGORIES

VEGETABLES
Baked aubergine with garlic and parmesan 239
Baked butternut squash, feta and mint 217
Beetroot, green beans and tahini dressing 282
Beetroot, orange, roasted hazelnuts 109
Caramelised cauliflower and almond salad 169
Cauliflower and celeriac soup 215
Cauliflower soup with dill and roasted cauliflower 82
Celeriac, savoy cabbage, apricot
and sunflower seeds 118
Fruit salad with fennel 277
Gazpacho with apple and yellow pepper 249
Goat cheese, figs and raspberries 69
Kale, red cabbage, apple and pistachios 182
Miso soup, carrot noodles
and wakame seaweed 157
Mozzarella, blackberries, marjoram
and apple 260
Pickled white asparagus, soft-boiled
eggs and caper vinaigrette 59
Ratatouille 270

Red cabbage, fennel and grapes 45
Roasted broccoli, blackberries and walnuts 46
Roasted celeriac, apple, spinach
and raspberries 85
Ruby grapefruit, avocado and pine nuts 192
Sugar snap pea and cabbage salad 155
Tomato, avocado, pine nuts and feta 34
Warm potato salad with broccoli and
cranberries 117
Watermelon, feta and black cumin 94

POULTRY
Duck
Duck breast, pan-roasted carrots,
orange and radicchio 198
Salad with duck, pickled shallots,
red currants and walnuts 38

Chicken
Balsamic and honey marinated chicken 89
Chicken and noodles in lime and ginger broth 106
Chicken casserole with butternut squash
and fennel 275
Chicken, cashew and sage with
lemon-steamed cabbage 110
Chicken in turmeric and lemon 185
Chicken meatballs with rocket sauce 133
Chicken teriyaki skewers 161
Chicken with peach, capers and tarragon 97
Chicken with pickled and roasted
mushrooms and sautéed leek 40
Chicken, quinoa, mandarin and
sunflower seeds 236
Chicken, red pepper salsa and
pearl barley risotto 196
Coconut chicken with ginger and lime 62
Danish style whole roast chicken, pear
compote and new potatoes 173
Lemon and rosemary chicken 245
Moroccan-style chicken with black olives 73
Peanut chicken kebabs 265
Poached chicken, leeks and fried apple 48
Salad with chicken, plum, cranberries
and hazelnuts 151
Soy-sesame chicken with buckwheat noodles 207
Whole roast chicken with apple
and hazelnut stuffing 121
Whole roast chicken with herbs 287

MEAT
Bolognese sauce 86
Braised lamb shank 186

Burger mania: burger with
goat cheese and beetroot 225
Caramelised onion soup 194
Charcuterie, fennel, red onion and caperberries 152
Cold veal, broccoli crudité and raw pickled onions 241
Lasagne 113
Leg of lamb with parsley, lemon
and crushed potatoes 51
Meatballs and sautéed cabbage
with fennel and blueberries 61
Meatballs in hazelnut pesto 242
Meatballs with coriander and spicy tomato sauce 273
Ossobuco 99
Pork cheeks, salt-baked celeriac,
beetroot and savoy cabbage 174
Roast veal, compote of sweet
potato and cooked onions 140
Salad with eggs, air-dried ham
and pickled tomatoes 232
Slow-roasted shoulder of pork with
white bean salad and ginger sauce 252

FISH
Baked cod with radish crudité, dill and samphire 74
Baked monkfish cheeks, spring
onions and pointed cabbage 285
Cod brandade, chervil and cranberries 93
Cured salmon, dill, apple and sheep's yoghurt 139
Eggs, tomato and baked salmon 148
Fish cakes with mango salad 263
Flounder with steamed cauliflower
and new potatoes 122
Salmon with orange and ginger 221
Sashimi 158
Sea bream with sweet corn and tarragon 134
Tuna salad with feta, yellow pepper and apple 235

EGGS
Eggs, tomato and baked salmon 148
Omelette with tomato and spring vegetables 311
Pickled white asparagus, soft-boiled
eggs and caper vinaigrette 59
Salad with eggs, air-dried ham
and pickled tomatoes 232
Scrambled eggs with asparagus and parmesan 311

QUINOA, BEANS, LENTILS
Chicken, quinoa, mandarin and sunflower seeds 236
Chickpeas, fennel, pineapple and mint 130
Quinoa, broccoli, apple and pomegranate 37
Red quinoa tabbouleh 203
White bean dip with baby vegetables 129

BULGUR WHEAT, COUSCOUS, PEARL BARLEY
Bulgur wheat salad with nectarine
and yellow pepper 70
Couscous with melon and orange 180
Pearl barley, roasted fennel, mango and mint 170

RICE
Brown rice, celeriac and figs 204
Sashimi 158

PASTA, NOODLES – AND A PIZZA
Bolognese sauce 86
Chicken and noodles in lime and ginger broth 106
Lasagne 113
Soy-sesame chicken with buckwheat noodles 207
Pasta puttanesca 218
Meatballs in hazelnut pesto 242
Fresh spring rolls with rice noodles,
mint and peanut sauce 250
Pizza and bubbly 292

SAUCES
Chicken stock 332
Hazelnut pesto 329
Mayonnaise 326
Parsley and lemon oil 328
Rocket sauce 328
Tomato sauce # 1: The quick one 330
Tomato sauce # 2: The slow one 331
Veal stock 333

DRESSINGS
Balsamic vinaigrette 324
Cider vinegar vinaigrette 323
Coarse-grained mustard vinaigrette 323
Elderflower vinaigrette 323
Hazelnut vinaigrette 322
Honey vinaigrette 324
Lemon vinaigrette 325
Lime vinaigrette 325
Mayonnaise 326
Mustard vinaigrette 322
Orange vinaigrette 325
Parsley and lemon oil 328
Raspberry vinaigrette 323
Soy sauce and sesame dressing 326
Yoghurt dressing with dill and lemon 327
Yoghurt dressing with smoked salt 327

PICKLING LIQUIDS
Pickling liquid #1 – Simple pickling liquid 334
Pickling liquid #2 – Spicy pickling liquid 334

Pickling liquid #3 – Balsamic pickling liquid 334

BREAD
Basic spelt bread 337
Burger buns 337
Focaccia 339
Gluten-free nut and seed bread: 340
Light gluten-free grain bread with nuts 340
Dark gluten-free grain bread with nuts 340
Gluten-free soda bread 341
Muesli bread 338

CAKES
Brownie 288
Carrot cake with vanilla yoghurt and apricots 77
Date brownie 101
Soft rice cakes 300

DESSERTS
Apple and blueberry crumble 255
Baked fruit with vanilla skyr 177
Brownie 288
Carrot cake with vanilla yoghurt and apricots 77
Chocolate mousse 70% 142
Cold buttermilk soup with beetroot 226
Date brownie 101
Mango, junket panna cotta and pomegranate 208
Old-fashioned apple cake 65
Poached pears, yoghurt and chocolate 266
Polkadot mountain jersey dessert 52

SMOOTHIES ETC.
Avocado and apple smoothie 308
Ginger shots 309
Raspberry and ginger smoothie 308
Strawberry and coconut smoothie 309

PORRIDGE, MUESLI, SPREADS
Hazelnut spread with 70% chocolate 316
Porridge with blueberries and chia seeds 307
Porridge with plums and almonds 306
Raw muesli with seeds 313
Rice milk-soaked muesli with fresh berries 315
Toasted almond spread with cinnamon 316
Toasted cinnamon muesli with seeds 312

RECIPE INDEX —
GLUTEN-FREE, NUT-FREE
AND DAIRY-FREE

Please be aware that some recipes contain nuts, gluten and dairy. They are therefore not included in this index. For a comprehensive index of recipes please consult the stage index or the alphabetical index.

Recipes that contain pine nuts, sunflower seeds and sesame are classified as nut-free.

Recipes that contain coconut (coconut milk or coconut oil) are not classified as nut-free.

Recipes that call for either milk or rice milk are classified as dairy-free recipes, since the milk can be substituted with rice milk.

Recipes that contain soy sauce are classified as gluten-free, but this depends on the particular soy sauce used. Check the sauces before using them. Tamari is always gluten-free.

Recipes with chocolate listed as nut-free do not account for traces of nut that may be in the chocolate you use.

GLUTEN-FREE RECIPES

Apple and blueberry crumble	255
Avocado and apple smoothie	308
Baked aubergine with garlic and parmesan	239
Baked butternut squash, feta and mint	217
Baked cod with radish crudité, dill and samphire	74
Baked fruit with vanilla skyr	177
Baked monkfish cheeks, spring onions and pointed cabbage	285
Balsamic vinaigrette	324
Balsamic and honey marinated chicken	89
Beetroot, green beans and tahini dressing	282
Beetroot, orange, roasted hazelnuts	109
Braised lamb shank	186
Brown rice, celeriac and figs (the recipe contains soya)	204
Caramelised cauliflower and almond salad	169
Caramelised onion soup	194
Cauliflower and celeriac soup	215
Cauliflower soup with dill and roasted cauliflower	82
Celeriac, savoy cabbage, apricot and sunflower seeds	118

Charcuterie, fennel, red onion and caperberries	152
Chicken and noodles in lime and ginger broth	106
Chicken, cashew and sage with lemon-steamed cabbage	110
Chicken casserole with butternut squash and fennel	275
Chicken in turmeric and lemon	185
Chicken meatballs with rocket sauce	133
Chicken stock	332
Chicken teriyaki skewers (the recipe contains soya)	161
Chicken with peach, capers and tarragon	97
Chicken with pickled and roasted mushrooms and sautéed leek	40
Chicken, quinoa, mandarin and sunflower seeds	236
Chickpeas, fennel, pineapple and mint	130
Chocolate mousse 70%	142
Cider vinegar vinaigrette	323
Coarse-grained mustard vinaigrette	323
Coconut chicken with ginger and lime	62
Cold buttermilk soup with beetroot	226
Cold veal, broccoli crudité and raw pickled onions	241
Danish style whole roast chicken, pear compote and new potatoes	173
Dark gluten-free grain bread with nuts	340
Date brownie	101
Duck breast, pan-roasted carrots, orange and radicchio	198
Eggs, tomato and baked salmon	148
Elderflower vinaigrette	323
Fish cakes with mango-pickled red onion	263
Fresh spring rolls with rice noodles, mint and peanut sauce (the recipe contains soya)	250
Fruit salad with fennel	277
Gazpacho with apple and yellow pepper	249
Ginger shots	309
Gluten-free soda bread	341
Goat cheese, figs and raspberries	69
Hazelnut pesto	329
Hazelnut spread with 70% chocolate	316
Hazelnut vinaigrette	322
Honey vinaigrette	324
Kale, red cabbage, apple and pistachios	182
Leg of lamb with parsley, lemon and crushed potatoes	51
Lemon and rosemary chicken	245
Lemon vinaigrette	325
Light gluten-free grain bread with nuts	340
Lime vinaigrette	325
Mango, junket panna cotta and pomegranate	208
Mayonnaise	326
Meatballs and sautéed cabbage with fennel and blueberries	61

Meatballs with coriander and spicy tomato sauce	273
Miso soup, carrot noodles and wakame seaweed	157
Moroccan-style chicken with black olives	73
Mozzarella, blackberries, marjoram and apple	260
Mustard vinaigrette	322
Old-fashioned apple cake	65
Omelette with tomato and spring vegetables	311
Orange vinaigrette	325
Ossobuco	99
Parsley and lemon oil	328
Peanut chicken kebabs (the recipe contains soya)	265
Pickled white asparagus, soft-boiled eggs and caper vinaigrette	59
Pickling liquid #1- Simple pickling liquid	334
Pickling liquid #2- Spicy pickling liquid	334
Pickling liquid #3- Balsamic pickling liquid	334
Pork cheeks, salt-baked celeriac, beetroot and savoy cabbage	174
Poached chicken, leeks and fried apple	48
Poached pears, yoghurt and chocolate	266
Polkadot mountain jersey dessert	52
Porridge with blueberries and chia seeds (the recipe is gluten-free if gluten-free oats are used)	307
Porridge with plums and almonds (the recipe is gluten-free if gluten-free oats are used)	306
Quinoa, broccoli, apple and pomegranate	37
Raspberry and ginger smoothie	308
Raspberry vinaigrette	323
Ratatouille	270
Raw muesli with seeds	313
Red cabbage, fennel and grapes	45
Red quinoa tabbouleh	203
Rice milk-soaked muesli with fresh berries	315
Roast veal, compote of sweet potato and cooked onions	140
Roasted broccoli, blackberries and walnuts	46
Roasted celeriac, apple, spinach and raspberries	85
Rocket sauce	328
Ruby grapefruit, avocado and pine nuts	192
Salad with chicken, plum, cranberries and hazelnuts	151
Salad with duck, pickled shallots, red currants and walnuts	38
Salad with eggs, air-dried ham and pickled tomatoes	232
Salmon with orange and ginger	221
Sashimi (the recipe contains soya)	158
Scrambled eggs with asparagus and parmesan	311
Sea bream with sweet corn and tarragon	134

Slow-roasted shoulder of pork with white bean
salad and ginger sauce (the recipe contains soya) 252

Soy sauce and sesame dressing
(the recipe contains soya) 326

Soy-sesame chicken with buckwheat
noodles (the recipe contains soya) 207

Strawberry and coconut smoothie 309

Sugar snap pea and cabbage salad 155

Toasted almond spread with cinnamon 316

Toasted cinnamon muesli with seeds 312

Tomato sauce #1: The quick one 330

Tomato sauce #2: The slow one 331

Tomato, avocado, pine nuts and feta 34

Tuna salad with feta, yellow pepper and apple 235

Veal stock 333

Warm potato salad with broccoli and cranberries 117

Watermelon, feta and black cumin 94

White bean dip with baby vegetables 129

Whole roast chicken with apple
and hazelnut stuffing 121

Whole roast chicken with herbs 287

Yoghurt dressing with dill and lemon 327

Yoghurt dressing with smoked salt 327

NUT-FREE RECIPES (N)

Avocado and apple smoothie 308

Baked aubergine with garlic and parmesan 239

Baked butternut squash, feta and mint 217

Baked cod with radish crudité, dill and samphire 74

Baked fruit with vanilla skyr 177

Baked monkfish cheeks, spring
onions and pointed cabbage 285

Balsamic vinaigrette 324

Balsamic and honey marinated chicken 89

Basic spelt bread 337

Beetroot, green beans and tahini dressing
(the recipe contains sesame) 282

Bolognese sauce 86

Braised lamb shank 186

Brown rice, celeriac and figs (the
recipe contains sesame) 204

Bulgur wheat salad with nectarine
and yellow pepper 70

Burger buns 337

Burger mania: burger with
goat cheese and beetroot 225

Caramelised onion soup 194

Cauliflower soup with dill and roasted cauliflower 82

Celeriac, savoy cabbage, apricot
and sunflower seeds 118

Charcuterie, fennel, red onion and caperberries 152

Chicken and noodles in lime and ginger stock 106

Chicken casserole with butternut squash and fennel 275

Chicken meatballs with rocket sauce 133

Chicken stock 332

Chicken teriyaki skewers (the recipe contains sesame) 161

Chicken with peach, capers and tarragon 97

Chicken with pickled and roasted
mushrooms and sautéed leek 40

Chickpeas, fennel, pineapple and mint 130

Chocolate mousse 70% 142

Cider vinegar vinaigrette 323

Coarse-grain mustard vinaigrette 323

Cod brandade, chervil and cranberries 93

Cold buttermilk soup with beetroot 226

Cold veal, broccoli crudité and raw pickled onions 241

Cured salmon, dill, apple and sheep's yoghurt 139

Danish style whole roast chicken, pear
compote and new potatoes 173

Duck breast, pan-roasted carrots,
orange and radicchio 198

Eggs, tomato and baked salmon 148

Elderflower vinaigrette 323

Flounder with steamed cauliflower
and new potatoes 122

Focaccia 339

Fruit salad with fennel 277

Gazpacho with apple and yellow pepper 249

Ginger shots 309

Gluten-free soda bread 341

Goat cheese, figs and raspberries 69

Honey vinaigrette 324

Lasagne 113

Leg of lamb with parsley, lemon
and crushed potatoes 51

Lemon and rosemary chicken 245

Lemon vinaigrette 325

Lime vinaigrette 325

Mango, junket panna cotta and pomegranate 208

Mayonnaise 326

Meatballs with coriander and spicy tomato sauce 273

Miso soup, carrot noodles and wakame seaweed 157

Mozzarella, blackberries, marjoram and apple 260

Mustard vinaigrette 322

Omelette with tomato and spring vegetables 311

Orange vinaigrette 325

Ossobuco 99

Parsley and lemon oil 328

Pasta puttanesca 218

Pearl barley, roasted fennel, mango and mint 170

Pickled white asparagus, soft-boiled
eggs and caper vinaigrette 59

Pickling liquid #1 – Simple pickling liquid 334

Pickling liquid #2 – Spicy pickling liquid 334

Pickling liquid #3 – Balsamic pickling liquid 334

Pork cheeks, salt-baked celeriac,
beetroot and savoy cabbage 174

Pizza and bubbly 292

Poached chicken, leeks and fried apple 48

Porridge with blueberries and chia seeds 307

Raspberry and ginger smoothie 308

Raspberry vinaigrette 323

Roast veal, compote of sweet
potato and cooked onions 140

Roasted celeriac, apple, spinach and raspberries 85

Rocket sauce 328

Ruby grapefruit, avocado and pine nuts 192

Salad with eggs, air-dried ham
and pickled tomatoes 232

Salmon with orange and ginger 221

Sashimi 158

Slow-roasted shoulder of pork with
white bean salad and ginger sauce 252

Soy sauce and sesame dressing
(the recipe contains sesame) 326

Soy-sesame chicken with buckwheat noodles
(the recipe contains sesame) 207

Sugar snap pea and cabbage salad
(the recipe contains sesame) 155

Tomato sauce #1: The quick one 330

Tomato sauce #2: The slow one 331

Tomato, avocado, pine nuts and feta 34

Tuna salad with feta, yellow pepper and apple 235

Veal stock 333

Watermelon, feta and black cumin 94

White bean dip with baby vegetables 129

Whole roast chicken with herbs 287

Yoghurt dressing with dill and lemon 327

Yoghurt dressing with smoked salt 327

DAIRY-FREE RECIPES (D)

Avocado and apple smoothie 308

Baked cod with radish crudité, dill and samphire 74

Balsamic vinaigrette 324

Basic spelt bread 337

Beetroot, green beans and tahini dressing 282

Beetroot, orange, roasted hazelnuts 109

Braised lamb shank 186

Brown rice, celeriac and figs
(the recipe contains soya) 204

Bulgur wheat salad with nectarine
and yellow pepper 70

Burger buns 337

Caramelised cauliflower and almond salad 169

Cauliflower and celeriac soup	215	Muesli bread	338	White bean dip with baby vegetables	129
Cauliflower soup with dill and roasted cauliflower	82	Orange vinaigrette	325	Whole roast chicken with apple	
Celeriac, savoy cabbage, apricot		Ossobuco	99	and hazelnut stuffing	121
and sunflower seeds	118	Parsley and lemon oil	328	Whole roast chicken with herbs	287
Charcuterie, fennel, red onion and caperberries	152	Peanut chicken kebabs	265		
Chicken and noodles in lime and ginger stock	106	Pearl barley, roasted fennel, mango and mint	170		
Chicken casserole with butternut squash and fennel	275	Pickled white asparagus, soft-boiled			
Chicken in turmeric and lemon	185	eggs and caper vinaigrette	59		
Chicken meatballs with rocket sauce		Pickling liquid #1 – Simple pickling liquid	334		
(unless you use milk instead of rice milk)	133	Pickling liquid #2 – Spicy pickling liquid	334		
Chicken stock	332	Pickling liquid #3 – Balsamic pickling liquid	334		
Chicken teriyaki skewers	161	Pork cheeks, salt-baked celeriac,			
Chicken with peach, capers and tarragon	97	beetroot and savoy cabbage	174		
Chicken with pickled and roasted		Poached chicken, leeks and fried apple	48		
mushrooms and sautéed leek	40	Porridge with blueberries and chia seeds	307		
Chicken, quinoa, mandarin and sunflower seeds	236	Porridge with plums and almonds	306		
Chickpeas, fennel, pineapple and mint	130	Quinoa, broccoli, apple and pomegranate	37		
Cider vinegar vinaigrette	323	Raspberry and ginger smoothie	308		
Coarse-grained mustard vinaigrette	323	Raspberry vinaigrette	323		
Coconut chicken with ginger and lime	62	Ratatouille	270		
Couscous with melon and orange	180	Raw muesli with seeds	313		
Danish style whole roast chicken, pear		Red cabbage, fennel and grapes	45		
compote and new potatoes	173	Red quinoa tabbouleh	203		
Dark gluten-free grain bread with nuts	340	Rice milk-soaked muesli with fresh berries	315		
Date brownie	101	Roast veal, compote of sweet			
Duck breast, pan-roasted carrots,		potato and cooked onions	140		
orange and radicchio	198	Roasted broccoli, blackberries and walnuts	46		
Eggs, tomato and baked salmon	148	Roasted celeriac, apple, spinach and raspberries	85		
Elderflower vinaigrette	323	Rocket sauce	328		
Focaccia	339	Ruby grapefruit, avocado and pine nuts	192		
Fresh spring rolls with rice noodles,		Salad with chicken, fresh plums,			
mint and peanut sauce	250	cranberries and hazelnuts	151		
Fruit salad with fennel	277	Salad with duck, pickled shallots,			
Gazpacho with apple and yellow pepper	249	red currants and walnuts	38		
Ginger shots	309	Salad with eggs, air-dried ham			
Hazelnut spread with 70% chocolate	316	and pickled tomatoes	232		
Hazelnut vinaigrette	322	Salmon with orange and ginger	221		
Honey vinaigrette	324	Sashimi	158		
Kale, red cabbage, apple and pistachios	182	Sea bream with sweet corn and tarragon	134		
Leg of lamb with parsley, lemon		Slow-roasted shoulder of pork with			
and crushed potatoes	51	white bean salad and ginger sauce	252		
Lemon and rosemary chicken	245	Soy sauce and sesame dressing	326		
Lemon vinaigrette	325	Soy-sesame chicken with buckwheat noodles	207		
Light gluten-free grain bread with nuts	340	Strawberry and coconut smoothie	309		
Lime vinaigrette	325	Sugar snap pea and cabbage salad	155		
Mayonnaise	326	Toasted almond spread with cinnamon	316		
Meatballs and sautéed cabbage with		Toasted cinnamon muesli with seeds	312		
fennel and blueberries (unless you		Tomato sauce #1: The quick one	330		
use milk instead of rice milk)	61	Tomato sauce #2: The slow one	331		
Meatballs with coriander and spicy tomato sauce	273	Tomato, avocado, pine nuts and feta	34		
Miso soup, carrot noodles and wakame seaweed	157	Veal stock	333		
Moroccan-style chicken with black olives	73	Warm potato salad with broccoli and cranberries	117		

THANKS

I could not have written this book without the amazing help of the many people involved:

First of all, I need to say: Hanspeter, you are the matchmaker from heaven – I'm truly grateful
that you have introduced me to my new business partner Ilya, without this connection no
one would have the chance to enjoy this book, from the bottom of my heart, thank you.

Ilya Katsnelson, there is not enough space in this book to describe how unbelievably happy I am
that you have chosen to believe in my projects and me. Thank you so so so so much, I am forever
thankful for everything that you have done and I can't wait to start our next exciting book adventure.

Bjarne and Anne Dorthe, thank you for believing that we can make a difference
and for introducing me to the delights of the cycling universe.

Thanks for, and to, the catering truck – my second home. Lars Williams, for being the
best support in the world throughout the whole genesis of the book. Jonathan and Rune,
my trusty apprentices, thanks for all the time spent with you guys in the kitchen.

Thank you to Restaurant NOMA, Peter Kreiner and Rene Redzepi,
for letting me use your kitchen for the photo shoot.

Thank you Hamilton for the incredible job you have done in absolutely no time!
Thank you Chris for your beautiful British eyes.

Thank you to Sarah Backer for being the best friend in the world and
tolerating me during the more stressed out periods of time.

Thank you to all our fantastic riders for eating my food and
sharing your thoughts of eating with the world.

Thanks to my mother Jette, who made sure that no desserts went to waste after the photo shoots.

Thank you to Rachel from Johannes Torpe Studios for your creative super mind.

Hannah

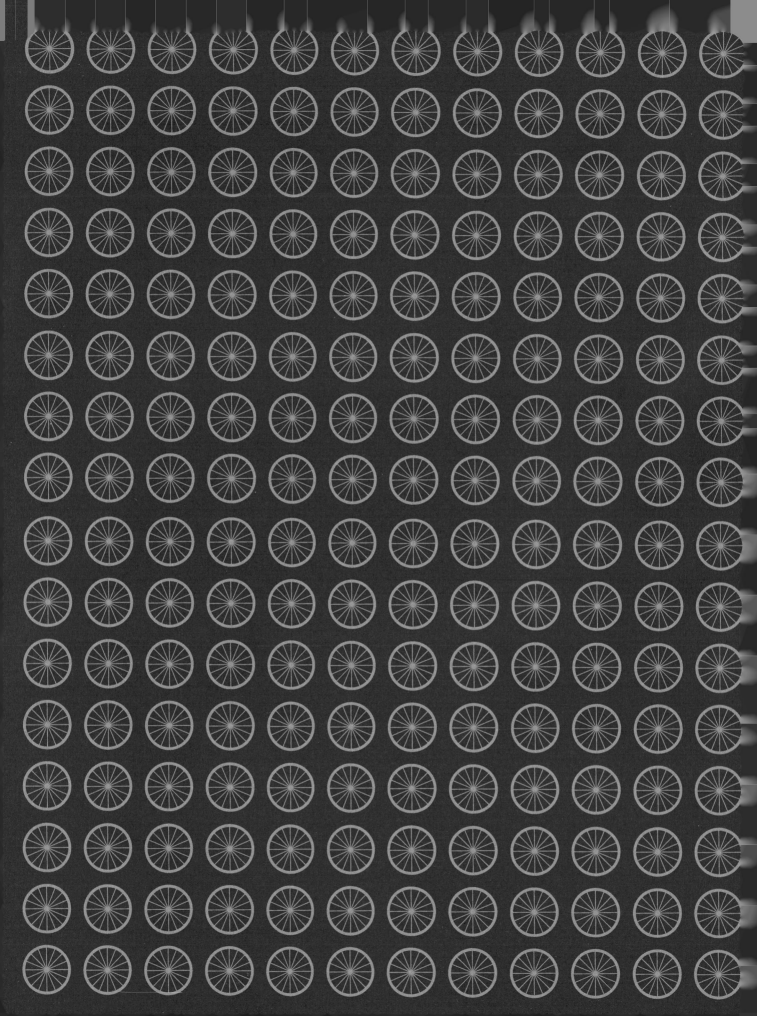